"*Yoga Therapy as a Whole-Person Approach to* teacher and therapist's professional library. Ananda and Lee bring together their decades of personal and professional wisdom and experience to create a comprehensive guide suited to both novices and the more experienced practitioner. The text acknowledges the many traditions that inform contemporary yoga therapy and is replete with extensive appendices of suggested practices including *yoga nidra* and *mudras*. This is a must-have!"

—*Leigh Blashki, Board of Directors IAYT*

"This book is the collaborative effort of well-known yoga therapists and practitioners Lee Majewski and Ananda Balayogi Bhavanani. Their intensive research and clinical experience working with persons afflicted with non-communicable disease (NCD) conditions have contributed to the development of a comprehensive, authoritative work on the process of yoga therapy. I consider this book to be valuable and timely to those who work in clinical and non-clinical set up in providing yoga support to people with NCD as well as those who work in preventive processes."

—*Dr. Latha Satish, Psychologist and Yoga Therapist and Researcher Chairman, Research Council Krishnamacharya Yoga Mandiram, Chennai*

"This is an exceptionally engaging, comprehensive, and, indeed, inspiring guide to the theory and practice of yoga therapy, well supported by the authors' depth and breadth of experience, as well as their extensive review of relevant modern yoga research. Cautions about an allopathic, symptomatic management approach to yoga therapy—called yogopathy—are balanced with principles and multiple examples for taking a whole-person approach to addressing the root causes of an individual's dis-ease. There is a practical focus on four major non-communicable disease areas yoga therapists work with: chronic respiratory diseases, cardio-vascular diseases, diabetes mellitus and cancer. Their articulation of how and why to adopt a holistic approach to each individual's personal situation will be helpful to the yoga therapist trying to explain what they do and why in a conventional healthcare context. This is may be especially important these days, as various physical and mental health disciplines are seeking to incorporate yoga into their therapeutic practices, but too often without deep personal training and experience in yoga and yoga therapy, and hence a tendency to simply fall back upon general protocols as opposed to a incorporating a wide range of unique individual considerations needed for healing."

—*John Kepner, Executive Director, the International Association of Yoga Therapists*

"As yoga rapidly gains popularity in the general population internationally, its use as a therapeutic intervention for diseases has grown apace. The authors, who are both deeply ingrained personally and professionally in the practice and application of yoga for health and healing, have delivered a comprehensive text on the theory, science, and application of yoga therapy. Their emphasis on the importance of the application of yoga practices in an integrative and holistic manner to address the whole person and not simply the disease or its symptoms is highly crucial to the success of yoga as therapy."

—*Sat Bir Singh Khalsa PhD, Assistant Professor of Medicine, Harvard Medical School and Editor in Chief,* International Journal of Yoga Therapy

YOGA THERAPY AS A WHOLE-PERSON APPROACH TO HEALTH

of related interest

Yoga as Self-Care for Healthcare Practitioners
Cultivating Resilience, Compassion, and Empathy
Aggie Stewart
Foreword by John Kepner
ISBN 978 1 84819 396 3
eISBN 978 0 85701 353 8

Yoga and Science in Pain Care
Treating the Person in Pain
Edited by Neil Pearson, Shelly Prosko and Marlysa Sullivan
Foreword by Timothy McCall
ISBN 978 1 84819 397 0
eISBN 978 0 85701 354 5

Yoga Therapy as a Creative Response to Pain
Matthew J. Taylor
Foreword by John Kepner
ISBN 978 1 84819 356 7
eISBN 978 0 85701 315 6

Yoga Therapy for Stroke
A Handbook for Yoga Therapists and Healthcare Professionals
Arlene A. Schmid and Marieke van Puymbroeck
Forewords by Matthew J. Taylor and Linda Williams
ISBN 978 1 84819 369 7
eISBN 978 0 85701 327 9

Yoga for a Happy Back
A Teacher's Guide to Spinal Health through Yoga Therapy
Rachel Krentzman, PT, E-RYT
Foreword by Aadil Palkhivala
ISBN 978 1 84819 271 3
eISBN 978 0 85701 253 1

Principles and Themes in Yoga Therapy
An Introduction to Integrative Mind/Body Yoga Therapeutics
James Foulkes
Foreword by Mikhail Kogan, MD
Illustrated by Simon Barkworth
ISBN 978 1 84819 248 5
eISBN 978 0 85701 194 7

YOGA THERAPY

AS A WHOLE-PERSON APPROACH TO HEALTH

LEE MAJEWSKI AND
ANANDA BALAYOGI BHAVANANI

FOREWORD BY STEPHEN PARKER

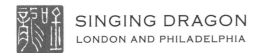

SINGING DRAGON
LONDON AND PHILADELPHIA

All photos in Chapters 13 and Appendix 3 and 6 are printed with
kind permission from Mr. Waldemar Borowiec.

First published in 2020
by Singing Dragon
an imprint of Jessica Kingsley Publishers
73 Collier Street
London N1 9BE, UK
and
400 Market Street, Suite 400
Philadelphia, PA 19106, USA

www.singingdragon.com

Library of Congress Cataloging in Publication Data
A CIP catalog record for this book is available from the Library of Congress

British Library Cataloguing in Publication Data
A CIP catalogue record for this book is available from the British Library

ISBN 978 1 78775 092 0
eISBN 978 1 78775 093 7

Printed and bound in the United States

My body is a house, I build for me,
Myself the architect shall be;
I cannot accept the stubborn fact
That I am fashioned by every act
Which I must determine with my own will,
And there I live, for good or ill.

(Author unknown)

Contents

Foreword

This work has been written by two authors with a profound respect for both scientific validation and for the depth and complexity of the yoga tradition, beyond what science can measure. Lee Majewski MA C-IAYT is a long-time yoga teacher and certified yoga therapist and a visiting faculty member of Kaivalyadhāma Yoga Institute, Lonavla, Maharashtra, India. Her personal experience of living with her cancer treatment provided the impetus for the design of the retreats described in the book. She is a frequent presenter in international conferences and has trained many therapists and yoga teachers in the conduct of the retreats. Ananda Bhavanani MD is a physician and certified yoga therapist who is also the successor of a venerable yoga lineage through his father, Swāmī Gītānanda Giri and their guru Kanakānanda Bhrigu, more familiarly known by his pre-monastic name as Ram Gopal Majumdar, "the sleepless saint" of Paramahansa Yogānanda's *Autobiography of a Yogi*. Dr. Bhavanani directs a yoga therapy training program, the Center for Yoga Therapy Education and Research of the Śrī Bālāji Vidyāpītha, a deemed university and medical school in Pondicherry in South India.

This book serves a number of important purposes. The first part of the book is an excellent introduction to the philosophy of yoga therapy from a yogic perspective. As such it is much-recommended reading for those with a general interest in yoga therapy. It serves as a corrective to the drift of this budding profession towards becoming a sub-discipline of medicine and physical therapy, where yogic practices are applied prescriptively, solely according to a medical diagnosis. This is what Bhavanani calls "yogopathy." Majewski and Bhavanani give a detailed account of what a "whole person," yogic process of diagnosis would look like. It is not enough to simply criticize, and these authors have gone the extra mile to fill out how a yogic perspective might approach the work of healing. It is significant to remember that in English, as well as many other Indo-European languages, the word "heal" comes from the same root as "whole" and "holy."

In addition to holding a respect for the depth of the practices of yoga, the book also maintains respect for the ancient *Āyur-vedic* medical system, authored, in part, by the same Patañjali who codified the yoga science. (This is the opinion of the oral tradition of yoga through my preceptors, Swāmī Rāma of the Himālayas and Swāmī Veda Bhāratī, not necessarily of Indological academics.) The practices of yoga have always been an important part of what an *Āyur-vedic* physician (*vaidya*) would offer people in addition to dietary prescriptions, herbal treatments and more. By looking at the whole person in context, the system provides not only holistic treatment, but, even more importantly, given the prevalence of chronic (habit-based) lifestyle illnesses today, a preventative focus that promotes long-term changes and improvement in the quality of life, particularly the cultivation of a resilient and joyful mind and heart.

One of the critical issues the authors tackle convincingly in conceiving holistic yoga therapy is the frequent disinclination of scientifically oriented yoga therapy to embrace the importance of spirituality to healing. This occurs despite a considerable body of empirical evidence which demonstrates that spirituality strongly potentiates healing. Here spirituality is understood as practices which facilitate a relationship with the highest levels of consciousness, rather than confusing it with religion, which comprises specific, culture-bound prescriptions for the nature of that relationship. This is particularly true in addressing the isolation, exhaustion, and hopelessness that patients are often left with at the conclusion of their prescribed medical treatment. In the case of Majewski's experience of her own cancer and that of retreat participants, she notes how often this isolation and hopelessness pushes patients towards ending their lives. The deeper one goes into the layers of embodiment presented by yoga through the system of *koshas*, the more extensive the spiritual healing effect can become. A similar argument was made by quantum physicist Amit Goswami PhD in his book, *The Quantum Doctor*, as he constructed a quantum model of healing that demonstrates how allopathy, homeopathy and *Āyur-veda* can all work in collaboration if one understands the levels at which those healing systems work.

The second part of the book describes four clusters of non-communicable illnesses which account for approximately 80 percent of deaths: chronic respiratory illnesses, cardiovascular diseases, diabetes mellitus, and cancer. This section provides evidence-based descriptions of what a holistic yoga therapy approach to these problems can offer. The most beautiful part of this section of the book is the personal account of Majewski's experience with her cancer treatment, which was effective in a medical sense, but which left her without a map for many of the exhausting, painful, and debilitating sequelae. This is important material for medical professionals to read because it details the patient experience of being left resourceless at the conclusion of the medical treatments, just when a person is at their most exhausted, depleted, and dis-spirited.

This inattention to the psychological side of illness, to the dis-ease which is the relationship every patient has to their illness, is a problem that appears wherever clinicians' fear starts running the show from the sidelines. It is very tempting in these circumstances to simply throw science and technology at the illness. This writer saw many similar examples of this in the early days of the HIV/AIDS epidemic. It may seem surprising to some that fear of cancer still exerts such an influence on treatment, but the fear of disembodiment, as Patañjali tells us, is ubiquitous in humans and the ultimate source of all our fears. The yoga system, which is about healing relationship at every level of practice from the first item in the list of limbs of yoga, non-violence, provides the ultimate permanent freedom from fear (for both patients and clinicians).

In the third section of the book, the authors provide a small-group residential retreat format that addresses each level of embodiment in the yoga system, which has never separated mind and body as medical systems have done in Western allopathic medicine. The three weeks of these retreats are packed with practices that refocus peoples' awareness of their mind-body and bring the whole person back together, as it were. Then there is a regular follow-up to help people to maintain the changes they have made. The measurement of these follow-up sessions to date validates the long-term effectiveness of the retreats.

The retreat format includes detailed descriptions of the practices used, so that the design is reproducible. These are taken from versions of *hatha yoga* and *pranayama* practice which come largely from the teaching of Kaivalyadhāma, one of the oldest modern yoga institutions in India and the first to conduct scientific research starting in the 1920s, from Richard Miller's version of practices for *yoga nidrā* (iRest) and from the Sikh tradition of Kundalini yoga. This creates an invitation to test these practices both in scientific experimentation and in personal experience, which is always the true test of any yogic practice. It also provides the opportunity to test practices from other traditions in which a given yoga therapist may be trained. My own guru, Swāmī Rāma, always encouraged us to test everything he gave us. "Don't just believe what I say—be a scientist!," he would say.

In summary, this is valuable reading on many different levels, providing a grounding in a traditionally yogic perspective on diagnosis and treatment, personal accounts of lapses in medical treatment from both retreat participants and the authors, the specific outline of a pair of residential retreats with first-hand accounts of participants, and a detailed account of the practices used. It is a work embodying careful thought about the nature of yoga therapy, a generous-hearted sharing of an approach that worked, and it shows a way of moving healing back towards the whole and holy person which, after all, is the goal of yoga writ large.

Stephen Parker PsyD, Licensed Psychologist and C-IAYT, Adjunct Assistant School Professor of Counseling and Psychological Services, Saint Mary's University of Minnesota, and author of *Clearing the Path, the Yoga Way to a Clear and Pleasant Mind: Patañjali, Neuroscience and Emotion* (Ahymsa Publishers, 2017)

PART 1

UNDERSTANDING YOGA AS THERAPY

As with any emerging field, yoga therapy is going through growing pains. The International Association of Yoga Therapists (IAYT) in the US, Australia Yoga Therapists, and other local organizations are doing valuable work in defining the scope and direction of this professional field, but there is still much confusion among the public about what yoga therapy is, and what it is not.

At one extreme, the general push for acceptance into existing healthcare systems and structures has created a reductionist definition of yoga therapy. Within the medical paradigm this results in yoga being limited to what fits neatly into such a system—working within a medical diagnosis and using *asanas* and *pranayama* to deal with the symptoms of disease in a prescriptive manner. This approach typically offers yoga for a certain symptom or diagnosis. It also often refers to meditation as existing outside of yoga, that is, yoga *and* meditation. For some, this is yoga therapy without the essence of yoga.

At the other extreme is the comprehensive definition of yoga therapy as a "psychospiritual technology,"[1] based on the process of enhancing or promoting the healing through empowering the client. This paradigm deals with the whole person, where the disease is understood as the lack of balance in the multilevel existence of humans. With its own assessment tools, such an approach "creates a safe environment for enquiry by the client, to empower them to create new responses, free of their former reactive patterns of behavior."[2]

And in-between these two extremes are all kinds of different shades and grades of approaches, depending on the yoga therapist's training, level of personal development, and professional experience. In other words, there is still much confusion and uncertainty or debate within this emerging field. For instance, I am often asked if spirituality and yogic counseling are within the scope of yoga therapy practice! Perhaps the biggest challenge for yoga therapists as well as for the public is to break out of the cultural paradigm of our understanding of what it is to heal and how to go about it. Therefore, in this first part of our book, we attempt to clarify the misconceptions around what yoga therapy is, and offer our understanding of the essence of yoga therapy.

Outline of Part 1

Chapter 1 begins with a brief overview of modern yoga therapy in traditional and contemporary models. We review the major living traditions of yoga therapy in India, since this is where this science first came from to the West. We also outline the different traditions. This is not a comprehensive presentation by any means, but it should give an idea of the major yoga therapy lineages.

In Chapter 2 we proceed to discuss the modalities of yoga therapy and its applications as a preventive measure, and outline its principles. We look at what yoga therapy is and what it is not, introducing the concept of "yogopathy" versus "yoga therapy." We also discuss a big concern of many contemporary therapists—how to keep yoga in yoga therapy, which includes the promise of spiritual transformation as a necessary part of the healing process.

Chapter 3 is dedicated to discussing the spiritual component of yoga therapy. In India this chapter would be unnecessary, as its cultural background is, in its essence, spiritual, with spirituality permeating the everyday life of the population. So quite naturally, the science of yoga is understood as the spiritual science. Unfortunately, the West still tends to treat spirituality exclusively as part of religion and not as part of everyday life, and there is much resistance, even fear, as we will see, in openly talking about it. (Perhaps this is the reason why yoga is often misunderstood as a form of religion.) There is also much misconception within the ranks of yoga therapists about spirituality, which many perceive as being outside of their scope. However, the body of research on spirituality as separate from religion is growing, with some researchers noting enhanced healing when the spiritual component is included. Even traditional healthcare systems are beginning to recognize the importance of the spiritual component in treating patients. Chapter 3 therefore looks at the existing research, and includes case records outlining the deep personal transformation of some of our patients on a healing journey. We propose that yoga therapy is the only secular complementary modality offering the promise of spiritual transformation as part of deep healing.

Yogic assessment lies at the core of yoga therapy. This fact is often not understood, especially by those who are limited to working only with a medical diagnosis. Yet the yogic way of assessing a patient should enhance, if not replace, medical diagnosis in our work. Chapter 4 is therefore dedicated to presenting a few different assessment tools. Although the appropriate assessment will depend on the nature of the therapist–client relationship and the environment in which the sessions are held, we hope you will find these helpful.

The assessment tools, among other factors, illustrate the level of knowledge and skill required of yoga therapists. And so, having a deeper understanding of what yoga therapy is and what tools we have at our disposal, we are ready, in Chapter 5, to look at who yoga therapists are, what makes them "good," and how they differ from yoga teachers.

CHAPTER 1

Beginnings of Modern Yoga Therapy

The origins of the philosophical and metaphysical teachings of yoga lie in a timeless history that is said to have originated in *Hiranyagarbha*, the causal germ plasm itself. This transcultural art and science of humanity grew from the roots of the traditional pan-Indian culture and way of life (*Sanatana dharma*), with a detailed codification presented by the great sage Patanjali through his *Yoga Darshana*, said to have been written more than 2500 years ago.

Today, yoga has become popular as a modality helping people to alleviate their physical, mental, and emotional imbalances. It is interesting to note that yoga as such was never meant to be a healing modality—yoga's goal for a human being is to reach enlightenment, or union of one's individual consciousness with Universal Consciousness. Yoga helps unify all aspects of our very being: the physical body, in which we live our daily life; the energy body, without which we will not have the capacity to do what we do; the mind body, which enables us to do our tasks with mindfulness; the higher intellect, which gives us clarity; and finally, the universal body, which gives us limitless bliss.

The three major time frames[1] of yoga history
Pre-historic (before 500 BC)
In the period before the written word, all spiritual teachings were transmitted orally from master (*guru*) to student (*sishya*) in forest hermitages. These are the teachings found today in the *Rig, Yajur, Sama,* and *Atharvana Vedas*.[2] The *Rigveda* talks about unity of the mind with the Divine in meditation (*yunjate man ut yunjate dhiyo vipraa viprasya brihato vipashchitah*; *Rigveda* Book 5 81:1); and the *Yajurveda* tells us that by regular yoga practice, we improve our

strength (*yoge yoge tavastaram vaaje vaaje havaamahe sakhaaya indramootaye*; *Yajurveda* 11:14).

Historic (500 BC–AD 1700)

In this period, the teachings were transmitted from master to student, using both oral and written traditions. These are the teachings found in the *Bhagavad Gita*,[3] *Upanishads*,[4] and Patanjali's *Yoga Sutras*[5] and *Hatha Yoga* texts. Even in ancient times, many types of yoga were taught, although the four main pillars were *Karma Yoga* (path of right action), *Bhakti Yoga* (path of devotion), *Jnana Yoga* (path of knowledge), and *Raja Yoga* (royal path to liberation). Feuerstein[6] has described 40 types of yoga ranging from *Abhava Yoga* (the unitive discipline of non-being) to *Yantra Yoga* (the unitive discipline of focusing the mind on the geometric representations of the cosmos). Of these, the main ones that have survived into the modern age are the *Ashtanga Yoga* teachings of Patanjali and the *Hatha Yoga* teachings of the *natha* yogis.[7]

Modern (after AD 1700)

In this period, the spiritual teachings were gleaned from many sources, often only through the written word and with or without the guidance of a living lineage of masters (*guruparampara*). During this time, yoga and its teachings moved from the East to the West, a phenomenon that is often attributed to the arrival of Swami Vivekananda in the US in 1893. Since then, various traditions, such as Tirumalai Krishnamacharya (B.K.S. Iyengar, T.K.V. Desikachar, and Pattabhi Jois), Swami Sivananda Saraswati (Satyananda, Vishnudevananda, *Satchitananda*), the Himalayan tradition (Swami Rama), the Self Realization Fellowship (Swami Yogananda), and the Rishiculture (Swami Gitananda) have spread worldwide.

Traditional basis of yoga therapy

In the *Hatha Yoga Pradipika*,[8] yogi Swatmarama states, "One who tirelessly practises yoga attains success irrespective of whether they are young, old, decrepit, diseased or weak." He gives us the guarantee that yoga improves the health of all and wards off disease, provided we properly abide by the rules and regulations (*yuvaa vrddho ativriddho vaa vyaadhito durbalo pi vaa abhyaasaat siddhimaapnoti sarvayogeshvatandritah*; *Hatha Yoga Pradipika* I:64).

The yogic view of health is exemplified in *Shvetashvatara Upanishad*, where it is said that the first signs of entering yoga are lightness of body, health, thirstlessness of mind, clearness of complexion, a beautiful voice, an agreeable odor, and scantiness of excretions (*laghutvam arogyam alolupatvam varnaprasadam svara sausthavam ca ganghas subho mootra pureesam Yoga pravrittim prathamam vadanti*; Shvetashvatara Upanishad II:13).

The *Hatha Yoga Pradipika* echoes these qualities: "Slimness of body, lustre on face, clarity of voice, brightness of eyes, freedom from disease, control over seminal ejaculation, stimulation of gastric heat and purification of subtle energy channels are marks of success in Hathayoga" (*vapuh krsatvam vadane prasannataa naadasputatvam nayane sunirmale arogataa bindujayogni diipanam naadiivishuddhir hatha siddhi lakshanam*; Hatha Yoga Pradipika II:78).

In *Gheranda Samhita*,[9] a classical treatise on *Hatha Yoga*, the human body is likened to an unbaked clay pot that is incapable of holding the contents and dissolves when faced with the challenge of water. It is only through intense heat generated by the practice of yoga that the human body gets baked, making it fit to hold the Divine Spirit (*aama kumbha ivaambhastho jeeryamanah sada gatah yoganalena samdahya ghata shuddhim samacaret*; Gheranda Samhita I:8).

In *Patanjala Yoga Darshana* we find an excellent description of the attributes of bodily perfection (*kaya sampat*). In Chapter 3 ("*Vibhuti Pada*"), that perfection of body includes beauty, gracefulness, strength, and adamantine hardness (*rupa lavanya bala vajra samhanana kaya sampat*; Yoga Darshana III:47). The effulgence that is characteristic of good health is also mentioned when it is said that deep concentration on the energy of digestion (*samana*) leads to radiant effulgence (*samana jayat jvalanam*; Yoga Darshana III:41).

Yoga emphasizes the importance of eating not only the right type of food, but also the right amount and with the right attitude. The importance of not eating alone, as well as the preparation and serving of food with love, is brought out in the yogic scheme of "right living." The inherent nature (*guna*) of food is taken into consideration to attain and maintain good health. The modern science of diet can learn much from this ancient concept of classification of food according to inherent nature, as it is a totally neglected aspect of the modern diet. The great Tamil poet-saint Tiruvalluvar offers sound advice on "right eating" when he says, "He who eats after the previous meal has been digested, needs not any medicine" (*marunthuena vaendaavaam yaakkaikku arundiyathu atrathu poatri unnin*; Thirukkural 942). He says that life in the body becomes a pleasure if we eat food to digestive measure (*attraal alavuarinthu unga aghduudambu pettraan nedithu uikkum aaru*; Thirukkural 943). He also invokes the yogic concept of *Mitahara* by advising that "eating a medium quantity of agreeable foods produces health and wellbeing" (*maarupaaduillaatha undi marutthuunnin oorupaadu illai uyirkku*; Thirukkural 943).

Living traditions of yoga therapy

Different regional and linguistic parts of India have been well served by the illustrious traditions of yoga. The visionary founders of these centers of excellence realized that in order to serve humanity in this modern day and age, the ancient traditional wisdom of yoga needed to work alongside modern medical science, with mutual respect and collaboration, leading to the wholesome integration of healthcare. Major centers flourishing in the new millennium include the tradition of Paramahamsa Madavdasji through the Kaivalyadhama Yoga Institute, the Krishnamacharya tradition through the Krishnamacharya Yoga Mandiram (KYM),[10] the Rishiculture Ashtanga Yoga tradition of Swami Gitananda Giri through the International Center for Yoga Education and Research (ICYER),[11] the Vivekananda Kendra tradition through the Swami Vivekananda Yoga Anusandhana Samsthana (S-VYASA or SVYASA),[12] and the popular Swami Ramadev Baba's work through the University of Patanjali.

Swami Kuvalayananda (1883–1966) founded the Kaivalyadhama Yoga Institute[13] in 1924 and began the first scientific research on yoga in the journal *Yoga-Mīmāṃsā*,[14] which is published to this day. Swami Kuvalayananda was also largely responsible for yoga becoming a subject in yoga colleges and universities, replacing traditional ashrams. Many eminent personalities such as Mahatma Gandhi and Jawaharlal Nehru used to take his advice regarding yoga and yoga therapy. Swami Digambarji succeeded him, and now Swami Maheshanandaji is the director while Shri O.P. Tiwari is the secretary—Shri O.P. Tiwariji is acknowledged as one of India's most senior yoga experts. Today, Kaivalyadhama is known worldwide for its research work on ancient yogic texts. Its college offers yoga training courses up to a Bachelor of Arts in Yoga Philosophy.

Shri Yogendra founded The Yoga Institute at Santacruz East in Mumbai in 1918. He was a pioneer in taking yoga to the West by founding probably the first ever yoga institute in the US, in Harriman State Park, New York, in 1919. A student of Paramahamsa Madhavdasaji, his emphasis was on "Householder Yoga," with "Yoga for the modern world" one of the teachings. The Yoga Institute has published many books on yoga, four of which have been preserved in The Crypt of Civilization at Oglethorpe University in Brookhaven, Georgia, to be opened after 6000 years, in 8113.

The Southern Peninsula of India has been the abode of a great many yoga masters. Yogacharya Shri Tirumalai Krishnamacharya (1888–1989) was a great master who lived in Mysore in Karnataka. A traditionalist to the core, he felt that yoga must be adapted to the individual. He had three main disciples, K. Pattabhi Jois, T.K.V. Desikachar, and B.K.S. Iyengar, and it is interesting that each one, although of the same lineage (Krishnamacharya), has codified quite different systems of yoga:

- His son and disciple, T.K.V. Desikachar, founded KYM in Chennai, and developed a system that adapts yoga to the individual (the *Viniyoga of Yoga*). T.K.V. Desikachar elevated KYM as the place of excellence in yoga therapy.

- K. Pattabhi Jois of Mysore codified the system of *Ashtanga Vinyasa Yoga*. It has become very popular in the West, with its challenging athletic nature, ideal for those who want to achieve something! His grandson is continuing his work in taking forward this system of vigorous *Hatha Yoga*.

- B.K.S. Iyengar founded the Ramamani Iyengar Memorial Yoga Institute in Pune in 1937. Today, his system of yoga is known as *Iyengar Yoga*. His book, *Light on Yoga*, remains one of the best instruction manuals for yoga still in print, and it is the standard textbook for *asanas*, translated into 28 languages.[15] He innovated the way students could attain precision in their practice of *asanas* by developing yoga props, including the now famous yoga mat. These props have helped those with an illness, those with a disability, older people, and weaker people to practice *asanas* efficaciously. There are about 75 scientific research papers from universities across the world about the efficacy of *Iyengar Yoga* as a therapeutic modality for health disorders.

Dr Swami Gitananda Giri, medical doctor and accomplished yogi, founded the Ananda Ashram[16] at Pondicherry, India, in 1968. Known as the Lion of Pondicherry, he also founded ICYER and Yoganjali Natyalayam, which are involved in teaching yoga to the young people of Pondicherry. His son and successor Dr Ananda Balayogi Bhavanani is continuing his work, and also currently serves as director of CYTER,[17] the Centre for Yoga Therapy, Education and Research, in Sri Balaji Vidyapeeth. Sri Balaji Vidyapeeth, a Deemed-to-be-University in Pondicherry, is rated in the top 100 universities of India in the NIRF (National Institutional Ranking Framework). It runs one of the rare yoga therapy centers operating from within a medical institution. CYTER offers yoga therapy to patients of the Mahatma Gandhi Medical College and Research Institute (MGMCRI); provides yoga training to all the university's medical, dental, and nursing students; and facilitates postgraduate courses in yoga therapy ranging from certificates and diplomas up to doctoral degree (PhD) level. CYTER is also a member school of the IAYT in the US, and the first university-based yoga therapy center in India to be on this list. It has completed two dozen research projects, with 106 papers published in high-impact journals.[18]

SVYASA is a university in Bangalore led by Dr H.R. Nagendra, and is based on the teachings of Swami Vivekananda. SVYASA specializes in yoga research and yoga therapy. Its research department has been associated with top organizations around the world, including the University of Texas MD Anderson Cancer Center, National Institute of Mental Health and Neuro-Sciences (NIMHANS), Indian Institute of Science (IISc), All India Institutes of Medical Sciences (AIIMS), KWA (Kuratorium Wohnen Im Alten), Karuna Trust, and many others. Since 1985 VYASA and S-VYASA have accounted for more than 350 papers on yoga in standard, peer-reviewed, and indexed national and international journals. SVYASA offers postgraduate courses and a Master of Science (MSc) in yoga therapy, as well as a PhD in yoga. In conjunction with the Indian government it offers special subsidized yoga teacher training for young Indian people from other countries.

Traditional models of yoga therapy

There are half a dozen major models of yoga therapy in India. These are based on concepts, principles, and practices that are prominent among specific centers, and one or more of these approaches would normally be used in Indian yoga therapy practice.

Krishnamacharya-Desikachar model

The Krishnamacharya-Desikachar model is based on Patanjali's *Yoga Sutras*. There is an understanding of the different stages of life and the different processes involved in each. By distinguishing needs and goals with reference to the individual, this tradition emphasizes the individualization of the approach to yoga and yoga therapy as a practice. The application is based on a broad segregation as follows: the growth process in children (*srsti karma*), the maturation process in older teenagers and young adults (*siksana karma*), a maintenance process preventing future complications (*raksana karma*), a spiritual process, especially in older people (*adhyatmika karma*), and as a healing modality and process in individuals with health issues (*cikitsa karma*).

In this classical tradition, yoga therapy is elevated to a highly sophisticated healthcare discipline. It is practiced as a client-empowering process, where the client is responsible for their healing process. It is done in an individualized, one-to-one setting with a multidimensional approach, often utilizing many tools of yoga. The client-centric process is context-sensitive and respects the age, occupation, ability, and other parameters of the individual. It is considered an evolving process, and is not used as merely a quick-fix solution. It is adopted as a personal and spiritual development path, as a process to develop one's own unique strengths, and hence it fits in ideally as a collaborative and complementary system of self-healthcare.

The four-pronged systematic arrangement (*vyuha*) model of yoga therapy is foundational to this tradition and is based on Maharishi Patanjali's *Yoga Sutras*. The steps involved in the process are: a complete and comprehensive understanding of the problem and the individual having the problem (*heyam*); establishment of the cause of the problem (*hetu*); the therapeutic goal of healing (*hanam*); and the selection and utilization of tools to bring about the desired goal (*upayam*). These are established through four ways of evaluation (*pariksha*) that involve: observational analysis of the client (*darsanam*); palpation and touch-based analysis (*sparsanam*); a detailed interview with the client (*prasnam*); and pulse examination (*nadi pariksa*).

Gitananda model

Swami Gitananda Giri claimed that *yoga therapy* is virtually as old as yoga itself—the "return of mind that feels separated from the Universe in which it exists" represents the first yoga therapy. *Yoga therapy* could be termed "man's first attempt at a unitive understanding of mind-emotions-physical distress and is the oldest wholistic concept and therapy in the world."[19] To achieve this yogic integration at all levels of our being, it is essential that we take into consideration the multidimensional aspects of yoga: a healthy life-nourishing diet, a healthy and natural environment, a holistic lifestyle, personal and social behavioral ethics (*yamas* and *niyamas*), bodywork through *asanas, mudras, bandhas*, and *kriyas*, breath work through *pranayama*, and the cultivation of a healthy thought process through *Jnana Yoga* and *Raja Yoga*.

Swamiji has written extensively, from the point of view of both a medical doctor and an accomplished yogi, about the relationship between health and disease:

> Yoga views the vast proliferation of psychosomatic diseases as a natural outcome of stress and strain created by desire fostered by modern propaganda and abuse of the body condoned on all sides even by religion, science and philosophy. Add to this the synthetic "junk food" diet of modern society, and you have the possibility of endless disorders developing...even the extinction of man by his own ignorance and misdeeds.[20]

He explained the root cause of disease as follows:

> Yoga, a wholistic, unified concept of oneness, is non-dual (or *adwaitam*) in nature. It suggests happiness, harmony and ease. Dis-ease is created when duality (or *dwaitam*) arises in the human mind. This false concept of duality has produced all conflicts of human mind and the vast list of human disorders. Duality (dis-ease) is the primary cause of man's downfall. Yoga helps return man to his pristine, whole nature. All diseases, maladies, tensions, are manifestations of divisions of what should be man's complete nature, the "Self" (*atman*). This "Self" is "ease". A loss of "ease" creates "dis-ease." Duality is the first disease, the unreasonable thought that "I am different from the whole… I am unique." It is interesting that the one of the oldest words for man is "*insan*." A return to sanity, "going sane," is the subject of real Yoga means of accomplishment (*sadhana*) and Yoga consistence spiritual practice (*abhyasa*). *Yoga therapy* is one of the methods to help insane man back onto the path of sanity.[21]

One of the specialities of the Gitananda tradition is the use of 12 diagnostic methods (*dwadasha rogalakshna anukrama*) in the process of yoga therapy assessment. These can be contemplated as a method of self-analysis (*swadhyaya*) that not only enables the therapist to understand the client better, but also enables the client to understand themselves better too. This is explained in detail in Chapter 4.

SVYASA model

This model is based on *Yoga Vashista*,[22] which describes the cause and manifestation of disease in detail—both psychosomatic as well as non-psychosomatic ailments. It attributes all psychic disturbances and physical ailments to the five elements (the *pancha mahabhuta*) in a similar manner to other systems of Indian medicine. Commonly seen diseases or disorders of a psychosomatic nature (*samanya adhija vyadhi*) are described as those arising from day-to-day causes, while the essential "disease" of being bound to the birth–rebirth cycle (*sara adhija vyadhi*) may be understood in modern terms as congenital diseases. The former can be corrected by day-to-day remedial measures such as medicines and surgery, whereas the essential disease of lifetime-to-lifetime bondage to human birth (*sara adhija vyadhi*) does not cease until knowledge of the Self (*atma jnana*) is attained.

It is interesting to note that traditional Indian thought views the very occurrence of birth on this planet as a disease and as a source of suffering! Tiruvalluvar reiterates this when he says, "It is knowledge of the ultimate truth that removes the folly of birth" (*pirappu ennum pedaimai neenga chirappu ennum chem porul kaanbadhu arivu; Thirukkural* 358).

Yoga understands that physical ailments that are not of a psychosomatic nature can be easily managed with surgery, medication, prayers, and lifestyle modifications, as required. Various yoga techniques may also be used to help prevent or correct physical ailments and restore health, with regeneration, recuperation, and rehabilitation as necessary.

Yoga Vashista gives an elaborate description of the mechanism by which psychosomatic disorders occur. It starts with mental confusion, which leads to agitation of the life force (*prana*) and a haphazard flow along life force channels (*nadis*), resulting in depletion of energy and/or clogging up of these channels of vital energy. This leads to disturbance in the physical body, with disorder in metabolism, excessive appetite, and improper functioning of the entire digestive system. Natural movement of food through the digestive tract is arrested, giving rise to numerous physical ailments. *Yoga Vashista* is many thousands of years old, and the concept of psychosomatic disorders in modern medicine has only recently been realized and accepted.

Iyengar model

"Yoga cures what need not be endured and endures what cannot be cured," said B.K.S. Iyengar. The approach to therapy in Iyengar's tradition is through the *asanas* and *pranayama*. The body, mind, breath, and emotions of an individual are closely integrated. A problem with one of these affects the other factors. So, through the body, we can also access and alter the condition of the breath, mind, and emotions.

The fundamental principle of yoga therapy in this system is to understand the alignment of the body, not only in the basic standing, sitting, and supine positions, but also in the range of *asanas*.

Iyengar created specific sequences of *asanas* for different conditions, which forms the basis of yoga therapy. Further individualized modifications are given depending on the age, health, and condition of the individual. "*Asanas* are not prescriptions or descriptions," said B.K.S. Iyengar, "thus, it is not just what *asanas* are done but how they are done that is important." This is the reason much emphasis is given in this system on precision and alignment in practice. For those who are unable to attain such precision, props or supports such as blankets, belts, pillows, chairs, bolsters, ropes, and other wooden props are used.

Kaivalyadhama model

According to Swami Kuvalayananda, founder of Kaivalyadhama, positive health does not mean mere freedom from disease but is a jubilant and energetic way of living and feeling that is the peak state of wellbeing at all levels—physical, mental, emotional, and social. He says that one of the aims of yoga is to encourage positive hygiene and health through the development of the inner natural powers of the body and mind. Thus, the adaptation and adjustment of the internal environment of man [sic] helps him enjoy positive health and not just mere freedom from disease. He emphasizes that yoga produces purification of all channels of communication (*nadi shuddhi*) and eradication of factors that disturb the balance of body and mind (*mala shuddhi*).

According to Swami Kuvalayananda, yoga helps cultivate positive health through three integral steps:

- Cultivating the correct psychological attitudes based on friendliness, compassion, cheerfulness, and indifference (*maitri, karuna, mudita, upekshanam*) towards those people, places, and events that are at ease, suffering, virtuous, and non-virtuous, respectively (*suka, duhkha, punya, apunya*).

- Reconditioning the neuromuscular and neuroglandular system—in fact, the whole body—enabling it to better withstand greater stress and strain.

- Laying great emphasis on appropriate diet conducive to such a peak state of health, and encouraging the natural processes of elimination through various cleansing processes (*nadi shuddhi* or *mala shuddhi*).

Swara Yoga model

According to *Shiva Swarodaya*,[23] a classical text on *Swara Yoga*,[24] disease develops when smooth and regular airflow (*swara*) in the nostrils does not adhere to fixed timings and days. Normally *swara* flows in the nostrils in a certain pattern according to phases of the lunar cycle. In the case of a disease developing due to the erroneous functioning of breathing (*swara*), a correction of that malfunctioning can cure that disease. The use of different techniques is also advocated for changing *swara* to relieve various disorders.

In summary, it is worth mentioning that India is leading the way in accepting and using yoga as a therapeutic modality. The Government of India is currently promoting indigenous systems of health through the recently formed Ministry of AYUSH.[25] Among other activities, it oversees research in yoga and yoga therapy through its Central Council for Research in Yoga & Naturopathy (CCRYN). A Yoga Certification Board (YCB) certifies yoga instructors and teachers at Level 1 and 2, while the Health Sector Skill Council has recently collaborated with the Indian Yoga Association to define and create vocational training for job roles in yoga therapy. The Morarji Desai National Institute of Yoga is currently the only government-run institute for yoga, and has brought together all the major traditions of yoga. It was awarded the status of a Collaborative Centre for Traditional Medicine (Yoga) by the World Health Organization (WHO) in 2013. The WHO recently held a Working Group Meeting with experts from all WHO regions to finalize a document regarding the setting of benchmarks for yoga training.

Most notably, however, AYUSH has recently (as of November 2018) announced a new initiative to address non-communicable diseases (NCDs, also called chronic psychosomatic diseases) that have become endemic with a large population of teenagers and a middle-aged population succumbing to lifestyle diseases. In an effort to implement lifestyle changes, AYUSH will include yoga and meditation and will teach certain *asanas* for patients with borderline diabetes, hypertension, and osteoarthritis.

The aim is to try to change the lifestyle of many who are becoming prone to diabetes and hypertension at an early age. It is mainly pre-diabetics and those suffering from borderline ailments who will be located and treated to prevent them from developing these diseases. There are 201 NCD centers across the state of Karnataka, one in each district, including 80 health centers and 121 community health centers. Besides diabetes, hypertension, and osteoarthritis, the centers also cater to patients with stroke, cardiovascular diseases, and cancer, with a focus on oral, breast, and cervical cancer.[26]

Another notable initiative is the Integrated Cancer Project (I-CAP)[27] submitted by the Network for AYUSH Cancer Care, Standing Research Committee, and Indian Yoga Association to the Ministry of Health and Family Welfare. In an 80-page document it recognizes the need to improve awareness, affordability, and access to care for Indian cancer patients. It further outlines detailed comprehensive strategies to deal with these challenges, and recommends setting up a center for excellence in yoga in oncology, with the mandate to further evaluate and understand the mechanism of interventions of yoga for cancer patients.

India is perhaps today the most advanced country in accepting yoga therapy by its government body and applying yoga therapy as a complementary modality in preventing or healing NCDs. In the West the approach is notably different, with the profession still not well recognized or regulated by government. There remains much confusion and many misconceptions around yoga therapy, and we will now attempt to clear these up in the next chapter, which is dedicated to yoga therapy, its principles, and its application.

CHAPTER 2

Yoga Therapy and its Application

Yoga therapy, part of yoga

"Oh, East is East, and West is West, and never the twain shall meet," said Rudyard Kipling in "The Ballad of East and West." This dichotomy, however, seems to have been overcome in recent times, as many Eastern healing traditions have slowly and steadily percolated through to the healthcare system worldwide. This is especially true of mind–body therapies that focus on the health-promoting intrinsic connections that exist between the human brain, mind, body, and individual behavior.

Yoga may be understood as the art and science of conscious living. This may, indeed, be as ancient as the universe itself, as these principles are truly transcultural, transcendental, and timeless in their universality.

In recent times, however, yoga has become more popular as a therapy, with the majority of people often coming to it seeking to alleviate their physical, mental, or emotional imbalances. This has been aided by a number of published studies and systematic reviews offering reliable scientific evidence of the potential of yoga in treating a wide range of psychosomatic conditions.

Illness, disease, and disorders are common in this world, and people everywhere are desperately seeking relief from their suffering. Yoga helps us to think better and to live better; indeed, it helps us improve ourselves in everything we do. Hence it holds out the promise of health, wellbeing, and harmony.

We must not forget that the use of yoga as a therapy is just a recent happening in its wonderful long history, which has historically served to promote spiritual evolution. Yoga helps us to unify all aspects of our very being: the physical body, in which we live our daily life; the energy body, without which we will not have the capacity to do what we do; the mind body, which enables us to do our tasks with mindfulness; the higher intellect, which gives us clarity; and finally, the universal body, which gives us limitless bliss.

Yoga as the original mind–body medicine

Yoga is one of the six reverential perspectives of the universe (*Shat Darshana*) as codified by the great seers (*Rishis*) of the pan-Indian cultural tradition. It provides us with a practical framework and perspective of the manifest universe (*prakruti*) and the pure consciousness that lies behind it (*purusha*). The moral and ethical foundations of yoga (*yama*, *niyama*) provide inner strength, conviction, and self-responsibility that manifest in both our personal and social life. They guide our attitudes with regard to what is right and wrong in our life and in relation to our Self, our family, and the entire social system. These changes in our attitude and behavior will go a long way in helping to prevent the root causes of stress in our life.

The five moral restraints of subhuman tendencies (*pancha yama*) include non-violence (*ahimsa*), truthfulness (*satya*), non-stealing (*asteya*), channeling of creative impulses in tune with the higher consciousness (*brahmacharya*), and non-covetousness (*aparigraha*). The ethical observances of a humane nature (*pancha niyama*) are purity (*saucha*), contentment (*santhosha*), leading a disciplined and minimalistic life (*tapas*), introspective self-analysis (*swadhyaya*), and attitude of acceptance of the Almighty (*Iswarpranidhana*).

Patanjali advocates adopting appropriate attitudes towards different situations, people, and events in our life. These include friendliness towards those who are at ease with themselves (*maitri*), compassion towards those who are suffering (*karuna*), cheerfulness towards the noble (*mudita*), and equanimity towards the non-virtuous (*upekshanam*). This enables us to have a clearer perspective on life and to deal with our problems more effectively. He further advises us to cultivate a contrary view (*Pratipaksha Bhavanam*) when faced with negative thoughts of a destructive nature that otherwise ultimately only lead to suffering.

The triple humor (*tridosha—vata*, *pitta*, and *kapha*)[1] theory of health and disease that developed during the late Vedic period is common to virtually all traditional Indian systems of medicine. Health is understood to be the balanced harmony of the three humors in accordance with individual predisposition, while disease results from an imbalanced disharmony. The *Tirumandiram of Tirumoolar*, the 3000-versed Tamil treatise by the Dravidian saint, prescribes the practice of yoga at different times of the day to relieve disorders arising from these imbalances. According to him, the practice of yoga at dusk relieves mucous, phlegmatic (*kapha*) disorders, practice at noon relieves gaseous, movement-based (*vata*) disorders, and practice in the morning relieves acidic, bilious (*pitta*) disorders.

According to the *Bhagavad Gita*,[2] yoga is defined as the disassociation from our tendency to attach to our suffering, pain, and illness (*dukkhasamyogaviyogam yoga samjnitham*; *Bhagavad Gita* VI:23). People with health conditions often tend to identify themselves with that condition and as a patient of that condition. This results in statements such as, "I am a diabetic" or "I am a hypertensive." In some cases this actually becomes a very strong identification and they claim ownership of that condition with statements such as, "My diabetes," "My hypertension," or "My cancer." Unless this mal-identification with their diseased state is broken, it becomes very difficult to actually bring about a "cure" for the individual.

One of the foremost concepts of yoga therapy is that the mind (*adhi*) influences the body, thus creating disease (*vyadhi*). This is the basis of psychosomatics and mind–body medicine, and is termed *adhi vyadhi* or *adhija vyadhi*, where the mind causes the disease in the physical body. In modern language, this is also termed psychoneuroimmunology, as modern health systems have started to realize that how we think and feel can positively or negatively influence our nervous, endocrine, and immune responses. One path leads to health while the other leads to disease and suffering.

Virtually every health problem that we face today either has its origin in psychosomatics or is worsened by the psychosomatic aspect of the disease. The mind and the body seem to be continuously fighting each other. What the mind wants, the body won't do, and what the body wants, the mind won't do. This creates a dichotomy, a disharmony, in other words, a disease. Yoga helps restore balance and equilibrium by virtue of the internal process of unifying the mind, body, and emotions. The psychosomatic stress disorders that are so prevalent in today's world can be prevented, controlled, and possibly even cured via the sincere and dedicated application of yoga as a therapy.

The yogic concept of health and disease enables us to understand that the cause of physical disorders stems from the seed in the mind and beyond. The disturbed mind (*adhi*) is the primary root cause while the physical disease (*vyadhi*) is only the final manifest effect in yogic philosophy. By paying careful attention to personal history, the origins of psychosomatic disease can nearly always be traced back to patterns of mental and emotional distress.

According to yogic thought, all diseases start not with the body, but from blockages in our subtler energy systems. All disturbances start at the psychic level beyond the mind (the psyche in Indian thought goes all the way up to the sense of Self), come down through a disturbed mind, and then manifest in the subtle energy channels (*prananadi*), and finally settle in the physical body. Therefore, the five-layered model of existence (*pancha kosha* or *pancha maya*) is one of the ancient Indian models that helps us to look for a root cause of the manifest problem or disease.

The five *koshas*

Anandamaya kosha

The *pancha kosha* model considers the human being to exist on multiple levels at the same time. According to this system of thought, the human being emerges out of "oneness," forming a sense of self-identity, just like the drop comes out of the ocean and has its outer membrane (*anandamaya kosha*). Each of the subsequent layers of existence (*koshas*) then represents the next level of separation, and their energy and vibration slows down and becomes grosser (see below). Note that in the figure below, although each *kosha* is represented by a separate circle, they are inseparable and completely interdependent, as they all exist at the same place at the same time. If we change something in one *kosha*, all other *koshas* also respond to that change.

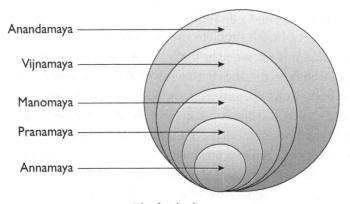

The five koshas

Vijnamaya kosha

Our wisdom, the non-judgmental witness, and our intellect manifest through the *vijnamaya kosha*. As this is a part of conscience in our higher mind, this *kosha* is responsible for discerning between good and bad, making us the master of our basic instincts, which lie in *manomaya kosha*. This *kosha* also represents the chemical activity at the cellular level of various organs in the body and maintains the optimum level of ingredients at tissue and blood level, that is, homeostasis.

Manomaya kosha

This is the energy of the basic mind (our core belief system, our conscious mind), and it is of denser energy. Our mind is what we think, feel, and express from our thoughts and impressions. The mind is working according to the signals it receives from the outside environment through the five sense organs. As the smell of a perfume that we recognize will give rise to a memory that reminds us of a person or an occasion, this memory will create emotions that get expressed in our gross body, such as happiness or dislike. In this way the mind has a great influence on our lower and denser *pranamaya kosha* and *annamaya kosha*, as the emotions that rise affect and change our normal breathing pattern and heart rate.

If such an emotional state continues over a long time, we will see vigorous affects in the *annamaya kosha* (gross body), initially as pain, and later on as more serious diseases. Here, the interstitial tissue fluid performs the important function of receiving an impulse from the brain and taking it from the cell to the sensory cortex. These strong affects of our mind through thoughts and emotions are the reason that we need to give importance to control and direct the movement of the mind towards the things that keep us balanced and healthy. As described by Patanjali, our identification with the mind and its movements is the cause of our suffering in life, and he describes how to overcome our miseries with the help of yoga. For many people, the claim that we are not the mind and that we can, in fact, manage our mind, is revolutionary.

Pranamaya kosha

The pranic *kosha*, the vital energy body, which is of even denser energy, engulfs our physical body—*annamaya kosha*. The *prana* is the life energy that stays in and around the *annamaya kosha* as long as the body is alive. It flows through the *nadis* (channels used for the *prana* to move within) to each and every cell in the body according to its needs. It will change the direction and quantity of flow according to the need—when we are running, we need more energy in the legs and lungs, and after eating food, we need more energy in the digestive system. If the *prana* does not move in its right direction or there are some blockages in its flow, we will experience it as a pain or disease in the *annamaya kosha* (physical body).

Annamaya kosha

The word *anna* indicates nourishing substances that enable survival at the physical level. Gross matter is something we can experience, see, and feel with our five senses. Our body is made out of cells, different tissues, bones, and muscles, and all of these need to be taken care of with a supply of energy and nutrients through eating, digestion, movements or exercise, cleansing, and giving the body rest. On this level we give importance to what is described in the texts about cleanliness of our body from inside and outside, eating appropriately, using our muscles in a good way, and having proper rest and sleep.

From the yogic viewpoint of disease, psychosomatic, stress-related disorders appear to progress through four distinct phases. These can be understood as follows:[3]

- *Psychic:* This phase is marked by mild but persistent psychological and behavioral symptoms of stress such as irritability, disturbed sleep, and other minor symptoms. It can be correlated with the intellectual (*vijnamaya*) and psychological (*manomaya*) aspects of one's existence, and yoga as a therapy can be very effective in this phase.

- *Psychosomatic:* If the stress continues, there is an increase in symptoms, along with the appearance of generalized physiological symptoms such as occasional hypertension or tremors. This phase can be correlated with the psychological (*manomaya*) and functional-physiological (*pranamaya*) aspects of one's existence, and once again, yoga as a therapy can prove very effective in this phase.

- *Somatic:* This phase is marked by disturbed function of organs, particularly the target, or involved, organ. At this stage the diseased state can begin to be identified. This phase can be correlated with the anatomical-physical (*annamaya*) and functional-physiological (*pranamaya*) aspects of one's existence. Yoga as a therapy is less effective in this phase, and may need to be used in conjunction with other methods of treatment.

- *Organic:* This phase is marked by full manifestation of the diseased state, with pathological changes such as an ulcerated stomach or chronic hypertension becoming manifest in their totality with their resultant complications. This phase can be correlated with the anatomical-physical (*annamaya*) existence as the disease has become fixed in the physical body. This is similar to the modern medical concept of target organ damage (TOD), and yoga as a therapy has a palliative and quality of life-improving effect in this phase. It also produces positive emotional and psychological effects, even in terminal and end of life situations. However, the early stages of the disease process are often overlooked, and the final stage is seen as an entity unto itself, having little relationship to one's living and thinking habits and patterns. This is because modern medicine only looks at the physical aspects and neglects the influence of existential (*pancha kosha*) and subtle manifestations (*trisharira*) on health and disease.

Yoga as a therapy works very well at both the psychic and psychosomatic stages. Once the disease enters the somatic stage, yoga therapy as an adjunct to other therapies may improve the condition. In the organic stage, yoga therapy's role is more of a palliative, pain-relieving, and rehabilitative nature.

The modern world is facing a pandemic of lifestyle disorders that require changes to be made consciously by individuals themselves. Yoga places great importance on a proper and healthy lifestyle, whose main components are:

- *Achar:* Yoga stresses the importance of healthy activities such as exercise, and recommends body–breath work (*asana, pranayama, kriya*) on a regular basis. Improved cardiorespiratory health, exercise tolerance, agility, and physical endurance are by-products of such healthy activities.

- *Vichar:* Healthy thoughts and a healthy attitude towards life are vital for wellbeing. A balanced state of mind is obtained by following moral self-restraints (*yama*) and ethical observances (*niyama*). As Mahatma Gandhi said, "The world has enough in this world for everyone's needs, but not enough for everyone's greed."

- *Ahar:* Yoga emphasizes the need for a healthy vegetarian diet that has an adequate intake of fresh water along with a well-balanced intake of fresh food, green salads, sprouts, unrefined cereals, and fresh fruits. It is important to be aware of the need for food to be prepared and served with love and affection (*sattvic*).

- *Vihar:* Proper recreational activities to relax the body and mind are essential for good health. This includes proper relaxation, maintaining quietude of action-speech-thoughts, and group activities wherein one loses the sense of individuality. Serving others in a selfless manner (*Karma Yoga*) is an excellent way to achieve inner peace and joy.

- *Vyavahar:* Healthy interpersonal relationships that enable us to be the best "we" can be, learning to adapt to other people in our life and create a sense of teamwork, enabling the sublimation of the ego into a positive energy that sustains relationships rather than harms them. When we learn to live with gratitude, respect, love, and acceptance, life becomes much better, and we grow as individuals.

Role of yoga as a preventive measure

While it is popular to look for the curative aspects of yoga, we must not forget that the major role of yoga is as a preventive therapy, preventing the painful suffering that is yet to manifest.[4]

If the practice of yoga is taken up during childhood, we can help so many conditions from occurring later on in life. This is primary prevention. Once the condition occurs, once the disease has set in, we have secondary prevention, which is more in the nature of controlling the condition, to whatever extent we can. Tertiary prevention is done once the condition has occurred, as we try to prevent complications, those that affect the quality of a client's life.

Clinical applications of yoga have been studied in pediatric and young adult populations with a focus on physical fitness, cardiorespiratory effects, mental health, behavior and development, irritable bowel syndrome, eating disorders, and prenatal effects on birth outcomes. Yoga has been suggested as an option for children to increase their physical activity and fitness, and may be a gateway for adopting a healthy active lifestyle in sedentary children who are intimidated by more vigorous forms of exercise. A detailed review[5] showed that yoga may benefit children with mental challenges by improving their mental ability, along with motor coordination and social skills, and that restoration of some degree of functional ability is possible in those with physical disabilities. A notable point mentioned by researchers was that, "Regardless of the goal, Yoga appears to be a multitasking modality that simultaneously treats both physical impairments as well as more global issues such as stress, anxiety, or hyperactivity."[6]

To achieve this yogic integration at all levels of our being, it is essential that we take into consideration the all-encompassing multidimensional aspects of human existence that include the following: diet, natural environment, holistic lifestyle, internal attitudes and thought processes, recurring negative emotions, adequate bodywork through conscious and steady postures (*asanas*), conscious channeling of energy through gestures and neuromuscular locks (*mudras, bandhas*), breath–body movement integrating practices (*kriyas*), and breath work through *pranayama*.

However, the most important point is that some responsibility for health, wellbeing, and healing lies in the hands of each individual. We, as therapists, empower our clients and facilitate their efforts towards self-healing. The *Purananuru*[7] says, "Life's good comes not from others, nor its gifts, nor ills. Man's suffering and its relief are both found within."

Principles of yoga therapy

When we set out to practice yoga therapy, it is vital that we understand and teach the principles of this unique system to our clients in the following way:

1. *Developing awareness of the body, emotions, and mind:* Awareness of the body can be achieved by conscious bodywork synchronized with breath and awareness in order to qualify as a psychosomatic technique. However, being aware of the emotions and thought processes is a challenge, and may take a lot of practice.

2. *Changing dietary habits:* Most disorders are directly or indirectly linked to unhealthy dietary patterns that need to be assessed and then addressed.

3. *Conscious relaxation of the entire body:* Relaxation is often all that most patients need in order to improve their physical condition. Stress is the major culprit and may be the causative, aggravating, or precipitating factor in many psychosomatic disorders. The relaxation part of every yoga session is important as it produces rest, rejuvenation, reinvigoration, and reintegration of all of the body's systems, down to the cellular level.

4. *Slowing down the breath, making it quiet and deep:* Rapid, uncontrolled, irregular breathing is a sign of ill health, hyperventilation, and an overactive mind. Slow, deep, and regular controlled breathing through the nose is a sign of health. Breath is the link between body and mind, connecting physical, physiological, and mental factors. When the breath is slowed down, the mind is calm and the metabolic processes are also slowed; anabolic activities begin the process of healing and rebuilding.

5. *Calming down the mind and focusing it inwardly:* Breath work is the most convenient and effective tool for training and management of the mind. Together with the practice of focused concentration during meditation, this will lead to bringing the mind under control.

6. *Improving the flow of healing "pranic life energy":* Prana is the energy of life and it can be used effectively for healing. The various energies driving different physiological functions of the body (*vayu*)[8] need to be assessed and corrected to bring about harmony. As an example, in those suffering digestive disorders, the focus may be more on balancing the functional energy of that area (*samana vayu*), whereas in pelvic conditions or in cases of constipation, it would be more on the functional energy centered in the pelvic region (*apana vayu*).

7. *Non-reaction to omnipresent stressors:* We have very little control over our surrounding environment and the stressors within it. So often the only way to reduce the impact of stress levels is by increasing our ability to deal with them. As the saying goes, "When face to face with the innumerable thorns in a forest, we may either choose to spend all our time picking them up or choose to wear a pair of shoes and walk through the forest." The difference is primarily in the attitude that is consciously chosen. Practicing points 1–6 will result in effective management of our reaction to stressors.

8. *Increasing self-reliance and self-confidence:* The challenges we encounter every day should be reframed and understood as opportunities for change. We must understand that we have the inner power to overcome each and every challenge that life throws at us.

9. *Facilitating natural elimination of wastes:* The natural elimination of wastes from the body is facilitated by cleaning practices such as the upper gastrointestinal cleanser (*dhauti*), lower gastrointestinal cleanser (*basti*), and nasopharyngeal cleanser (*neti*). Accumulation and stagnation of waste materials in either the inner or outer environment always causes problems. Yogic cleansing practices help to wash out the impurities (*mala shodhana*), helping the process of regeneration and facilitating healing.

10. *Taking responsibility for our own health:* Perhaps this is the most important principle. This requires the client to examine their life and change the disease-forming factors that are in their reach. The current healthcare system fosters an attitude of victimhood and disempowerment, with the power and responsibility for our health entrusted completely to the medical profession. This relieves us from taking responsibility for our disease-forming habits. Yoga empowers clients with tools so they can experience their own power.

Scientific basis of using yoga as a therapy

Numerous studies have been done in the past few decades on the psychophysiological and biochemical changes occurring following the practice of yoga. A few clinical trials have also shown promise, despite yoga not being ideally suited to the scientific gold standard of "double-blind" clinical trials.

The difficulty of finding the right methods and apparatus to study the higher aspects of yoga is still to be overcome. The subtle aspects of yoga are yet to be scientifically measured, and may only be understood when more sensitive equipment and methods of research become available. Most of the research done on yoga to date focuses on its bio-physio-psychological levels.

Some important physiological benefits of yoga

Yoga produces a stable autonomic nervous system equilibrium, with a tendency toward parasympathetic nervous system dominance rather than the usual stress-induced sympathetic nervous system dominance. This is of great potential in psychosomatic stress-related illnesses. Cardiovascular and cardiorespiratory efficiency increases. Heart rate and blood pressure decrease, leading to a reduced load on the heart. Respiratory rate decreases with improved respiratory efficiency. The amplitude and smoothness of respiration increases, along with all parameters of pulmonary function such as tidal volume, vital capacity, and breath-holding time. EEG alpha waves increase. Theta, delta, and beta waves also increase during various stages of meditation. Gastrointestinal and endocrine functions normalize, with improvement in excretory functions. Musculoskeletal flexibility and joint range of motion increase. Posture improves with improvement in strength, resiliency, and endurance. Body weight normalizes and sleep improves, with increased energy levels, and immunity increases with improved ability for pain tolerance.

Some important psychological benefits of yoga

Somatic and kinesthetic awareness increase with better self-acceptance and self-actualization. There is better social adjustment with a decrease in anxiety, depression, and hostility. Psychomotor functions such as grip strength, balance, dexterity and fine motor skills, eye–hand coordination and reaction time, steadiness and depth perception, and the integrated functioning of body parts improve. Mood often improves and subjective wellbeing increases while cognitive functions such as attention, concentration, memory, and learning efficiency improve.

Overall biochemical effects of yoga

The biochemical profile often improves, indicating an anti-stress and antioxidant effect, which is important in preventing degenerative diseases. There are decreased levels of blood glucose, total white blood cell count, total cholesterol, triglycerides, low-density lipoprotein (LDL), and very-low-density lipoprotein

(VLDL). At the same time, following yoga, it has been reported that there are increased levels of high-density lipoprotein (HDL) cholesterol, ATPase, hematocrit, hemoglobin, thyroxin, lymphocytes, vitamin C, and total serum protein.[9]

Therapeutic modalities of yoga therapy

There are numerous therapeutic modalities used in the application of yoga as a therapy. It is important to remember that yoga therapy is not a prescriptive modality and we always start from assessing the client and their disease and keep the assessment process throughout the length of the therapy. As different traditions of yoga emphasize using different methods for yoga therapy, it is therefore beneficial for a therapist to be familiar with the different lineages that offer specific practices. The more we know, the more research we study, the more tools we have at hand to help our clients. As therapists our loyalty is with the client and not the lineage—we should always use the best tool for the client's benefit, no matter what lineage the tool comes from.

In general terms, however, we can divide a vast array of yogic practices into the following:

Physical therapies

Consciously adopted static postures (*asanas*), systematic and managed breathing coordinated with movements (*kriyas*), and seals and locks for neuromuscular energy (*mudras* and *bandhas*) gently stretch and strengthen the musculoskeletal system in a healthy manner. They improve the mobility and flexibility of the different joints and groups of muscles. There is also concomitant improvement in the systemic function such as respiration, circulation, digestion, and elimination. A general sense of health and wellbeing is also promoted by these aspects of yoga that help release "feel good" hormones such as endorphins and encephalin.

Emotional and mental therapies

Yoga addresses the deeper aspects of emotional wellbeing and introspectional self-analysis (*swadhyaya*), breath-based techniques of vital energy control (*pranayama*), practices enabling mastery and withdrawal from sensory reactivity (*pratyahara*), intense concentration (*dharana*), and contemplative oneness (*dhyana*). Chanting, devotional music (*bhajana*), and *yoga nidra* are very effective in managing emotions, attitudes, and thought processes.

Development of healthy psychological attitudes

Yoga encourages us to step back and take an objective view of our habitual patterns of behavior and thoughts. This enables us to cope better with situations that normally put our bodies and minds under strain. Patanjali emphasized the need to develop the following qualities in order to become mentally balanced human beings: a non-attached and objective meta-cognitive attitude (*vairagya*), balanced acceptance of life (*chitta prasadanam*), friendliness towards those who are at ease with themselves (*maitri*), compassion for those who are suffering (*karuna*), cheerfulness towards the noble and virtuous (*mudita*), and indifference towards those who stray from the noble path (*upekshanam*), and so on. Conscious adoption of the right attitude towards the situation, person, place, and/or event is one of the most important aspects of yoga as a therapy. If this is not done, we practice yogopathy, and not yoga therapy.

Mental therapies

There are a great many useful techniques of relaxation and visualization, and these are found in the higher introspective aspects of *Jnana* and *Raja Yoga*[10] as well as *yoga nidra*. There are also practices such as concentrated gaze (*trataka*).

Spiritual therapies

Scriptural study and self-introspection (*swadhyaya*), spiritual community seeking knowledge of the reality (*satsangha*), devotional singing (*bhajana*), and chanting sessions and yogic counseling are important aspects of yogic therapy that are often neglected in favor of physical therapies alone. These are described in more detail in a separate chapter dedicated to yoga therapy and spirituality (Chapter 3).

The correct use of these modalities according to the condition and needs of clients can enable us to strike at the root cause of the disease. If this is done properly and early enough in the process of disease, the manifestation of the disorder can correct itself, and health and harmony can manifest once again.

Managing the breath

The vital life force acts as a catalyst in all our activities, and yoga, through the enhancement of this energy, attempts to help achieve optimal health and healing. *Pranayama* may thus be defined as the art and science of controlled, conscious expansion of such vital energy through managing the breath. Masters of ancient (Vedic) times placed great importance on *pranayama* and advocated its practice in order to unleash the inner potential energy (*kundalini*). Indian culture lays great emphasis on *prana* and *pranayama*—ancient Vedic literature says, "God is breath" as well as "Breath is life and life is breath."[11] *Atharvana Veda* even goes on to state, "*prana* is the fundamental basis of whatever is, was and will be."

In the *Prasnopanishad* we can find the following statement: "All that exists in all the three worlds is under the governance of *prana*." It is said in the *Shiva Swarodaya*, "The life force (*prana*) verily is one's greatest friend, companion and there is no greater kinsman than the life force."[12] In the *Yoga Vashista*, sage Vashistha says that when the energy of the life force (*prana*) is restricted, then the mind dissolves, like a shadow of a thing when the thing is absent.[13]

In the *Hatha Yoga Pradipika*, Yogi Swatmarama says, "When respiration is disturbed, the mind gets disturbed. When breath is steady and undisturbed, mind is also steady and undisturbed. By consciously controlling respiration, the Yogi attains steadiness of mind" (II:2).[14] He also says, "Mind is the master of the senses, while the breath is its Lord. Mastery of the breath lies in its absorption that depends on conscious vibrations induced during smooth, steady inhalation and exhalation" (IV:29). He lists the important breath-based energy practices (*kumbhaka*) such as skull shining breath (*kapalbhati*), sun-cleaving breath (*surya bhedana)*, victorious breath (*ujjayi*), hissing breath (*sitkari*), beak tongue breath (*sitali*), bellows breath (*bhastrika*), and bee-sounding breath (*bhramari*), among others.[15] He also warns us that, although *pranayama* can eradicate all diseases, it may cause a multitude of problems if performed improperly (II:16).

According to the *Hatha Yoga Pradipika*, when the nerves are purified by *pranayama*, the body becomes slender and lustrous, gastric fire increases, inner sounds are heard, and excellent health is attained. Chapter II, verses 36–68 describe the benefits of each *pranayama*:

- *Kapalbhati* balances *kapha*, stimulates blood circulation, slows peristaltic movement, and improves digestion.

- *Surya bhedana* cures *vata* disorders, purifies the sinuses and blood, removes parasites, and rejuvenates cells.

- *Ujjayi* is said to remove the disorders of phlegm and structural elements (*dhatus*), increases stamina and agility, and alleviates nerve disorders, stress, and depression.

- *Sitkari* alleviates hunger, thirst, the need for sleep, or lassitude.

- *Sitali* balances *pitta*, relieves colic, spleen disorders, fever, tumors, and bile disorders, and neutralizes even the most dangerous of poisons.

- *Bhastrika* balances all three *doshas* (*vata, pitta, kapha*), pierces three *granthis*, has the capacity to cure phlegm, bile, and gas disorders, infuses vigor, stamina, and alertness, improves memory, removes depression, and helps increase the gastric fire.[16]

The practice of *pranayama* helps to regulate our emotions and stabilize the mind, which is said to be as restless as a "drunken monkey stung by a scorpion." Emotions and breath are known to have a deep relationship. When we get angry, we can experience that our breathing becomes rapid, and it is slower when we are cool and relaxed. Thus the slow, rhythmic, and controlled breathing in *pranayama* leads to the emotional control seen in dedicated yoga practitioners. Conscious, deep, and regular breathing can synchronize and reinforce inherent cardiovascular rhythms and modify baroreflex sensitivity, which may be attained by practicing *ujjayi* and *pranava*.[17] The sound-based vibrational breaths (*pranava* and *bhramari*[18]) enable the manifestation of an inner harmony that results in the attainment of a state of mental calmness.

According to Dr Swami Gitananda Giri, the inherent message of *pranayama* can be summarized as follows: "There is an absolute and direct correlation between the way the man breathes and his energy level, the length of his lifespan, the clarity and subtlety of the thoughts, and the quality of the emotions."[19]

Deep, slow breathing is economical[20]

Many novices have a false notion before they begin *pranayama* as they think that slowing down the breath will limit the air they take in, and hence reduce the amount of gaseous exchange! This is, however, totally wrong as in fact we increase the efficiency of gaseous exchange by enhancing ventilation during deep breathing. The table below illustrates this concept, that shallow breathing makes us work a lot (30 breaths/minute) for very little (1500 ml volume of gas exchange) while slow, deep breathing gives us 40 percent more alveolar ventilation (5100 ml with just 6 breaths/minute). We must also remember that *pranayama* is concerned with much more than just alveolar ventilation; it also deals with the enhancement of subtle energies that will be proportionately enhanced by such slow and deep conscious breathing.

	Normal	Shallow	Deep
Volume (ml)	500	200	1000
Rate (/minute)	12	30	6
Ventilation (ml)	6000	6000	6000
Dead space (ml)	150	150	150
Dead space volume (ml)	1800	4500	900
Alveolar volume (ml)	4200	1500	5100

Shifting from individuality to universality

Yoga, which emphasizes the universal, is a perfect foil to those human activities that glorify the personal experience. The process of yoga therapy helps the individual to shift from an "I"-centric approach to a "we"-centric approach. Transformation from "I-ness" to "we-ness" is the core of spiritual healing.

The *Bhagavad Gita* says, "Yoga is skill in action" (2:50). The real yogi is conscious and aware at the physical, mental, and emotional levels of their being. They gain great control over all aspects of life, thus developing a real skill in living. They realize that their duty is to do their best, but that the ultimate result is not in their hands. The yogi performs the needed action not for the sake of the fruits of that action, but because it is good and necessary to do so for everyone's benefit.

This belies the Western belief that the competitive spirit produces the highest skill. To this the yogic answer is: detachment from the fruits of the action produces the greatest efficiency. The beauty of yoga is that these abstract principles become concrete in the daily practice of the techniques available in the yoga system. Once the client practices yoga with discipline and consistency, these concepts grow naturally, slowly but surely taking root in all aspects of the client's life.

"Yogopathy"[21] vs. yoga therapy

We are part of the "instant" culture. We are used to instant food and instant solutions. These are attitudes we have grown up with in our life—as yoga teachers, yoga therapists, and clients. When we go to the doctor we are focused on solving physical problems with medicine—we then get medication that suppresses the symptoms and allows us to go on living the lifestyle that caused the problem in the first place. When we go to a therapist our focus is on fixing our mental or psychological problems through different techniques, so that we can feel better without changing anything. Our focus is on the problem, on the illness—this lies at the heart of pathogenesis. In pathogenesis we want to know what can we do to avoid the problem or cure the symptoms. Our stance is reactive—we only act when there is a manifestation of the problem. Most of us do not think of our health when there is no pain or loss. This is the majority of people's state of awareness.

The word "-pathy" is the postfix to stress "feeling" or "suffering," and is used in words such as antipathy or sympathy. In modern language it is often used with the meaning of morbid affection or disease, such as neuropathy, psychopathy, or arthropathy, and hence it is also used in the names of systems of treating disease symptoms—allopathy, homeopathy, hydropathy, osteopathy.[22] Yogopathy describes the use of yogic techniques in treating the symptoms of the disease. It is based on pathogenesis, focusing on dealing with symptoms.

Modern yoga therapy's focus on the physical symptoms can be useful at times. If facilitated skillfully, the client will experience to a certain degree the transformative power of yoga. This can be a stepping stone to motivate the client to accept more encompassing applications of yoga therapy, rather than simply recommending yogic techniques following the philosophy of "a pill for every ill."

Managing and suppressing the manifested symptoms with yoga techniques is just as good or bad as modern allopathic medicine managing symptoms with pharmaceuticals. In such cases the focus is primarily on symptomatic management without ever getting close to the "real" cause of the disorder. How many doctors look at the emotional and psychological issues that are the primary cause of the problem in so many of their patients? The concept of psychosomatics in modern medicine is no older than a hundred years and few doctors think about how the mind induces disease in the body.

When today we find our yoga therapists making the same mistake in merely treating manifesting symptoms without remedying the "real" cause, Dr Bhavanani prefers to call this yogopathy! It may be useful in some cases, but it misses the true strength of yoga therapy—the opportunity to address the root cause of the problem.

An example of this yogopathy trend is when we use *shavasana* (Corpse Pose) to manage patients with hypertension, quoting research that has shown that it reduces blood pressure. We seem happy just to bring the blood pressure down for the time being! The transformative yoga therapy would first assess the primary cause of the patient's hypertension. Based on such an assessment, it would recommend multilevel solutions suitable for this particular client, choosing from lifestyle changes, and yogic techniques to move and cleanse the body and manage the mind and thought processes, for the client to practice over time. Without an attempt to find and deal with the root cause, it remains merely yogopathy.

Another common example is using left nostril (*chandra nadi*) *pranayama* to lower blood sugar or right nostril (*surya nadi*) *pranayama* to relieve bronchospasm without looking for the real cause of the patient's diabetes or asthma. When we do this, how are we any different from the modern doctors who prescribe anti-diabetic and sympathomimetic agents for these patients? Where is the true potential of yoga therapy in this type of approach? Where is the effort to find and deal with the primary cause? Without a transformation of attitude or lifestyle, can it be yoga therapy?

Sometimes inexperienced yoga therapists are so taken by the available tools— from *asanas*, *pranayama*, chanting, meditation, *mudras*, etc.—that they lose the view of the person in front of them and get lost in choosing the best "option for the given disease/or symptom." This was very apparent in my discussions with yoga therapy students where I had to repeatedly steer them towards the client as a person rather than the condition the client suffered from.

If we want to use the transformative potential of yoga therapy, we need to shift our paradigm from a focus on disease to health promotion, from pathogenesis to salutogenesis. *Salus* (Latin) means health and *genesis* (Greek) means source, hence *salutogenesis* means the source of health. In order to move our habitual pathogenic orientation as yoga teachers, therapists, and at the same time as clients, to a salutogenic orientation, we need awareness to change:

- The goal, from better medical intervention to improvement of our natural and created environment.

- Focus, from curing chronic disease to client ownership, to act in a way helps cause health.

- Norms, from paternalism and entitlement, to empowering clients to cultivate health.

- Orientation, from fixing parts of the system, to healing by bringing all systems into harmonious coherence.

According to Antonovsky,[23] at the heart of salutogenesis lies a sense of coherence (SOC), "a pervasive, long lasting and dynamic feeling of confidence" that:

- One's internal and external environments are predictable.

- There is a high probability that things will work out as well as can be expected.

SOC has a strong positive correlation to perceived physical and mental health and quality of life. It has three main components:

- Cognition—"my world is understandable."

- Coping skills—"my world is manageable."

- Motivation—"my world has meaning."

Salutogenesis, as the health-promoting approach, lies at the core of yoga therapy. When we do an initial assessment of the client, we focus on multilevel functioning in harmony. We identify disharmony at each level of functioning (according to *pancha kosha, doshas, gunas,* and *vayus*), and create a protocol specific to this client's goals to help them move from disharmony to harmony, from disease to health. Together with the client we keep evaluating the progress towards reaching their potential. We facilitate a proactive stance in the client—where they take ownership and responsibility to move forward to grow on a wellness continuum. This helps the client to discover how to live fully.

Yoga has a term for such a dynamic state of wellness—*swastha*—defined by Sushrut[24] as: "a dynamic balance of the elements and humors, normal metabolic activity and efficient elimination coupled with a tranquil mind, senses and contented soul."

Unless we aim to treat the whole individual on all levels, as per *pancha kosha, doshas,* and *vayus,* including underlying psychosomatic disassociation and ignorant perception of reality, we are not practicing real yoga therapy. Therefore, in the application of yoga therapy it is vital that we take into consideration all the following aspects that are part of an integrated approach to the problem. These include the code of personal and social ethics (*yamas* and *niyamas*), diet, environment, attitude, lifestyle, bodywork through *asanas, mudras,* and *kriyas,* breath work through the use of *pranayama,* and the management of a healthy thought process and attitudes through the higher practices of *yoga nidra,* chanting, and meditation.

However, we must remember to look for and assess the root cause of the problem because if not, we are practicing yogopathy, and not yoga therapy!

Contemporary trends and thoughts on the future

The limitation of modern medicine in managing stress-induced psychosomatic, chronic illnesses is the strength of yoga therapy. Hence a holistic integration of both systems enables the best quality of care for clients. It is imperative that advances in medicine include the holistic approach of yoga to face the current challenges in healthcare. The antiquity of yoga must be united with the innovations of modern medicine to improve quality of life throughout the world. This approach is becoming more acceptable with time, and a great proponent of such a method is Dr Dean Ornish, who has just published, with his wife Anne, *UnDo It! How Simple Lifestyle Changes Can Reverse Most Chronic Diseases.*[25] They describe in detail lifestyle medicine that they have been practicing and researching for the last 40 years, which is based on such an integrated approach, and has successfully reversed cardiovascular disorders and other NCDs.

Lately, Dr Bhavanani has actually begun to question the very scientific research itself that makes up the foundation of "evidence-based" yoga therapy. Many excellent scientists are researching yoga and its effects on different populations and in different conditions, yet their understanding of yoga is too limited to produce meaningful results. This is because they try to fit the grand design of yoga into the limited box of scientific methodology, and end up not studying "yoga" at all. The research that is published is excellent from a scientific perspective, but truly very limited from a yogic perspective. We need to continue working on keeping the yoga in yoga therapy, and especially in yoga research, where it tends to get lost in the tight limitations of "standardization" and "study protocols." Yoga therapy, by its definition, cannot be standardized or limited, as it is carefully crafted to the need of each client.

A brief qualitative survey on the utilization of yoga research resources by yoga teachers found a general lack of awareness of yoga research among practicing yoga teachers and therapists.[26] Although a majority of respondents agreed that research was important, few were seriously updating themselves on such research findings through scientific channels. Most were updating themselves through general articles on the internet, and in most cases such information seemed to have minimal influence on their day-to-day teaching and practice.

At the individual level, when we acknowledge that yoga demands consciousness in every moment, we need to be living yoga in its highest and truest sense. Unless we live a life of yoga, or at least attempt to do so, how can we understand the inherent spirit of "wholeness" that joins all things together? Unless we lead by the example of our lives, how can we convince others to follow us? A good teacher teaches more by example than by words, and so does a good therapist, who heals more by "being" the therapy than by just assessing and prescribing techniques. The acquisition of a degree in yoga does not guarantee that the therapist will be a good yoga therapist. Conversely, someone's lack of an academic qualification doesn't mean that they will be a bad yoga therapist. Intelligence, empathy, compassion, and understanding are not necessarily by-products of an academic career or institutional status.

The need of the hour is for a symbiotic relationship between yoga and modern science. To satisfy this need, living human bridges combining the best of both worlds need to be cultivated. It is important that more dedicated scientists take up yoga and that more yogis study science, so that we can build a bridge between these two great evolutionary aspects of our civilization. Yoga is all about becoming "one" with an integrated state of being. Yogopathy, in contrast, is more about "doing" than "being." When viewed from this holistic perspective, yoga can never really be an intervention, as this role must be left to yogopathy. We, as yoga practitioners, teachers, researchers, and therapists, must make a sincere and determined attempt to strengthen that one important link in the chain of yoga, the link of our personal, "every moment practice" (*sadhana*). This is imperative, for the very strength of the "chain of yoga" depends on it. We write about this further in Chapter 5.

A note of caution

As yoga therapy starts to be introduced into mainstream healthcare, we must not fall into the dangerous trap of claiming that yoga is a miracle that can cure everything. Such statements do more damage than good—this "puts off" the modern medical community more than anything. They then develop a stiff resistance to yoga instead of becoming more open to this health-restoring science. As the use of yoga therapy in medical centers is still in its infancy, we must be cautious with our conscious and unconscious thoughts, words, and actions.

This is not to downplay the potentiality of yoga because it *does* have a role in virtually each and every condition. We must realize, however, that although yoga can improve the condition of nearly every client, it doesn't necessarily translate into words such as "cure." Modern medicine doesn't have a cure for most conditions and so, when yoga therapists use such words, it creates a negative image that does more harm than good.

The need of the modern age is to have an integrated approach, one that is open to using the best from all traditional and modern forms of therapy. We must try to integrate concepts of yoga in coordination and collaboration with other systems of medicine such as traditional, complementary, and integrative

(TCI) medicine, allopathy, Ayurveda, siddha, and naturopathy. Physiotherapy, osteopathy, and chiropractic practices may also be used with yoga therapy, as required. The advice on diet and adoption of a healthy lifestyle is very important irrespective of the mode of therapy employed for the client. US longitudinal research confirms this.[27] Eleven thousand people were tracked for over 20 years, concluding that a healthy lifestyle can give women an additional ten years and men seven years of life free of cancer, heart problems and type 2 diabetes.

We need to always be rational and sensible in our approach to health, and realize that yoga therapy is not a magic therapy! It is not "one pill for all ills." There should be no unsubstantiated claims made in this field. Yoga therapy is also a science and must therefore be approached in a scientific, step-by-step manner. It should be administered primarily as a "one on one" therapy that allows the therapist to modify the practices to meet the needs of the individual. It is not a "one size fits all" or "one therapy fits all" approach!

As human beings, we fulfill ourselves best when we help others. Yoga is the best way for us to consciously evolve out of our lower, sub-human nature into our elevated human and humane nature. Ultimately, this life-giving, life-enhancing, and life-sustaining science allows us to achieve in full measure the Divinity that resides within each of us.

In summary, yoga therapy is much more than a common yoga class. We have looked at the principles and modalities of yoga therapy and discussed its applications. We have touched on the yogic assessment of a client and how this differs from the medical model. Finally, we have pointed to the spiritual component of this ancient science. Spirituality today is still generally misunderstood as belonging to religion, and is an aspect of yoga therapy that is often underestimated or even neglected in a client's journey to health. We feel that it is very important to start the discussion on the role of spirituality and the promise of spiritual transformation in yoga therapy as an important component of a client's healing. So the next chapter is dedicated to spirituality in yoga therapy.

CHAPTER 3

Yoga Therapy and Spirituality

In 2015 Kelly Turner PhD, a onco-psychologist, published her research in a book titled *Radical Remission: Surviving Cancer Against All Odds*, which quickly became a *New York Times* bestseller.[1] She examined over 1000 cases of spontaneous remission from advanced cancer, talked to over 50 non-Western alternative healers from Brazil, China, England, and Zimbabwe, and interviewed over 100 cancer patients who had had spontaneous remission from terminal cancer. After collating all the data, Turner found over 75 healing factors, the following nine of which were mutual to all the cases and were the key to spontaneous healing:

- Deepening spiritual connection
- Having a strong reason for living
- Taking control over one's health
- Releasing suppressed emotions
- Increasing positive emotions
- Following one's intuition
- Embracing social support
- Using herbs and supplements
- Radically changing diet.

Turner's research on spontaneous healing points to what ancient yogis knew thousands of years before: transformation needs to happen on all levels of human existence in order for healing to take place. *Pancha kosha* points to our existence on five levels simultaneously and homogenously. If we are to start healing, we need to stop looking just at the body and start looking at all levels of human existence. All nine factors mentioned by Turner correlate with the *pancha kosha* model:

- Three are connected to our spiritual being (*anandamaya kosha*):

  - Deepening spiritual connection

  - Having a purpose in life

  - Embracing social support.

- Two are connected to our mental being (*vijnamaya kosha*):

  - Taking control over one's health

  - Following one's intuition.

- Two are connected to our emotional being (*manomaya kosha*):

  - Releasing suppressed emotions

  - Increasing positive emotions.

- And finally, two factors necessary for healing on Turner's list are connected to our physical and energetic body (*pranamaya* and *annamaya koshas*):

  - Using herbs and supplements

  - Radically changing diet.

Some of these findings had already been confirmed earlier by other researchers, who had also looked at the immune system and other factors—for example, moving away from our community and "not belonging" can make us ill and increase our mortality by two to three times.[2] Relationships of any sort (good or bad) improve our odds of survival by 50 percent, with the effects of isolation equivalent to smoking 15 cigarettes per day or being an alcoholic, and twice as harmful as being obese.[3] Another study[4] concluded that the number of groups to which we belong, particularly if we have strong relationships within them, is more vital than any diet or exercise program, and protects us against the worst toxins and greatest adversity.

Sir Martin Brofman postulated that the physical body is influenced by the subtle energy field (emotions and thoughts), which are determined by our consciousness.[5] By the same token he suggested that our perception creates our reality. There is no question that today's scientists and researchers acknowledge the importance of the mind in the health equation. The WHO went even further, defining health as a "state of complete physical, mental and social wellbeing and not merely the absence of disease or infirmity."[6]

All of these point to our mind as a source of disturbance and disease. Hence Western scientists assume that there is a problem in the mind. On the other hand, Eastern philosophy states that the mind itself is the core of the problem. Although the healing needs to start with the mind, this is not enough.

It is interesting to see such a correlation between Turner's findings and ancient Indian wisdom. We may also note that this is totally outside of the traditional medical healthcare paradigm. As we will see, there are more correlations between health, contemporary research, and yoga sciences.

What does research say about yoga?

Right from its inception in 1924, the pioneering Kaivalyadhama Yoga Institute (India) initiated contemporary scientific research on the effects of yoga. In 1924 it also set up the first ever yoga research magazine journal by the name of *Yoga-Mīmāṃsā*, which is still published today.[7] In their first ever laboratory they conducted many leading experiments on yoga, studying its effects on the body's functioning.

Today, the total body of research is now outside the scope of this book. Suffice to say that a comprehensive analysis of yoga therapy from 1967 to 2013[8] shows a three-fold increase in the number of publications from 2003 to 2013. Most publications originated from India, followed by the US and Canada. The top four disorders addressed by yoga intervention are: mental health (depression and anxiety), cardiovascular disease (hypertension and heart disease), respiratory disease (asthma and chronic obstructive pulmonary disease, COPD), and diabetes. The report concluded that the use of yoga as a complementary therapy in clinical practice led to health benefits beyond traditional treatment alone.

Over time researchers have confirmed the importance of *asanas* but also the effects of yogic breathing techniques, which have beneficial effects for the cardiovascular and autonomic nervous systems,[9, 10] and cancer-related fatigue.[11] Furthermore, yoga practices are shown to increase heart rate variability and enhance vagal tone while decreasing the sympathetic tone in those with hypertension[12] as well as decreasing blood pressure.[13] Another review[14] postulates that slowing down the breath to six breaths per minute induces rhythms of autonomous physiological functions (heart rate, blood pressure, blood flow to the brain) to act in coherence, reinforcing each other, and resulting in better functioning of the immune system, reduction of inflammation, regulation of blood sugar levels, induced calmness and clarity of mind, and a feeling of inner peace.

The following is a summary of some of the benefits of yoga therapy and its physical and psychological effects understood through modern research.

Physiological benefits

- Improved general health, posture, muscle tone, sleep quality, immunity, and pain tolerance.

- Stable autonomic nervous system with better orthostatic tolerance and neuromuscular coordination.

- Increase in alpha rhythm, inter-hemispheric coherence, and homogeneity in the brain.

- Decreased EMG activity.

- Normalized gastrointestinal tract and endocrine function.

- Improved cardiorespiratory efficiency, musculoskeletal flexibility, range of joint movement, physical endurance, strength, and energy levels.

- Decreased heart rate and blood pressure.

- Healthier and safer pregnancy—an increase in birth weight and decrease in preterm labor.

Psychological benefits

- Improved mood and interpersonal relationships.

- Increased subjective wellbeing and self-acceptance.

- Increased somatic and kinesthetic awareness.

- Increase in self-actualization and social adjustment.

- Decreased stress, hostility, irritability, anxiety, and depression.

Cognitive functional benefits

- Improved memory, attention, focus, concentration, depth perception, and learning efficiency.

Biochemical changes after yoga practice

DECREASED

- Glucose

- Sodium

- Cholesterol

- Triglycerides

- LDL

- VLDL

- Catecholamines

- Lipid peroxidation.

INCREASED

- HDL

- ATPase

- Hematocrit

- Lymphocytes

- Thyroxin

- SR protein.

One of Swami Gitananda Giri's American students had joined his course in Pondicherry in the early 1970s. She had left the US after some preliminary tests and while in India received news through the post that she had been diagnosed with cancer. A young, famous ballerina, and someone who had immense determination and dedication to being healthy, she decided to immerse herself in intensive yoga practices for a full year at the Ananda Ashram and to take things as they came when she returned home. To her surprise, when she returned and was re-tested, there were no signs of any cancer at all. When asked about this amazing miracle, all her doctor would say was, "Maybe the results of the preliminary tests were wrong in the first place!"

The healing power of yoga is unquestionable. In the words of a client,

> Today, 14 months later after starting yoga therapy, I am in a very different place. Despite living with a chronic illness, I am mentally and emotionally much stronger. My mind is steadier and I am more in touch with my body and my emotions. I try to ride the waves rather than sinking. I have the ability to return far more quickly and easily back to stability when I go out of kilter. Yoga therapy is and continues to be a major part of my healing journey. (S.L.)

Another client wrote:

> I stopped taking insulin in the second week of [the] Beyond Cancer retreat. Now, after [a] due medical test doctors confirmed that my diabetes has been reversed. I am not taking any medicine or insulin for the last…6 months and sugar level is absolutely well under control. Credit for this also goes to your wonderful retreat at Kaivalyadhama Yoga Institute. (R.T.)

What about spirituality and health?

More research has also emerged on spirituality since 2000. Three systematic reviews of academic literature identified more than 3000 empirical studies on spirituality and health.[15, 16, 17] One of the obstacles to defining the protocols of research on spirituality is the difficulty of separating spirituality from religion. "Spirituality traditionally was regarded as a core part of religion. However in [the] last decades spirituality definition became much broader," writes Harold Koenig.[18] On the other hand, the general population at large still regards spirituality exclusively as an inherent part of religion. This is reflected in the following. The WHO wanted to modify its 1948 definition of health—"*Health is a state of complete physical, mental and social well-being and not merely the absence of disease*"—and add "spiritual wellbeing." However, due to many protests, the definition stayed as it had originally been created.

There are many proposed new definitions of spirituality that attempt to separate it from religion. In their review article, Alexander Moreira-Almeida and colleagues[19] propose the following division between spirituality and religion:

- "Spirituality is a personal quest for understanding answers to ultimate questions about life, about meaning and about relationship to the sacred or transcendent [which may or may not be connected to religion or religious community]."

- "Religion is an organized system of beliefs, practices, rituals and symbols designed to facilitate closeness to the sacred or transcendent."

Despite a growing body of research, "the spiritual concerns continue to be one of the most overlooked aspects of research, while the importance of physical and psychological factors are routinely acknowledged."[20] In a critical review on coping with heart failure, Clark and Hunter propose, "spirituality is expressed through beliefs, values, traditions, and practices."[21] They further stress that "the quantitative evidence also confirms that spiritual needs and/or distress contribute to greater individuals' experiences of suffering."

On the other hand, addressing aspects of spiritual wellbeing, a study by McCabe and colleagues found significant improvements in pain intensity, physical function, mood, and cognitive function.[22]

In 2015, Koenig[23] published a systematic and thorough review of quantitative research in which he studied findings from over 3000 studies of the effects of religion and spirituality on mental health, health behaviors, and physical health. All 3000 were positively affected by spirituality and religion. It will be exciting to see the results of a new and as yet unpublished study conducted by Duke University in the US examining the effects of religiosity on the length of telomeres (related to the process of wear and tear of the body).

Emerging research confirms the connection between spirituality and lives, our physical, emotional, and mental wellbeing and functioning. Yet spirituality continues to be so closely related to religiosity that it is often used synonymously. In our opinion, although religion and yoga both strive to lead humanity into spiritual transformation, there is a significant difference between the two. Religion demands faith as it is based on dogma passed down from "authority." That is its starting point. On the other hand, yoga is entirely existential, experiential, and experimental. "Yoga is known through yoga. Yoga arises from yoga."[24] It has to be lived, experienced, and experimented with, with the helping hand of a teacher. Yoga depends on testing hypotheses in experience and in this sense it is scientific, even though the domains of that experience extend beyond the objectively measurable.

But is there any difference in the effects of religiosity and spirituality on our health factors? This was the question Daaleman and colleagues[25] considered when they looked at 277 geriatric outpatients living in the community and the interaction between religion, spirituality, and the perception of health status. Interestingly, the results showed that there is a difference. The findings confirmed that greater spirituality, *but not greater religiosity*, is correlated with patients' appraisal of good health. *So higher spirituality, but not necessarily religiosity, means better health.* It also confirmed that we perceive ourselves as healthier when we are more spiritual.

What about spirituality and yoga?

And what about spirituality and yoga? We know that it brings about better health, but does yoga relate to spirituality? How relevant is it? Does the research confirm the correlation between the effects of yoga and the *pancha kosha* model—the multilevel of existence, which incorporates the spiritual level as well?

Despite a wide body of research, we still do not know the mechanism by which yoga produces these effects in the body and in our psyche. Yoga therapy is a young discipline in the West, and the research so far is applying scientific methods that exclusively focus on the discrete effects of particular practices and biochemical changes. As Michael Lee suggests, "exclusive focus on discrete effects ignores the reality of the yoga of Patanjali… This limited view gives rise to the second, and perhaps more significant, impact. The focus on the evaluation of yoga using a cause-and-effect model tends to discount the potential of yoga to address the complex issues underlying the condition being studied."[26] Yet "the reason why yoga therapies are so effective, both in preventive medicine and in assisting conventional treatment, is because Yoga addresses all 3 aspects of wellness—physical, mental and spiritual," writes Dr D. Sarkar,[27] vascular surgeon and certified yoga therapist.

Swami Kuvalayananda writes in *Yogic Therapy*, "Yoga regards no disease as a local affection [sic] but as a critical change in the body system as a whole."[28] He writes further, "no disease, according to Yoga, can be completely cured by the practice of one single posture (*asana*) or even *mudra*, nor, for that matter with the performance of these yogic exercises (*asanas*) alone. All these are part of a composite treatment." The reality of Patanjali's Yoga (as outlined in the *Sutras*) is "clearly defined as a transformational process," claims Michael Lee, in his recent article.[29]

This last statement resonates to my core. I always struggled with expressions such as "Yoga for cancer," "Yoga for back pain," or "Yoga for hormonal balance." In my understanding, yoga does not heal specific diseases. Yoga restores balance to the human multilevel existence. It heals by transforming the human being and thus may heal the human being, although it may not cure them from the disease. So often I would receive a plea from a distraught family member—"My mother has cancer and doctors say they cannot help any more. Can your retreat heal my mother's cancer?" It pains me to disappoint them and explain at length that we do not treat the disease; we treat human beings suffering from a disease.

On the other hand, although there is an intrinsic value to have a small group of clients afflicted with the same disease such as cancer, diabetes, or cardiac problems, the group then becomes cohesive and creates a strong support and resource for each other. It also helps the therapist create more specific, targeted yoga therapy for such a group, with individual adaptations.

However, we need to keep in mind that *yoga therapy is not a prescriptive science*. No specific prescription can be made for yoga for cancer or yoga for diabetes or yoga for X for that matter, although this kind of thinking is very common as we have been brought up in a culture of "a pill for every ill." Such an attitude defies the essence of yoga therapy. When we consider applying yoga therapy, we need to change the paradigm completely in two respects. First, we have to stop focusing on a medical diagnosis of disease with just its symptoms. We need to consider and assess a deeper cause of the imbalance of human existence that resulted in the manifestation of disease in the body. We describe this process in detail in Chapter 4.

Second, following our assessment, we need to consider the whole human being and focus on health—what can bring balance back to this particular client? It may be yogic tools dealing with attitudes and ethics (*yamas* and *niyamas*). It may be higher practices like *yoga nidra*, chanting, or meditation. It may be breathing management and techniques, *kriyas*, or *asanas*. It may be diet and the way food is consumed. It may also be an irregular circadian rhythm. Or it may be all of the above. The determination of the most appropriate path will entirely depend on the client, their goals, and the level of ownership of responsibility for their own health, and how much they are prepared to implement. I often get asked about what yoga (usually meaning *asanas*) I use for cancer. Invariably I will answer—none! I use yoga therapy tools to assist human beings to heal the disease conditions by bringing balance to their life.

The great T.K.V. Desikachar[30] taught that the spirit of yoga starts from where you find yourself. As everyone is different and changes from time to time, *there can be no common starting point, and ready-made answers are useless*. Yoga (therapy) should be offered according to aspirations, requirements, and the culture of the individual, and in stages, progressively.

Ancient yogis knew experientially how to deal with all levels of human existence and passed on this science verbally through generations, until, in 300 CE, Patanjali noted it all down in what is considered today the bible of yoga—Patanjali's *Yoga Sutras Darshana*. Throughout millennia this and other ancient yogic texts became a roadmap for adepts in yoga to follow on the path to enlightenment.

But what exactly is yoga?

It seems that many people have many answers to this question. A great yogi from the last century, Paramahansa Yogananda, gave the following answer in his book *The Essence of Self Realization*: "Most people in the west, and also many in India, confuse Yoga with Hatha Yoga—the system of bodily postures. But Yoga is primarily *a spiritual discipline*." Another great teacher, Shivananda, stressed,

> Yoga means union. Although many people think this term refers to union between body and mind or body, mind and spirit, the traditional acceptance is union between the *Jivatman* and *Paramatman*, that is, between one's individual consciousness and the Universal Consciousness. Therefore Yoga refers to a certain state of consciousness as well as methods that help one reach that goal—or state of union with the divine.[31]

Shri Aurobindo said, "Yoga is [the tool for] condensed [human] evolution."[32] And so we, as yoga therapists, are assisting in our clients' evolution—a huge responsibility!

And yet, although yoga does not require the adoption of religious beliefs or dogmas, its practices aim at the experience of contemplative states of consciousness and offer a promise of spiritual transformation. We believe yoga can rightly be categorized as a practically applied philosophy within the philosophical discipline of mysticism, whose primary goal is the experience of a transcendent, unitive state of consciousness.[33] "The evolution of one's awareness is an integral aspect of yoga as a transformational process," writes Mark Stephens, "…this process is one of awakening and integrating on the path to more holistic, congruent and healthy experience in being alive."[34]

It is interesting to note that yoga as such was never meant to be a healing modality. Yoga's goal for a human being is to reach enlightenment, or union of one's individual consciousness with Universal Consciousness. Yoga sets out tools to work with one's nervous system and brain to expand its capability for higher states. Perhaps, however, such a union cannot be obtained without reaching mastery over the body, over life energy within (*prana*), over emotions, and over one's mind or thought processes. And perhaps the process of getting there compels us to correct disturbances on all these levels of our existence. And so, by consistently practicing yogic techniques daily, we can create transformation on *all* levels—physical, emotional, mental, and *spiritual*. According to Turner's research, that composite transformation, on all levels—physical, emotional, mental, and spiritual—is what needs to be included in the process if radical healing is to take place.

Unfortunately, it seems that when yoga was introduced to the West at the end of the 19th century, it was only partially adopted—more as physical exercise than the philosophical and practical science of personal transformation. Perhaps in translating yoga from the deeply spiritual culture of India into the highly individualistic culture of the West, slowly, generations were not able to prevent the dilution of the tradition. The spiritual component of practice became very weak and the emphasis of yoga became more aligned with getting fit and the body image-conscious middle-class Westerners. It's enough to see yoga depicted in printed media to understand this. (To break this pattern, we have included pictures of *asanas* performed by a 69-year-old female in what follows!)

When we hear someone saying, "I have a yoga class today," we tend to see in our minds a studio with yoga mats and people doing all kinds of different poses. The common understanding of "yoga" nowadays, in the West and in some parts of India, seems to have been reduced to an exercise practice with perhaps some controlled breathing. Even meditation is usually mentioned separately from yoga or in addition to yoga.

This general reductionist misconception of what yoga is, paired with mistaking spirituality for religion, creates much confusion in yoga practitioners. Even some yoga therapists seem to think that spirituality is beyond the scope of yoga and yoga therapy. It seems that even we, practitioners, yoga teachers, and therapists, cannot agree on this subject. This was the question an anthropologist, Caroline Nizard, tried to answer in her paper titled "Is Yoga a Spiritual Path?" during the recent Annual Conference of the European Association for the Study of Religions (EASR) in June 2018 in Bern, Switzerland.[35]

In her fieldwork through 2013–2017, Nizard gathered the accounts of 56 long-term yoga practitioners of mixed religions (including some agnostics) from France, India, and Switzerland. She found no significant difference between cultural identities in the practitioners' understanding of yoga, but she did find significant differences in their relation to the spirituality of yoga, although all participated in the same practices. So even we, as professionals, cannot agree on what yoga is offering us.

An interesting study from Smith and colleagues[36] looked at the different effects of an *asana*-only yoga class and more comprehensive yoga practice (including ethical and spiritual components). Eighty-one students over the age of 18 at one university in the US participated in the study, and over time participants in both studies showed a decrease in depression and stress and an increase in a sense of hopefulness compared with the control group. However, *only the comprehensive yoga group experienced a decrease in anxiety-related symptoms and decreased salivary cortisol from the beginning to the end of the study.*

In other words, the spiritual component in the yoga protocol created additional and measurable healing value. This is in line with Daaleman *et al.*'s study on a geriatric population quoted earlier, in which spirituality increased the positive effect on health.[37] The importance and additional benefit of the spiritual component in the yoga protocol has been confirmed in the latest meta-analysis from the Mayo Clinic.[38] It concluded that yoga is a viable anti-hypertensive lifestyle therapy and produces the greatest blood pressure benefits when breathing techniques and meditation or mental relaxation are included.

This also correlates with research presented in *Radical Remission* in which Kelly Turner quotes two factors each in the physical, emotional, and mental domains.[39] But in the spiritual domain she lists three factors that are needed for radical healing: deepening spiritual connection, having a purpose in life, and embracing social support. Thus the significance of the spiritual component, as stressed by Turner, becomes vitally important in the process of healing. It is also in line with *pancha koshas*—the Ayurvedic model of the multilevels of human existence—that healing is most effective when it includes the spiritual factor (*anandamaya kosha*).

But can yoga therapy create spiritual transformation?

A recently published ethnographic study[40] asked, "*Is yoga a possible vehicle for experiencing transcendence?*" In Catalonia, Spain, in 2011, a yoga non-governmental organization (NGO) and the Department of Justice signed an agreement that opened the door for yoga classes and intensive courses for all Catalonian inmates. The research project was designed as a multiple case study at a number of prisons. A total of 54 inmates, male and female, engaged in intensive daily yoga practices for 2 to 3 hours over a 40-day period. Most of the participants who volunteered for the study already practiced yoga in weekly classes.

When the inmates were asked what they valued most about doing yoga, the majority referred to the possibility of transcending their constrained "here-and-now." They described feelings of "connectedness," "self-awareness," and "flow." Smith postulates that "encountering oneself" is the key component in such spiritual experience. This encounter with the "embodied self" brings about a moment in *asana* practice that practitioners identify as "spiritual."[41] Such acts of transcendence, singular to yoga, were seen as the most appreciated component of practicing yoga in prison.

Griera, however, mentions one more important factor—the social and intersubjective character of transcendence experiences.[42] She noticed the importance of the group in favoring and sustaining the shift to another reality. That "collective energy" became a decisive factor for experiencing transcendence or, as the inmates describe it, "really doing Yoga." "Yoga connects me with my divinity," reports the practicing inmate. "Years ago I used to do drugs…and with yoga I have felt similar sensations… However, this comes from inside of me, comes from my own serenity and I feel happy with myself." Based on the outcomes, Griera suggests that yoga is not only physical work but also, in some cases, a doorway to spiritual knowledge. For some inmates the practice of yoga can even be the starting point for a spiritual journey.

The importance of the group setting and intensity of practice was also stressed in another study that compared members of a yoga ashram with another group of non-ashram residents (the control group).[43] The ashramites showed a higher percentage of positive responses on a number of factors, including "felt personality change," "experience resulted in change in life," "experience of oneness," and being "in touch with divine or spiritual."

Likewise, a study of yoga interventions in cancer patients reported improvements in measures of spirituality relative to the control group. In particular, the meaning or peace component of spiritual wellbeing increased within 10 weeks in the yoga groups.[44, 45]

More probing questions regarding intensive yoga practices and spirituality were asked in a study by Büssing *et al.*[46]—such as, what specific aspects of spirituality did yoga help to develop? The researchers looked at 160 students who had signed up for two years of yoga teacher training. They measured conscious interaction, compassion, lightheartedness, and mindfulness. The intensive yoga practice significantly increased these specific aspects of the practitioners' spirituality, but the changes were dependent on their original spiritual self-perception. In other words, the intensity of change was dependent on the practitioners and their attitudes towards spirituality.

We see this confirmed at our retreats—Beyond Cancer and Chronic Solutions. Both incorporate six hours of yoga practice daily for 21 days. The protocol includes meditation, *yoga nidra*, chanting, mantras, *mudras*, *pranayama*, and *asanas*, and lectures on how these practices affect the body and mind (with an informal introduction to basic philosophy during lectures). Such intensity often produces dramatic and lasting transformations in the participants' lives, when they are ready.

With time we noticed that the deeper the spiritual transformation in the client during the three-week retreat, the more profound the healing was on many levels—physical, emotional, mental, and spiritual. One of the traits we noticed in retreat participants was the existence of a deep, often unconscious, negative emotion that was hidden and had not been dealt with in the past. Commonly this was anger or hurt or some kind of emotional pain.

Practicing yoga intensely over a three-week retreat tends to bring all these emotions to the fore. In order to heal, people have to become aware of the feeling, accept it, feel it, and by the sheer fact of being accepted, such feelings tend to dissolve. But it requires courage to face yourself and your own pain. The small group setting is helpful in supporting each and every participant in their journey—they become a family supporting and watching each other go through difficult transformations. The long-term follow-up with clients also attested to the sustained nature of these shifts. In general, they were able to exercise an increase in objective judgment, take unselfish action, and were willing to accept "what is."

But we also noticed over the seven years of running these retreats that the more the participant was "closed" and "resistant" or even "defiant" in their attitudes, the lesser were the improvements in their healing. What is perhaps more significant is that it was more likely that the disease, such as cancer, would come back. As we watch our clients working (or not) through their issues during our retreat, it becomes clear to what extent the participant may (or may not) benefit from the retreat. We believe that our life attitude is indicative of the potential level of our healing. But at the same time, we, as yoga therapists, are never able to predict the end result of our intervention. We can only assist our clients at every step and facilitate the healing to the degree the client is ready and able to heal. As Hippocrates recommended, "Before you heal someone, ask him if he is willing to give up the things that made him sick."

The benefits of intensive yoga therapy, which include a spiritual component in small group treatment, are illustrated by the following two case records taken from our retreats. The first one is about Harry, who was referred to us by a medical doctor only two days before we began the Beyond Cancer retreat.

Harry was a quiet 65-year-old man from Canada, of Indian descent, who had never practiced yoga before. He had Stage 4 lymphoma, and had just finished chemotherapy and radiation two months ago, which had proved unsuccessful. Doctors could give him no more treatment. Although he was in constant pain (for which he had morphine), he was determined to attend as much of the program as he could. Right from the beginning his will to live was very apparent.

The results of a test on the first day of the program showed much tension, depression, and anger. I was not surprised—he was told he had only six months to live. Sujaya, one of the co-participants, wrote: "We each had our stories but his was the most painful as his cancer had not been contained by traditional medicine. He was in debilitating pain caused by the spreading tumor. His eyes reflected the pain and hopelessness he felt and my heart went out to him. I could not imagine what it must feel like when you are waiting to die."

Harry had great difficulties with *asanas* and *yoga nidra* because of the physical pain. But he faithfully attended all classes and did as much as he could. As we went on to the second week of the retreat, with each passing day Harry developed a definite sparkle in his eye and a lightness in his walk. He was changing his attitude to the medical prognosis. He began to talk about the future.

One day Harry asked me for a counseling session. He talked about his life, about those he loved and had hurt, and about his regrets. His guilt and shame was almost palpable. I asked him to put his story on paper for the next session. We met again after a few days and he read aloud to me what he had written on eight pages. It was a difficult read for him and he stopped a few times to hold the tears back. We then built a little fire and he burned page by page while we held hands, chanting "Trayambakam," his favorite healing mantra we use at the retreat. The next day his smile became much bigger as he said, "I left a lot of burden in that fire and I feel much lighter!" Later on we heard him humming an Indian raga he remembered from his childhood.

By the end of the program the tests confirmed improvement on all fronts: his tension had gone down from 17 to 8 (on a scale of 0–36), depression down from 22 to 9 (on a scale of 0–60), anger down from 13 to 5 (on a scale of 0–48), vigor increased from 5 to 13 (on a scale of 0–32), fatigue went from 16 to 10 (on a scale of 0–28), and confusion from 13 to 7 (on a scale of 0–28). When we reviewed the results together, Harry said, "Yes, that's about how I feel, at peace with myself and the world. And one more thing…when I came to the program I was afraid of death; now I am not. I will live as long as I can and spend as much time with my sons as possible."

Four weeks later we learned that Harry had passed away peacefully, surrounded by his family and friends. The referring medical doctor commented, "This Beyond Cancer retreat was the best present we could give him before passing on." A few days later, Harry's family came to visit us and were grateful that we had helped Harry. He manifested peacefulness and a sense of acceptance at the time of his passing, which they attributed to yoga.

Such a deep transformation in three weeks was mainly possible due to intensive daily yoga practice and the client's eagerness to apply himself to the program. Six hours of daily yogic practices in a small group for 21 days had, indeed, produced a deep spiritual transformation. At the end of his life Harry transformed his guilt, shame, and deep fear of imminent death into acceptance and inner peace. This is a good example of yoga as a deep transformational practice, which heals, but doesn't always cure.

The second story is perhaps less dramatic but also speaks about profound spiritual transformation. As a participant in the Chronic Solutions retreat, this client's situation was completely different—his disease and discomfort was of much lesser magnitude than Harry's. The 72-year-old psychotherapist from England had never practiced yoga before, and knew very little about it. He also considered himself to be a sworn atheist. Here we quote verbatim, with his permission, the story as he wrote it, about six months after attending the retreat.

I had decided to attend the three-week course in October 2014 run by Lee Majewski at Kaivalydham Yoga Institute in India, [in the] South East of Mumbai, as I was recovering from some severe arthritis following a period of feeling really unwell after food poisoning in Sri Lanka. Well, that was one demonstrable symptom but perhaps also, just getting older was another, having passed my seventy-second birthday and deeply conscious that for the last lap of this race we all run, I needed to pay closer attention to my body and to my mind. I had at that stage not really thought about my heart.

The course was a daily program of very gentle yoga postures, *pranayama* breath routines, awareness, study, and chanting, not to mention lovely simple food day after day. A nice cocktail! The first week is of course always the hardest and I duly struggled while at the same time noting an almost immediate increase in general vitality, which I ascribed to *pranayama*. Looking back on the experience I now see just how deeply significant and necessary this practice of breath work really is. I had for years tried to meditate but it was not really until I started working with the breath that I realized that to watch the breath is to meditate.

The second week seems to be the week when "the stuff rises" so to speak, and in my case this was most certainly the case. It took the form of finding myself almost uncontrollably angry at our course leader...poor Lee. This exploded one day and I attacked her verbally, an assault in the face of which she stood calmly firm and looked at me with increased attention. We subsequently had a chat about it and I realized I was projecting an old hatred born of fear onto her, and having seen it, as is the way with these things…it collapsed and I was free of it, important in what was to happen next.

Kindly, I think partly as a result of this, Lee started in our meditation sessions to direct us to working on the heart center (heart chakra as it's called in the Indian Tradition). This for me was the crowning experience of my whole visit and I came to realize just how helpful the whole chakra system really is in helping us to unblock old wounds. I suppose I have here to own that, on reflection, in spite of many attempts to be otherwise, my heart still remained closed. This is a terrible condition and one I suspect very common in the West, for if the heart is closed, then "loving" is not really possible. We may seek "love" as hard as we like but "loving," loving life, loving people, loving all experience, eludes us. A most painful condition that arises I suspect from very early birth or childhood traumatic experience in which the heart closes in order to survive. And when the heart closes out of these traumatic contacts with the world it builds around itself a hard casing like an old walnut that has sat beside the fire all winter. Hard and very difficult to crack open.

Working with the heart center for us meant repeatedly bringing our attention to bear on the heart, imaginary breathing in and out of the heart, evoking in the heart positive emotions such as gratefulness, kindness, appreciation, mercy, and finally perhaps love itself. When I commenced this I have to say I was a bit suspicious. Was this just a new age dream? Did it actually do anything?

In one session quietly concentrating on my heart it suddenly burst into flame. I could not believe it; I suddenly had a veritable bonfire going in the area of the heart. Small to begin with, it began to flower until my whole interior horizon was ablaze. The session finished and I was left dumb with wondering, weepy, slightly shaken, unsure of what had happened but realizing something big really had happened. We dispersed for lunch and I wandered off on my own towards the kitchens.

As I entered the courtyard a clear intuition came over me that I had not quite finished this piece of work and so, seeking out a chair under a tree, I re-entered my interior world and brought my attention back to the fire in my heart. Almost immediately I saw the fire glowing deep down inside me and my attention was taken by one small specific coal that seemed to glow more brightly than the others. In my imagination I picked this glowing coal up in my fingers and stared at it deeply. In a flash I immediately vanished deep, deep inside myself, deeper than in any meditation I had ever done before and

I swam around inside myself like this for some minutes, head "deep under water" so to speak. I suddenly popped out again and went and had lunch!

This experience has stayed with me when I returned to the UK and it's as if a whole new dimension has arisen in my experience of being alive. I find it the most potent antidote to negative feelings and emotions. Should these crowd in upon me (as they are wont to do in grey old January London!?) I simply bring my attention to the heart and circle around it with positive affirmations of emotions such as joy, loving gratefulness for what I have, rather than what I do not have and lo and behold my negative feelings evaporate. As I usually do this in the early morning I come down to breakfast and my wife says, "Why are you so damn cheerful?"

Also I think once we re-open this center in ourselves a compulsion seems to arise, and it certainly did in me, to be more honest with ourselves and more straightforward and honest with others. I found myself being much more critical of myself in terms of relationships, wanting things straightforward, nothing concealed, a higher integrity as if the heart could not stand anything not quite right, not straight and authentic. Finally it seemed to me as if one other essential faculty was restored to me through this heart center work and that was that my gratefulness heart meditations turned into what I can only describe as praise. This did not seem to be praise to a specific God, or even an idea like it, but to something out and beyond my small self, something altogether larger and more powerful than myself, to which the only right attitude seemed to be praise. This has given my life a new sense of direction in this respect and it is a joyful thing.

So having completed this retreat and having been able to keep my practice going on my return to England my advice would be, chuck the anti-depressants away, stop rushing around trying to distract yourself with ever finer distractions, breathe, meditate and bring your attention to the heart again and again until it fills you up. You may be surprised!

NAMASTE.

Nick P.

This dramatic spiritual transformation opened "a whole new dimension...in the experience of being alive" for our client, changing his attitude towards life and "wanting things straightforward, nothing concealed, a higher integrity as if the heart could not stand anything not quite right not straight and authentic." Although an atheist, Nick suddenly found something more—"something out and beyond my small self, something altogether larger and more powerful than myself, to whom the only right attitude seemed to be praise. This has given my life a new sense of direction in this respect and it is a joyful thing."

This experience motivated him after going back home to dive deep into studying yoga and especially Patanjali's *Sutras*. A few years later, Nick wrote to me:

> I run study groups now on *Patanjali* because I think he, more than anyone else I know, articulates so well the difference between psychical and spiritual. The intense first priority is to get ourselves free from psychical enmeshment *then* we begin to get an idea of how it actually binds us and *how* we can become freer. Good psychotherapy! It seems to me this is the best way to deal with the various demons hanging on to our toes so we may get a glimpse of what the spiritual is… we do so love to take short cuts!

These two examples speak to the promise of true healing (but perhaps not always curing) through profound spiritual transformation, a promise that yoga therapy holds for our clients. Perhaps because of the intensity and duration of our program we witness many profound spiritual shifts in our clients after every retreat. Typically the attitudes are changed and the spark in the eye and spring in the step are back.

But not everyone goes through such profound transformations. Not everyone is ready or even sometimes willing to let go and risk exploring the territory outside their psychological and mental comfort zones. We, as yoga therapists, do not really know the deeper layers of our clients and their readiness for spiritual transformation. I found out how deeply Nick was transformed only after receiving his letter.

What is perhaps more interesting is that clients may not know themselves if they are ready for spirituality and transformation! This knowledge comes out only after they start intensively practicing yoga themselves. And either the client allows the new experiences to take them forward, reaping the positive effects, or they resist and hold on to the safety of the "known." Here is the account of a 45-year-old female, an executive in a big financial firm in the US, with whom I worked over a few years:

I had a few different physical symptoms that were causing me unrest (vertigo, forgetfulness, anxiety, to name a few). Since modern medication wasn't providing me with the relief and the best of doctors were unable to give me diagnoses, I decided to try a different path. At the end of 2012 I spent three weeks at Kaivalyadhama in Lonavala turning to yoga therapy.

I recall one of our early conversations and Lee asking me if the unrest in my body could be part of my spiritual journey to finding my peace. I was scared of the word "spirituality" and wanted to run from the conversation. To me it meant being religious, having blind faith, something to do with ghosts and after-life, general voodoo, and not taking things in my own control. I think in logic and purpose, and there was no room for something called spirituality.

Lee helped me uncover my fears, and my journey of being myself vs. living by expectations started. I returned home from my three-week trip with tools like breathing, meditation, and yoga practice that helped me deal with my physical symptoms. It was not like they disappeared—I was just not letting them control me. My family and friends noticed a sea change. I was calmer, nicer, took better care of my self, resisted situations and people that didn't make me happy.

This is how my journey of finding myself, staying centered started! In 2015, I saw Lee again and told her that now I feel I'm on my spiritual path!… It is about being open to where life takes me, being comfortable with myself, being grounded and centered (and spiritual) that has helped me face life and its curve balls—fighting breast cancer, seeing my dad battle liver cancer and losing him…and so much more.

In this case we had daily two- to three-hour sessions throughout her three-week stay in Kaivalyadhama. She then went back home and continued to practice prescribed yoga techniques daily and regularly. I had sporadic contact with her in person and follow-up over the phone. But she was obviously ready to venture into transformation through her regular yoga practice (*sadhana*), as over time she made a great shift and progress in her spirituality and healing. Today she is able to understand why and when the symptoms re-appear, and is able to manage them accordingly.

The research data on yoga, spirituality, and health supports the notion that yoga enhances transformational processes, including spiritual and transcendent states. Furthermore, that these transformational states and processes may be singular to yoga practice and philosophy. Yoga is unquestionably a spiritually transformational discipline. It may also be the only secular science and complementary discipline offering a spiritual roadmap, which is beneficial and vital to the transformative healing of human beings.

Modern medical sciences have recognized the importance of the spiritual component in healing.[47] In recent years, we have seen the emergence of tools for spiritual assessment, such as the FICA-Spiritual History Tool or HOPE-Questions for Spiritual Assessment.[48] For those who are connected to religion, spiritual guidance is accessible through the chaplaincies available in many hospitals or through churches. However, those who are not connected to any particular religion usually have no means to improve their spiritual health as part of healing. Yoga therapy's capacity to influence spiritual well-being presents a unique opportunity to offer the solution within a medical setting, where there is none offered to non-believing patients at the moment.

This data also points to the importance of a few other factors:

- The extended length and intensity of yogic practices seems to create more profound spiritual shifts.

- The social and intersubjective character of transcendental experience— the collective energy of the group—is helpful in creating and sustaining these shifts.

- The changes depend on the individual's spiritual self-perception.

- It is necessary to revive spirituality in yoga by reinforcing the spiritual component of yogic practices such as *yamas* and *niyamas*, chanting, *yoga nidra*, use of *mudras* and *bandhas*, meditation, and understanding philosophy through yoga courses and discussions.

The ancient yogi knew that the intensity of practice over time speeds up the goal of furthering the development of the student. The *gurukul* system was based on the student or disciple staying with the *guru* for longer periods of time, with daily spiritual discipline and study, as per the *guru*'s direction. Today, only a few ashrams are left to fill this role, places where you can immerse yourself in longer intensive yogic practices. The role of the *guru*, however, became less accepted after revelation of the many power and sexual abuses around even the most respected names.

"The reason Yoga therapy is so effective in both preventive medicine and in assisting conventional treatment methods is because Yoga addresses all three aspects of wellness—physical, mental and spiritual."[49] This sums up the opinion of serious practitioners and students of yoga—yoga encompasses the art of self-realization, self-transformation, and self-healing.

Patanjali compiled the tools for such profound transformation in 300 CE in what is called "*Ashtanga Yoga*,"[50] or the eight limbs of yoga. This first, most translated and commented-on classic Indian text, which organized and synthesized yoga—Patanjali's *Yoga Sutras Darshana*—provides the roadmap to healing and spiritual transformation. The collection of 196 short aphorisms outlines the tools and results of practicing them, of which spiritual transformation is at the core. The *Sutras* clearly explain the process and practical methods of raising levels of awareness, gaining deeper wisdom, exploring the potential of the mind, and eventually going beyond the mind. If this is not spirituality, then I do not know what is… Sadly this has sometimes either been either ignored or misunderstood by the growing population of contemporary young yoga teachers and yoga therapists.

It seems that we have been so taken in the West by our need to be forever young and to have perfect-shaped bodies that the body postures (*asanas*) have completely dominated our understanding of yoga and anything else has fallen off the radar. Yet in Patanjali's *Yoga Sutras* only 3 out of the 196 *Sutras* deal with postures! Even the majority of research tends to be focused on the biomedical effects on the body, which excludes the much wider impact of yoga on human existence. With once- or twice-a-week *asana* classes, the deep transformative value of yogic science and the promise of spiritual transformation eludes us.

But new voices are beginning to point back to the richness of the ancient science. In their 2015 book, *The Eight Limbs of Yoga: A Handbook for Living Yoga Philosophy*, Stuart Sarbacker and Kevin Kimple point to the "great potential for self-transformation through Yoga" and its capacity "to transform one's relationship with others and the world in profound ways."[51] As Michael Lee mentions in his recent article, "The gold nugget of Yoga therapy—its capacity to be a catalyst for meaningful and lasting transformational change—remains largely hidden."[52]

We hope that the future can be changed in a positive way, and the maturing of professional organizations such as the IAYT in the US, Japan Yoga Therapy Society, or Yoga Australia can be the catalyst we need. These organizations must work towards the creation of a healthy and wholesome image of yoga and yoga therapy. Only by educating members as well as the public about the true essence of yoga and yoga therapy can we do this.

CHAPTER 4

Yogic Tools for Assessment and Health Evaluation

Yoga has its own traditional and cultural system of assessment, diagnosis, and health evaluation. However, as it does not seem to have a "standardized tool," many in yoga therapy practice claim (mistakenly) that it doesn't have its own system. This misconception often fosters an unhealthy dependency on the modern medical diagnosis alone. We need to be clear that we cannot move out of our scope of practice (SoP) and "borrow" assessment tools from other professions, and furthermore, it will not be correct to create therapeutic yogic plans based on the results of such borrowed assessment tools. It follows that both the assessment and therapeutic plan should be based on knowledge from the ancient texts, and should, as far as possible, merge together seamlessly.

The development of these yoga therapy tools for clinical assessment is, as we speak, a work in progress worldwide. What we can do today, however, is set the standards for assessment tools in the field of yoga therapy. We can show examples of this work in progress. We can encourage others to read the ancient texts and then find ways to bring this knowledge into the modern-day clinical setting. Perhaps at the end we will not be limited to one standard assessment tool. Perhaps there will be as many tools developed as the situations and environments in which the assessment takes place. Nevertheless, we need to be aware of the standards and frameworks of yoga therapy in order to create adequate tools.

Need for yogic assessment tools

Yoga therapy must never be limited to a mere treatment of an externalized diagnosis or to symptoms. Hence, it is imperative we have tools to "tailor make" individualized protocols or modules, that take into account a thorough search for the "root cause" of the disease and then try to find a way out of it with awareness.

It is also important that an attempt be made to help the client understand and accept the root cause of their problem and further familiarize themselves with factors causing, aggravating, or mitigating it. Self-awareness of the client is often the only way to prevent worsening of the condition and its relapse, and to facilitate self-reliant conscious measures towards the adoption of a healthier lifestyle by the client.

Of course, the inference drawn from such a detailed yogic analysis can assist us in forming a baseline for pre-treatment and post-treatment comparisons. This also acts as a reference to assess progress in therapy at various points of time in order to make modifications or advancements accordingly.

Framework of yoga therapy

The often-quoted traditional basic framework for the application of yoga as therapy is usually based on a derivative of the teachings of Maharishi Patanjali as codified through his *Yoga Sutras*.[1] Verses 16 to 26 of the second chapter ("Sadhana Pada") elaborate the concept of addressing the problem, finding its cause, and then applying the therapeutic remedy (the goal of therapy) through use of appropriate tools (*heya-hetu* and *hana-upaya*).

- The first and foremost step in this comprehensive template of yoga therapy is to try and understand as completely as possible the nature of the problem/issue/challenge/manifest suffering (*heya*). It is important to focus on how long the problem has been in existence, how severe it is, and how it impacts the client's daily life. We need to assess together with the client the physical, emotional, mental, social, financial, and spiritual aspects, to have a holistic picture of the current "state" of the individual who is seeking our help.

- The second step attempts to find the possible causes of the problem (*hetu*). This must not stop at a superficial level of symptoms but try to unravel the potential root causes that are causing the manifest signs and symptoms of disease. It is important to make a complete search for internal causes, which could include genetic predisposition, maladapted stress responses, energy imbalances, distorted perceptions, as well as negative emotions and self-image. On the other hand, external causes could be infective, accidental, environmental, or traumatic in nature. Finally, we need to address in detail the role of an unhealthy lifestyle, as this is often the main cause of the whole problem. An example would be two clients with the same symptoms—both obese and both depressed. However, one may be depressed because they are obese, and the other one may be obese because they are depressed.

- In the third step, a joint understanding is developed between the client and the therapist towards setting the target goals for the therapeutic process (*hana*). The client may have a certain goal in mind while the therapist has another. These goals may be different and hence a joint discussion and collaborative and realistic plan needs to be made to avoid disappointment later. An example would be a cancer patient seeking yoga therapy to enhance energy, improve sleep, reduce fatigue, and deal with pain while the therapist may be more focused on "preventing an occurrence of" the cancer.

- The final step in this process is the adoption of concrete concepts and practices that then contribute to the development of a comprehensive individualized protocol (*upaya*). This is the stage where the actual tools are determined in order to achieve the goal set in the third stage. This may include a combination of any or all of the techniques in our therapeutic armory including counseling, shifts in attitude (*bhavana*), lifestyle modifications, and practices of *Ashtanga Yoga*, *Kriya Yoga*, *Hatha Yoga*, mantras, *yoga nidra*, and most importantly, relaxation. It is only during the relaxation phase that healing truly manifests, and hence we should never forget the importance of this often-neglected aspect in yoga therapy.

Understanding the issues that brought the client to us

In order to properly understand the client and their problem, we need to make sure that we keep our ego in check and that we are conscious of any projections or transference that may occur as the result of our own experiences. Our own history affects our judgment and we need to be *very* aware of this fact in order to prevent mis-assessment. Very often we have "blind spots" around our own issues, and it is always good to have some kind of supervision set up to be able to verify our own projections getting in the way of assessment.

In Lee's case this manifested in a peculiar way. She noticed that after finishing a three-week intensive retreat, Beyond Cancer, she would be completely depleted of energy and had to spend two to three days resting in bed to slowly regain her vitality. One day she was discussing the retreat with a friend—a yogi scholar and psychotherapist—and she mentioned her affliction. He listened carefully and then said, "Most likely you have unresolved issues around the work you are doing with cancer patients." It took only a second to realize that she had never grieved the death of her father from lung cancer when she was 15. That night she let it all surface and had a deep release. Since then she tends to be tired, which is to be expected after leading three weeks of an intensive retreat, but never so depleted as before.

Here are a few suggested check points for yoga therapists before they face a client:

A SUGGESTED PERSONAL CHECKLIST FOR YOGA THERAPISTS

1. Do not bring your personal problems into the assessment process.

2. Let go of your prejudices and do not let that influence the assessment.

3. Patience and perseverance are key qualities if you are to do justice to the assessment process.

4. Intelligence and empathy guide an objective and logical assessment.

5. Do not judge the client, and never condemn them for choices they may have made. Remember, it is their life!

6. Always remember that your role is limited to facilitating their inherent healing mechanisms and not to impose your will on them.

7. This should be a bidirectional interactive process and their choices should be accepted and respected, even if they are contrary to your own personal views.

For the purpose of assessment it is always useful to use the five-layered existential model (*pancha kosha*) as it enables us to develop a thorough understanding through processes of observation (*darshanam*), touch (*sparshanam*), detailed interview (*prasnam*), and assessment of energy flows (*nadi pariksha*) the issues that may be of a physical, functional, psychological, intellectual (frustrations and conflicts), or even spiritual nature.

Evaluating physical or structural (annamaya) issues

Yoga therapy evaluation of physical wellbeing starts the moment the client enters the office, as keen observation can provide immense clues about many aspects of their health. We look at the body type (endomorphic, ectomorphic, or mesomorphic) and deposition of body fat (apple, pear, or hourglass body forms). This enables us to have a better understanding of the constitutional aspects of the individual (*dosha*), and helps in the selection of practices as well as the adaptations that may be required for different body types. Taking it even further, body mass index (BMI) may be evaluated by measuring weight and height and calculating it in kg/m². This objective measure is always useful as it gives a clear baseline for pre and post comparisons, and also gives us a clue to metabolic and cardiovascular risks that increase proportionately with BMI.[2] Medical practitioners are always more comfortable with yoga therapists who speak their language and use standardized metrics. So it is always better to indicate BMI rather than just saying, "My client is overweight," "They have a huge tummy," or worse, "They have a huge stomach."

The need to obtain consent for physical examination is something that cannot be stressed enough, as no yoga therapist should ever touch their client without clear verbal or even preferably written consent. This should be obtained in the initial stage itself, as later it may take a nasty turn, especially if the client is not satisfied with the results of their therapy. This warning percolates into the practices and hands-on assistance that may be given by the therapist in the sessions. Many people are very sensitive of their personal space, and we need to respect this.

During the focus on the physical aspects of the client, it is important to create a constitutional (*dosha*-based *prakriti*) analysis by an inferential approach. Individuals with a movement-predominant constitution (*vata*) usually have a thin and light frame. They often complain of sudden bouts of fatigue. They typically have dry skin and hair with cold hands and feet. When this becomes imbalanced, they may complain of weight loss, constipation, joint pain, muscle weakness, restlessness, and indigestion.

Individuals with a metabolism-predominant constitution (*pitta*) are usually of medium size and weight and complain of early greying, baldness, or thinning hair. They claim that they can eat anything and usually have a warm body temperature. When in balance, a lustrous complexion, abundant energy, and a strong appetite manifest, but when out of balance, skin rashes, burning sensations, excessive body heat, heartburn, and indigestion predominate.

Large, soft eyes are often the first thing we notice in clients with a cohesion-predominant constitution (*kapha*) who manifest smooth and radiant skin with thick abundant hair. When *kapha* is in excess, they tend to be overweight or obese with fluid retention. The signs and symptoms of allergies often manifest on the surface of their body.

It is desirable that therapists obtain sufficient competency and the necessary skills of observation and manual palpation to assess the client's spine for any abnormalities such as lordosis, kyphosis, or scoliosis. This would also include an assessment of gait through observation of the length and pace of steps, stiffness of body, swiftness, unequal weight bearing, swing of the arms and legs, as well as an open or closed stance.

They should watch for any tremors in the body region such as the limbs, and note their duration, speed, severity, and presence at rest or during movement. In the yogic perspective these tremors are an externalized manifestation of internal emotional and mental imbalances (*angamejayatva*). Disharmony at a higher psychic level induces imbalances in neurochemical transmitters and psychophysiological pathways, resulting in these physical tremors. Through the slow and steady practice of *asana* we can help our clients attain a better state of inner balance (*sthria-sukham*), and this may help them to transcend the pair of dualities (*dwandwa*) that are viewed as the essential cause of these tremors.

Therapists should be observant of any lumps and if found, their presence should be noted, with details of the region, size, shape, consistency, and tenderness. The client may often know of such masses of tissue and may already have been getting treatment for them. If it is a new finding, such information should be shared through professional referral with a healthcare professional for further medical evaluation.

Yoga therapists should be conversant with the basic clinical signs of anemia such as fatigue, pale conjunctiva, skin and tongue, as well as observing brittle nails and any shortness of breath. Anemia is often a cause of breathlessness and a rapid heartbeat, as well as fatigue, and hence this initial finding enables us to better understand issues that come up when we consider alterations in physiological function.

Diet plays a vital role in health and disease, and therapists should obtain details about the type of food and frequency of eating as well as the nature of the food taken. A word of warning: although yoga stresses the need for a life-enhancing (*sattvic*) diet, we must not be judgmental about the client's choice of food, and listen to them patiently. Once we get the information, we can slowly make appropriate suggestions about changes that can be brought into their life, depending on their cultural, social, and religious value systems. In the process we should understand the situational aspects of the client's life, and find ways to change what is within their means and reach. A commonsense approach to diet having appropriate levels of fiber and adequate nutritional benefits obtained from seasonal local produce is often more beneficial than any "hard and fast" approaches that only result in no one ever following them! Sensible statements such as, "Eat to live; don't live to eat" and "What you eat becomes you, so be careful what you eat" are more useful than loads of advice. Perhaps a most often overlooked factor is how we eat, how much we eat, and when we eat. Changing the "fast food on the go" to mindful eating, the regularity of meals, and eating to two-thirds of capacity is also important. Finally, appropriate levels of hydration are also very important—at least 2 liters of water should be consumed daily to make sure that we keep our body hydrated.

Joint mobility and stability requires thorough observation. Therapists should evaluate the range of movement and note the presence of any limitations, hyper-mobility, or instability, looking for pain, swelling, redness, raised temperature, tenderness, and the presence of any deformities or scarring. If any abnormalities are present, a detailed inquiry should be made into its history and manifestation, with a stress on the factors that aggravate or mitigate the issue.

All of these observations should be substantiated with taking a detailed history, either in a passive, receptive manner or a focused one. A passive manner means letting the client talk about their physical problems as they will. A focused enquiry is when the therapist guides the conversation towards verifying the observations they have already made.

Pain is something that is very personal, and therapists must never doubt it when a client talks about it. However, its severity can always be determined by asking probing questions about how it affects the individual's day-to-day life and also whether it impacts their quality of life and so on. We must not forget that more often than not, the client would have consulted numerous healthcare professionals before coming to us.

This is especially pertinent if no one had been able to find a specific cause for the client's pain, as they may start to become very defensive about it, and at times may be in a state of confusion. Professor K.R. Sethuraman[3] often talked about medically unexplained symptoms (MUS).[4] He reiterated that the client definitely had symptoms impacting their life, because otherwise they would not have sought help from a healthcare professional in the first place. However, many of these MUS are psychosomatic in nature, and a "cause" is often not readily found after initial investigations.

It is often useful to ask the client to demonstrate their physical issues by asking them to stand up or stretch their limbs, or by showing you where the issues manifest. This gives them a sense of empowerment because they are involved in the process. It helps us understand how aware they are of the body.

Becoming aware of the body, emotions, and mind is one of the principles of yoga therapy itself.

One of the most important aspects of health is a sense of physical wellbeing. This needs to be dealt with as a priority because even a small improvement in this dimension makes the client more conducive and receptive to further efforts.

Evaluating physiological or functional (pranamaya) issues

As yoga therapists, it is important we honor the sentiments of our clients when they talk about the limitations they experience with regards to their normal day-to-day functioning. We need to assess with empathy how such issues impact their day-to-day life. We need to have intelligence and empathy to be good yoga therapists. Modern medicine was originally an art (that had a heart); it then became a science (that had a head).

The great Yogamaharishi Swami Kanakananda Brighu used to say, "God breathed into man the breath of life; and then expected him to keep it going!"[5] The breath is the key to good health as all systems are influenced by healthy or unhealthy patterns of breathing. When assessing our client, we must observe their breathing, both while they are unconscious of it and also when we bring their awareness to it. Normally most people have no awareness of their breathing at all, and it's only when their respiration is compromised that they even start to think about it. This is an unhealthy awareness of the breath, or rather, a dire lack of it. Yoga, on the other hand, brings about a healthy consciousness of breathing through awareness of the whole process, thus shifting from brainstem-led automatic reactivity to cortical-guided conscious responsiveness.

We need to observe the client's breathing and note whether it is shallow or deep, regular or irregular, and whether there is a harmonious pattern. The rate should be counted for a full minute through passive observation, as once they realize we are watching them, they will become self-conscious, and numerous changes occur. The average amount should be under 14 breaths per minute.

We need to watch and see if it is paradoxical, that is, a reversal of the normal pattern. Usually the abdomen expands during inspiration and comes back during expiration. However, in paradoxical breathing, the reverse is happening. Determining which areas of the lungs are being used is important as we wish to help them learn to breathe into all 10 of the bronchopulmonary segments of each lung. We also need to ask them and determine whether they are suffering from dyspnea or have a difficult and labored breathing as this is a sign of impaired oxygen transport that could be either cardiac or pulmonary in origin. Whether such dyspnea is present on exertion, normal activity, or even at rest is useful in determining the severity of their condition. If they experience a sense of tightness and breathlessness while lying down (orthopnea), they surely need an expert medical consultation, as this is a sign of heavy cardiorespiratory compromise. Watch for the presence of a cough, as aggravating and mitigating factors should be understood to help us guide them in their recovery to good health.

In yogic philosophy, irregularity in breathing patterns (*shvasaprasvasa*) is understood to be one of the main physical manifestations of mental and emotional upsets. Ancient yogis contemplated this deeply, and realized that mental disturbances cause irregularity and instability of respiration. Through their experiential perspective they realized that by stabilizing the breath, we can concomitantly produce stability of emotions and mind. This knowledge is used by yoga therapy today in the practice of *pranayama*, when it is used as a means of altering the higher (mind) through the lower (body). This is one of the best examples of the numerous somatopsychic applications found in the practices of *Hatha Yoga*, the physical science of balancing equal and opposite energies.

Another physiological function we need to assess in our yoga therapy session is that of circulation. This dynamic manifestation of the subtle energy flowing throughout the body (*vyana vayu*) is vital. Any impairment leads to unhealthy congestion, as well as insufficiency of oxygen transport. A healthy circulation manifests through warmth in the body while the lack of it leads to cold extremities. Of course, stress-induced sympathetic over-activity leads to the typical cold, clammy hands due to the excessive sweating accompanying such moments of tension.

The heart rate may be ascertained by taking the pulse (*nadi pariksha*), and by noting the rate, rhythm, and regularity we can get a good idea of the heart and its function. In addition, if the yoga therapist is working in a medical setting, they should be able to measure the pulse and also, if possible, train in the procedure to record blood pressure. These vital parameters give us a clue about circulatory imbalances that are often symptomless, and hence known as silent killers. Using the pulse we can also determine dominant *dosha* and its deregulation, and thus choose an appropriate *pranayama* protocol. This, of course, requires extra yogic training in understanding the pulse in relation to *doshas*.

When we do various yoga practices, the gentle warmth that manifests in the limbs may be understood as a manifestation of healthy life energy (*prana*) flowing in that area. Conversely, when any particular area is cold, lack of such a healthy energy flow may be inferred. The level of relaxation during practice can be evaluated by the peripheral flow, as when the sympathetic drive is reduced and the parasympathetic drive becomes dominant, enhanced tissue perfusion and opening up of the capillary bed happens. The extremities are often felt, in such a case, as filled with a sense of warmth through the "warm golden energy" of *prana*. The yogic saying, "Where the mind goes, there the energy flows"[6] holds good, and the circulation is often a physiological manifestation of the mindfulness of various body parts.

The principle that is involved here relates to the "improvement of the flow of healing life energy." This is vital for good health, as such an improvement induces relaxation, regeneration, and rejuvenation. Relaxation is often all that most patients need in order to improve their physical and physiological condition. Stress is the major culprit of many NCD ailments, and may be the causative, aggravating, or precipitating factor in many psychosomatic disorders. Doctors often tell their patients to relax, but never tell them how to do it! The relaxation part of every yoga session is most important because the benefits of the practices done will seep into each and every cell.

Normally one shouldn't be aware of the heart beating during rest. However, if the client expresses such a symptom, you will need to go deeper into the complaint, as it may be a rhythm disorder or a manifestation of stress. The heart center is an important energy vortex (*anahata chakra*) and enables us to manifest empathy and compassion and have a sense of understanding in various social and interpersonal relationships. It is also important in helping us to develop a healthy intrapersonal relationship with our own self as well as a transpersonal relationship with the Divine. This then manifests as social and spiritual health.

Yoga therapists should investigate by asking questions about any changes in appetite, changes in body weight, and heat or cold intolerance. The back of the hands can be used for a generalized evaluation of body temperature at the forehead, neck, etc. that helps in this assessment. Increased temperature is reflective of higher metabolic activity while a colder body temperature is indicative of lower metabolism. This is important in creating the yoga therapy protocol as practices, especially of *pranayama*, are then chosen accordingly. All of this enables us to understand the energy of digestion, assimilation, and metabolism (empowered by the *samana vayu*). If this energy is found to be overactive, cooling practices may need to be used, whereas an inactive state will require invigorating practices.

Another area that needs to be evaluated by yoga therapists is the sleep pattern, and this should include a focus on both its quality as well as quantity. Questions such as, "Do you fall asleep easily?" and "Do you feel refreshed when you wake up or do you feel tired?" are more useful than just a mere detailing of hours spent asleep. The presence or absence of daytime sleepiness is also important as it may indicate inadequate quality of night sleep. Sleep is the time when we heal best, and the lack of this vital need will hinder the whole healing process. An improvement in sleep after starting yoga is one of the most important benefits leading to a better quality of life for individuals. This may, in fact, be the most important factor from the perspective of those suffering terminal illnesses, and is often expressed by them as the best benefit they have got from yoga.

Therapists should inquire about the client's bowel movement as all traditional systems consider constipation a major cause of most diseases. Changes in color, amount, or timing and regularity are important. If a client mentions the presence of blackened stools or blood in the fecal matter, urgent medical referral is warranted to rule out any gastrointestinal bleeding. Loss of the normal color with whitening of fecal matter may imply liver issues. Facilitation of natural elimination of wastes is one of the principles of yoga therapy, and this aspect of assessment enables us to plan appropriate yogic cleansing practices. Stagnation always breeds disease, and hence, unless toxins are cleaned, many of the practices may not have the desired effects.

The elimination process and its energy (*apana vayu*) inquiry should also cover bladder habits and sweating that may be more or less than usual. Further inquiry (*prashnam*) about increased thirst, discolored or decreased urine output, altered odor of urine, or headache can give us an idea of whether the individual is hydrated or not. This also enables us to rule out any renal malfunction, as decreased urine out is a sign of such disorders while an increase could suggest diabetes. A darker coloration of urine would be a sign of gross dehydration while complaints of blood in the urine warrant medical referral.

An aspect that is often not forthcoming is the nature of reproductive function, and this may require some direct questioning or may only manifest in subsequent sessions. This may be especially true in some cultures where a female client may not be comfortable talking about such private issues with a therapist. However, we need to evaluate menstrual function, its regularity, any excessive flow, presence of pain, and infertility, as these will influence the protocol. It is safer to avoid some of the inversions during the actual menstrual flow and instead focus on relaxation and restorative practices. As the downward-flowing energy (*apana vayu*) is responsible for reproductive function, a healthy focus on this area and usage of practices that enable loving care should be encouraged. This would also apply in cases of male sexual dysfunction, and this may often not be forthcoming too.

From a yogic perspective the evaluation of the energy flows (*prana vayu*) is very important, and all the inputs we get from observations, history taking, and examination will ultimately help us form a yogic assessment. This would be based on subtle energy flow (*vayu*) and constitutional (*dosha*) imbalances etc., and will have nothing to do with a medical diagnosis such as diabetes or hypertension. Making such a "yogic assessment" is very much within our SoP, whereas attempting to make a medical one is not. As yoga therapists, our choice of practices for the individual client will be based on a yogic assessment, and the practices will aim at rectifying any imbalances rather than treating the medical diagnosis. However, as we proceed in this approach, there can also be expected subtle and later even discernible improvements in the medical diagnosis.

We also need to focus on assessing the lifestyle (*jiva karma*) of our client, as many NCDs prevalent today are due to unhealthy lifestyle. Yoga places great importance on a healthy lifestyle, and we need to evaluate the client on the basis of the main components of such a lifestyle by inquiring into the physical activities of their daily life (*achar*), their dietary choices (*ahar*), modes of relaxation and recreation preferable to them (*vihar*), the nature of their social and interpersonal relationships (*vyavahar*), and their habitual thought patterns (*vichar*). The findings of this investigation will help apply the basic yogic principles that are useful in managing lifestyle disorders including developing appropriate attitudes, stress management, normalization of metabolism, relaxation, visualization, and other contemplative (*dharna/dhyana*) practices.

As yoga therapists we should develop a broad understanding of the various body rhythms (*jiva vrittis*) such as the circadian (24-hour cycles, such as sleep–wake), infradian (longer than a day, such as the menstrual cycle), and ultradian (shorter than 24 hours, such as the nasal cycle) rhythms that are a manifestation of our inner and outer harmony with nature (see the end of this chapter for a template). Irregularities in these biorhythms imply a loss of harmony, and hence a more detailed further search for the cause should be made.

Evaluating psychological (manomaya) issues

An important factor in this category is the assessment of the client's general awareness, and self-awareness in particular. We need to observe if they are aware of their surrounding, of what they are doing, whom they are with, and how aware they are of themselves, etc., as we interact with them in an interview. Their level of awareness will indicate to what extent we can accept their views at face value. We also need to assess if their focus is on the lack of health and disease or on getting well. Are they focused on the problem, or looking towards a solution? Are they identifying with their disease or not? This sets the stage for introducing self-inquiry (*swadhyaya*)-based practices. It will also indicate their ability in daily life to adopt a strong contrary and responsive attitude (*pratipaksha bhavanam*) towards negativities or habitual destructive tendencies (*samskaras* and *vasanas*).

Often many of our clients identify with their diseased state and start to introduce themselves as a patient of that condition—"I am a diabetic" or "I am a cancer patient." Sometimes they even start to subconsciously make a claim to their disease by saying, "My diabetes," "My hypertension," or "My cancer." Such mal-identification needs reframing during yogic counseling to help them detach from such tendencies; otherwise, a real change may never manifest despite the best of therapies. It is often useful to ask them to start rephrasing their statements by referring to the condition as a third person, such as, "the diabetes" or "the cancer." This sets an important foundation for the dramatic changes that can manifest once we stop clinging onto the diagnosis and label. As Swami Gitananda Giri would say, "Are you sick to get sicker, or to get better?" If the disease is being used as a crutch for social and/or emotional support, it is tough to bring about a change.

As yoga therapists, we need to address the sense of painful suffering (*duhkha*) felt by our clients, especially at the emotional, social, and mental level. A useful way of approaching such a situation is to help the client realize that often the greatest teachings are given in moments of great despair. Yoga understands that this may be the best "teachable" moment, and hence we find the highest teachings of the *Bhagavad Gita* and *Ramayana* coming at such points for Arjuna and Lord Rama. Swami Gitananda Giri used to say, "A nervous breakdown is actually an opportunity for a spiritual breakthrough if we can realize the positive implications in our moment of despair and dejection." The teachings of the *Yoga Vasishtha* and the *Bhagavad Gita* seem to be the first recorded "psychological yogic counseling" sessions in human history. They were delivered when both Lord Rama and Arjuna were in the depths of their depression. If we can help the client to see the moment of pain, difficulty, or despair as an opportunity for growth, we can help our client achieve a better state of health.

Healing manifests best when we are relaxed, and hence we need to determine whether our client is capable of relaxing or not. This may seem outright funny as we expect everyone to be able to relax easily, but this is not true. Very often people are so stressed that the very relaxation seems too stressful for them. Keep evaluating the client, and see whether they can relax or not. Are they able to be still? Can they sit still? Can they lie down without fidgeting and looking around? These are open-ended questions that are not limited just to the initial consultation but also continue during therapy sessions.

You can also check whether they are able to close their eyes and "let go" while relaxing. So many of our clients, especially those with mental health issues, get tense if they are asked to close their eyes during the session. In such situations we may need to introduce relaxation initially with eyes open, and then, once we gain their trust and confidence, introduce the closing of the eyes later. We need to observe their breath and notice if there is any change during relaxation. Does it go faster or slower? Is it deeper or shallower? Someone falling asleep during relaxation is just a sign that they really need the relaxation. All of these questions enable us to understand better the current psychological status of our client, a reflection of the *manomaya* existence.

We need to passively observe their facial expression and see whether they can smile or not, and take note of how well they can laugh. If someone can at least force a smile and laugh a bit, we will be able to help them much more than when both are completely absent. "Fake it till you make it" often seems to work. We also need to observe the unconscious physical twitches and movements (tics). If present, we should further inquire about how aware the individual is of these.

It is important to evaluate the mental makeup and level of thoughts (*chetana*) of our clients through a *guna*-based evaluation.[7] We need to determine whether the nature of our client is influenced primarily by dull and passive (*tamasica*) patterns, or by dynamic and passionate ego-centric activity (*rajasica*), or by pure and kind noble aspirations (*sattvica*). According to the *Bhagavad Gita*, the food we eat, the way we worship, the austerities we undertake, and the charity we perform may all be sub-classified under the *Trigunas* according to the spirit and inner nature of the act itself.[8]

Tamasic manifestations often include addiction, depression, dishonesty, and self-destructive behavior including sexual perversion (*viparita buddhi*). This could further manifest as hate, vindictiveness, and violence. In extreme cases it could lead to criminal behavior, but often less drastic manifestation includes carelessness, dullness, and lethargy.

Rajasic manifestations, on the other hand, could be inferred through anxiety, hyperactivity, indecision, and unreliability. Often such individuals are extremely ambitious and aggressive, and may or may not realize that their anger is harming relationships. They may have a tendency towards impulsiveness, manipulation, and self-aggrandizement, with an expressed or unexpressed desire to control everything.

The goal of such an assessment is not to be judgmental and condemn the client, but to help them to have an objective view of where they are and to understand how they can develop inner stability and a sense of ease. We can introduce to them the *sattvic* qualities as something to aspire and grow into, rather than mere abstract philosophical concepts that seem beyond human reach. An ability to comprehend in a positive manner with clarity and self-esteem is a very valid goal (*hanam*). Such aspirations when seeded into the mind at a receptive state will, with appropriate practices, develop and manifest calmness, compassion, faith, forgiveness, and love.

After we build a close and trusting relationship with a client we need to probe even deeper to understand the habitual patterns (*samskaras*) and inherent tendencies (*vasanas*). These are the root of the action–reaction (*karma*) cycles and are linked to the inborn affiliations (*kleshas*) according to yogic psychology, as codified by Patanjali in *Yoga Sutras*. Attachment to position in life (*lokha vasana*), attachment to level of education and knowledge (*jnana vasana*), and attachment to the body (*deha vasana*) are the most ingrained of all human conditions. These color our perspective and make us err in our judgments. It is often said, "We see things not as they are, but as we are." Unless we understand the deeper matrix distorting the client's perceptive, we cannot help them realize how much they are skewing reality. We often find that the client may hold a conscious or subconscious strong negative emotion towards another person or people. Helping the client to realize that, and then resolving such emotion through yogic practices, lies within the promise of yoga therapy.

We should also check for the presence of any previously diagnosed psychiatric condition that may or may not have been treated. This is very important as often such diagnoses are considered a stigma and hence clients may not be forthcoming with the details. If the mental diagnosis is currently being treated with a prescription, we will need to understand the possible side effects of the medication and address these as well. A general question about any prescriptions the client has may start such a difficult conversation.

Evaluating intellectual (vijnamaya) issues

Many a time the client comes to us with issues that don't really seem to be discernible at the gross levels. However, when we investigate deeper, we realize that something is just "not right" at a deeper level of the mind. This may be understood as the subtle root cause (*adhi*) often mentioned in yogic pathophysiology. If we set out to evaluate this "higher mind" or intellect (*buddhi*) level, we often come upon a sense of disassociation, a sense of being "out of sync" or a sense of "not being in the right place at the right time." It is as if all the different layers (*koshas*) have gone out of alignment. This was often discussed in detail by Swami Gitananda who termed it *nara*, or a disassociation of the five *koshas*, resulting in a cascade of manifestations in the grosser layers.

The client may say that they are always late to places or events, and so miss buses, trains, and even important appointments for job interviews. They may state that while walking towards a doorway, instead of walking through the door, they end up bumping into its side frame. Many accidents are narrated where they "knew" it was "going to happen" and yet "couldn't stop it." Swamiji taught that unhealthy habits, lifestyle, breathing, emotions, and negative thought patterns were the cause of this disassociation leading to various somatic and psychosomatic disorders. In modern terms this may be understood as stress. Virtually every disease or disorder is caused, precipitated, or aggravated by stress.

We need to inquire into the deeper conflicts and frustrations that are part of the client's life. They may not be forthcoming initially as these are often very personal, but such deeper issues start to surface only after we gain the client's confidence. Are they at ease with themselves or not? Do they often find themselves caught in the midst of a dilemma and "between a rock and a hard place"? Does their conscience seem to prick a lot, and does this lead them to ruin many aspects of their life? All of these are vital if we are to find the root cause of the sense of uneasiness (*dwaitham*) that is preventing our client "feeling themselves."

We need to determine if they are aware of and how well they understand their own problem and how they choose to communicate it (*vacha*). Is it more verbal or non-verbal communication? And when we give them any suggestions, do they listen or merely hear? How well they adapt to the stressors in their life and the choices they make is very much part of this level of existence. Are they in a reactive mode for the most part of the day, or are they responsive? Do they realize when they are reactionary and reflexive rather than responsive and reflective? All of these questions enable us to understand the *vigjnanamaya kosha* aspect of our client. Unless we help them overcome and rectify any subtle imbalances at this level, with a proper protocol, our mutual efforts towards healing may not be very effective.

The principles of yoga therapy involved in this part of the process are the awareness of emotions, thoughts, and choices, the calming down of the mind, focusing it inwardly, and the ability to fortify oneself against omnipresent stressors. Assessment of these and of the spiritual level of existence will only be possible with time, when the relationship between the yoga therapist and client grows into deep mutual respect.

Evaluating spiritual (anandamaya) issues

Each and every living being is endowed with amazing self-healing potential, but we are often ignorant of this. As yoga therapists, it is important that we address this and try to understand how well the client is connected to their "own self." Are they "at ease" with themselves or is there a sense of duality or separation between their own mind and body? Often people identify themselves with their mind—"I am my thoughts," we hear often.

We need to search for the cause of their problems by addressing the core of the afflictions (the root *klesha*, *avidya*). The hold of this primary distorter of our perspective is often very tight and influences everything through ignorance.

This is then compounded by the false sense of ego (*asmita*). What are the client's sources of hope, strength, and comfort? What does the client hold on to during difficult times? Do they belong to a supportive community? What things do they believe give meaning to their life? Do they believe in a greater power or god? Are they religious? Are they spiritual? What does spirituality (or religion) mean to the client? What role do their beliefs play in regaining their health? As we develop our relationship with the client we can start such conversations. This will help us to assess this layer of existence.

The need to survive at any cost (*abinivesha*) induces the exaggerated stress response. The diametrically opposite pulls of the attraction (*raaga*) to some things and the aversion (*dwesha*) to other things may create deep inner conflicts. How attached are they to their likes and dislikes? Are they able to balance them or not? Without the client's awareness and understanding of the necessity of detachment, the tranquility and equanimity of mind will remain unattainable, until the client realizes that we can introduce Maharishi Patanjali's concepts through the practice of self-purification (*Kriya Yoga*). Otherwise, the importance of discipline, self-analysis, and acceptance (*tapa, swadhyaya, ishwar pranidhana*) as the means to overcome these afflictions may never be realized.

Once an understanding is gained, we can then work to increase the client's self-reliance and self-confidence, and help them take responsibility for their own health—as Swamiji would say, "Regain their birthright of health and happiness."

A summary of pancha kosha assessment
ANNAMAYA ISSUES

- Type of body and deposition of fat

- Stress in the body

- BMI

- Posture—lordosis, scoliosis, kyphosis

- Assessment of movement:

  - Gait

  - Limitation of limb movements

  - Tremors

  - Scarring

- Signs of anemia—pale, breathlessness, rapid heartbeat, fatigue

- Diet—eat to live or live to eat, regularity, *sattvic*

- Pain—area, duration, severity, aggravation

- Medical diagnosis—single or multiple, medications and their side effects.

PRANAMAYA ISSUES

- Breathing patterns:

  - Shallow or deep

  - Ratio of exhale to inhale

  - Patterns—smooth, interrupted inhale or exhale

  - Depth—clavicle, intercostals, abdominal

  - Breaths per minute

- Pulse reading for *doshas—vata, pitta, kapha*

- *Vayus* assessment:

  - *Vyanavayu*—blood circulation problems, cold or warm extremities

  - *Samanavayu*—digestive issues, urinary and reproductive issues

  - *Apanavayu*—elimination, sweating

  - *Pranavayu*—hyperventilation, sighing or yawning, breath per minute

  - *Udanavayu*—thyroid issues, self-expression, metabolism, sleep patterns

  - Subsidiary *pranas*—belching, sneezing, etc.

MANOMAYA ISSUES

- Any mental medical diagnosis

- Mental side effects of medicaments

- Focus on disease or health

- Level of awareness

- Level of emotional suffering

- Ability to relax

- Facial twitches or unconscious movements

- *Guna* assessment—*tamasic, rajasic, sattvic*

- Strong or weak—likes and dislikes

- Daily routines, habits

- Deep negative emotions.

VIJNAMAYA ISSUES

- Strong or weak belief system, convictions

- Lifestyle, daily routines, habits

- Sense of being in the right place, at the right time, being on time

- Habitual thought patterns

- Stress levels and adaptation

- Strength of ego

- Awareness and self-introspection.

ANANDAMAYA ISSUES

- Sense of religion and/or spirituality

- Sense of "self"

- Sense of life purpose

- Sense of connection to the universe

- What does the client hold on to during difficult times?

- Do they believe in a greater power or god?

- Do they have a supportive community?

- What brings the meaning to their life?

- What role do their beliefs play in regaining their health?

All of these layers of our existence have been addressed separately in this section, yet all are one and the same as they belong to the same individual. We, as yoga therapists, must never forget to look at the bigger picture. This can only be done with time and the trust we build with the client. If this is done efficiently and with competence, we, and the client, will be able to understand the problem and its cause, and find the remedy that needs to be applied.

In short:

- Treat the client with respect and always obtain explicit consent, especially before any hands-on examination or corrections.

- Observe the client's body, its proportions, unconscious and conscious movements, function, and their level of body awareness.

- Observe their breath, how slow or quick it is, and how it changes when consciousness is brought into play, such as when you ask them to breathe as opposed to when they are passively breathing.

- Listen to the client and try to understand their thoughts and expressions. Look out for hidden aspects that may have been left unsaid.

- Gain their confidence and then you will find the whole "box" opens up and you get to see the real cause of the problem.

- Witness how they relate to themselves and others and be aware of how they distort the perspective (*kleshas*). Slowly help them also "see" this, and then witness if changes occur or whether they just go into denial. If so, more sessions may be needed.

- Try and put all the pieces of habitual patterns, conditioning, inherent tendencies, and latent desires together to understand where the source of the problem is. As you get to know them better, the assessment will be shifting.

- Keep working from the gross to the subtle and to the causal, and then evaluate the changes as they manifest from the causal through to the subtle and finally the gross levels of existence.

- Do not give up, even if it seems tough, as this is the golden opportunity we have to truly help another human being out of suffering and into ease. However, always walk "half a step behind" the client, watching for an opening to the next step.

- Be prepared that some clients may come to you to hear what they want to hear. They may be not open to any suggestions that do not agree with their preset ideas. You may find that they have already visited a few care workers before and "didn't receive any help." Very likely they were given a solution but were not ready to accept it. It is up to you to evaluate how set the person is in their expectations of what they want to hear, and to decide whether to continue with the sessions.

Examples of assessment tools

We understand that perhaps there will be many tools of assessment, depending on your work environment and your type of client. If you work within the healthcare system in a team with other medical personnel, most likely you will use more "healthcare"-friendly language and tools. If you work independently in private practice, there is more freedom to use yoga therapy tools and language in communication with a client. Maybe you need to assess clients ahead of time for longer, intensive, therapy retreats. Perhaps instead of a standardized assessment tool you will end up with many tools, filling different needs and ways of evaluating a client's state of health. Here are a few different assessments as examples used for different applications.

Swami Gitananda Giri's assessment tool

Swami Gitananda Giri[9] developed one such tool, detailing 12 diagnostic points (*dwadasha rogalakshna anukrama*). Not only does it enable the therapist to understand their client better, but it also enables clients to understand themselves better too (*swadhyaya*). The 12 points are:

- *Triguna* (individual nature): Which of the *trigunas* are they? Are they *tamasic* (dull and inactive, inert), *rajasic* (over-active, always doing something, busy), or *sattvic* (calm, composed, with a quiet personality)?

- *Tridosha* (personal constitution): What is the predominant *dosha*? Are they *pitta* (fire/bilious), *vata* (air/movement), or *kapha* (water/earth); or a combination?

- *Trivasana* (inherent tendencies): Which of the *trivasanas*, the three vanities, is predominant? What are the inherent tendencies? What drives the person? Are they caught up in family, status of life, titles after their name, vain knowledge, a "know-it-all attitude"?

- *Prana* (energy flows): What is the flow of *vayus* like? How is the *prana*? *Apana*? *Samana*? *Udana*? *Vyana*? Are there disturbances in the flow?

This also includes energies used in uploading and downloading thoughts (*akasha* and *chitra prana vayus*).

- *Abhyasa* (personal discipline, self-effort): Will they be able to keep up the yogic tools you give them? Do they have the self-discipline? How does this manifest in their lives? Are the disorders caused by their lack of willpower or *abhyasa*?

- *Jiva karma* (lifestyle): What is the person's lifestyle? What type of activities do they do during the day? Or night? Are these building *karmas*, are their actions producing reactions?

- *Chetana* (quality of thoughts): Are their thoughts negative, about themselves, disturbing?

- *Vacha* (communication): How do they communicate? Rapid, slow, broken, flowing, clear?

- *Ahara* (diet): What are their dietary habits? Are their meals regular? How many a day? What food do they eat? Is it nourishing for the mind, body, and soul? Do they share with others? Is there emotional over-eating? Do they eat junk food (the quality of *gunas* and *doshas* are manifesting here)?

- *Viparita buddhi* (destructive habits): What negative self-destructive habits do they have? Smoking? Drinking? A sedentary lifestyle? Indulging in unsafe practices that may bring disease? Are they indulging in dangerous activities that may result in an accident?

- *Jiva vrittis* (biorhythms): How are their biological rhythms? Digestion, elimination, bladder functioning, heart rate, blood pressure, respiratory rate? How are they breathing? In females, how are their menstrual cycles?

- *Sankalpa* (aspirations): What are their aspirations? Do they want to get better or stay sick? The pay-off is attention. Do they have the power to follow their desire and manifest it? Perseverance? Are they satisfied with where they are? Is their intent working with action (*kriya*), and do they have the power to bring their thoughts into action?

This helps to understand the client, where they are now, and where they want to go, and then for the therapist to be able to work on how they may get there. Yoga therapy is about recognizing where the person is, helping them understand where they are, why they are there, and what they can do to get to where they want to be. Our role is to facilitate this process of self-empowerment and self-actualization.

Optimal State assessments (Amy Wheeler et al.)

Another example of an assessment is Amy Wheeler and her colleagues' Optimal State. The Optimal State Assessment System tools[10] are based on a model of the *gunas*, sourced from Patanjali's *Yoga Sutras* and Ayurveda. This assessment system includes the ten classical pairs of opposites from Ayurveda, the five-element theory from Samkhya, and the three *gunas* of the mind from Patanjali. It is a practical and simple way for the teacher and student to begin a dialog around habitual thoughts, mental habits, emotions, and physical sensations in the body, all based on the *gunas*. From this dialog, the therapist can negotiate with the client which daily practices from yoga and Ayurveda might bring the student back into balance. The suggestions for daily practices are also based on the ten pairs of opposites, five elements, and three *gunas*. This is an excellent example of an assessment and treatment plan protocol that stays within the SoP of yoga therapy, yet it is very intuitive and accessible to clients who have no understanding of yoga. There is no other field of study that uses these concepts to assess and give lifestyle guidance.

Here is one of the sample assessments:

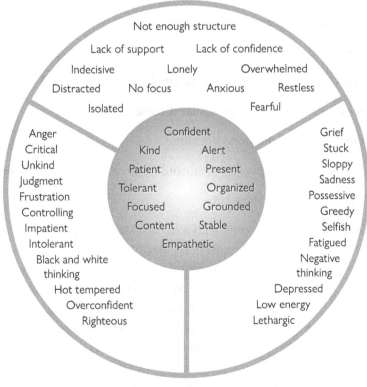

Mental emotional state assessment

Yoga for Health Institute's case records

In the Beyond Cancer and Chronic Solutions retreats, the Yoga for Health Institute uses "case records" (see below) that participants submit at the time of registering. Please note that in the case records silhouettes are used for clients to indicate the level of pain and place of radiation (if applicable). This is done with those participants in mind who have chemo brain and who find it difficult to express themselves in words (an excellent suggestion from Andre Haralyi, a yoga therapist with extensive experience working with cancer patients). It is much easier to point to the place of radiation or pain than to describe it in words when you are suffering from severe brain fog (or chemo brain).

This assessment is amended during individual sessions at the beginning of the retreat. We also use a circadian rhythm assessment (see below) in the first days together with *pranic* pulse reading, which we do regularly throughout the retreat.[11] Circadian rhythm regularity and *pranic* pulse reading allow us to assess the *pranic* and nervous system of the clients, which indicates the effects of the practices on individuals during the retreat.

Deregulation of the circadian rhythm is a lifestyle problem and has been shown to, among other factors:[12]

- Contribute to inflammatory diseases

- Weaken the immune system

- Increase the risk of cancer and metabolic syndrome

- Increase the risk of cardiovascular diseases

- Increase levels of the stress hormone

- Increase the risk of psychiatric disorders or neurodegenerative diseases

- Accelerate the aging process.

We find that all our clients come with a deregulated circadian rhythm, and so part of our retreat function is to bring regularity back to our clients' circadian rhythm in the three weeks. In the process clients then start sleeping more deeply, getting better rest, and to feel their metabolic functions coming back to a regular rhythm. In the following table clients observe and note their nostril blockages at specific times during the day for five days. This, together with reports on their sleep, gives a picture of how deregulated their systems are.

Circadian rhythm assessment: nostril check

	Day 1	Day 2	Day 3	Day 4	Day 5
Upon rising					
Before lunch					
Before dinner					
Bed time					
Notes: L, left open, R, right open, B, both open, LP, left partially, RP, right partially.					

The following case records are used in qualifying potential participants in our three-week intensive retreats. The detailed assessment is done in person on arrival, including the standardised tests.

Yoga for
Health Institute

CASE RECORD—CANCER

1. Personal details

Last name: . . . . Middle name: . . . . First name: . . . .

Date of birth (DD/MM/YYYY). . . . . Occupation: . . . .

Address: . . . .

. . . .

Email: . . . . Mobile number: . . . .

Tel. no.: . . . . Next of kin: . . . .

Family members: . . . .

Who lives with you? . . . .

. . . .

Dates of the course you want to attend: . . . .

2. History of the disease

a. What type of cancer were you diagnosed with? . . . .

b. Dates of diagnosis: . . . .

c. Dates of last treatment: . . . .

d. What kind of treatments did you have? (Please list all) . . . .

. . . .

e. Surgery type: . . . .

f.   Chemotherapy? Yes ☐ No ☐; if yes, how many sessions? . . . .

g. Radiation? Yes ☐ No ☐; if yes, how many days? . . . . Pre/post surgery:

. . . .

h. Other relevant information: . . . .

. . . .

i. Mark on the drawing the place where radiation was applied:

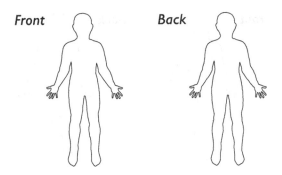

Front   *Back*

3. Side effects

a. Do you still suffer from side effects? Yes ☐ No ☐; if yes, please choose from the following list of symptoms:

Physical symptoms

Osteoporosis ☐ Constipation ☐ Nausea ☐ Neuropathy ☐ Insomnia ☐ Anemia ☐

Mental symptoms

Feeling of hopelessness ☐ Anxiety ☐ Depression ☐ Forgetfulness ☐ Fear ☐

Chemo brain

Have difficulty multi-tasking ☐

Confuse dates and appointments ☐

Misplace objects ☐

Forget details of recent events or conversations ☐

Struggle for the right word or phrase ☐

Have difficulty focusing on one task ☐

Feel mentally "slower" than before ☐

Any other:

. . . .

. . . .

b. If you have pain, please indicate where on the drawing:

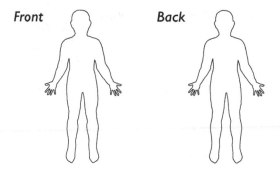

Front   *Back*

On a scale of 1–10 (10 is the most severe pain), please mark the level of the pain you feel:

●--●

1   2   3   4   5   6   7   8   9   10

c. Do you have any physical disability since the treatment? Yes ☐ No ☐; if yes, please describe: . . . .

. . . .

d. On a scale of 1–10, please mark the level of your physical disability (10 is your physical ability before cancer):

●--●

1   2   3   4   5   6   7   8   9   10

4. Current status

a. Are you currently doing any type of physical exercise? Yes ☐ No ☐; if yes, please describe: . . . .

. . . .

How many times a week?: . . . .

b. Are you doing yogic practices? Yes ☐ No ☐; if yes, how many times a week? . . . .

c. Do you have any food allergies? Yes ☐ No ☐; if yes, please describe . . . . . .

. . . .

d. Do you have any other allergies that you know of? Yes ☐ No ☐; if yes, please describe . . . .

. . . .

e. Do you have any other diagnosed physical/mental condition? Yes ☐ No ☐; if yes, please describe . . . .

. . . .

f. Any particular instructions/recommendations given by your surgeon/doctor?

. . . .

g. Any contra-indications noted? Yes ☐ No ☐; if yes, please describe . . . .

. . . .

h. What, if any, medicine/drugs/herbs are you currently taking? . . . .

. . . .

i. Have you seen an Ayurvedic or traditional Chinese medical practitioner? Yes ☐ No ☐; if yes, what advice were you given? . . . .

. . . .

j. Have you been recommended any special foods or supplements? Yes ☐ No ☐; if so, by whom? . . . .

k. What resources have been most useful throughout your cancer care/treatment/recovery (social, physical, mental/emotional, and spiritual)?

. . . .

l. What attitude would you say was most useful for you to have throughout your treatment and recovery? . . . .

. . . .

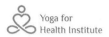
Yoga for
Health Institute

CASE RECORD—NON-COMMUNICABLE DISEASES (NCDS)

1. Personal details

Last name: . . . . Middle name: . . . . First name: . . . .

Date of birth (DD/MM/YYYY): . . . . Occupation: . . . .

Address: . . . .

. . . .

Email: . . . . Mobile number: . . . .

Tel. no.: . . . . Next of kin: . . . .

Family members: . . . .

Who lives with you? . . . .

. . . .

Dates of the course you want to attend: . . . .

2. History of the disease

a. Have you been diagnosed with a chronic problem? Yes ☐ No ☐

b. Dates of diagnosis: . . . .

c. Date of last treatment . . . .

d. What kind of treatments did you have? (Please list all) . . . .

. . . .

e. Surgery types and dates: . . . .

. . . .

f. Other relevant information: . . . .

. . . .

3. Side effects

a. Do you have any physical disability? Yes ☐ No ☐; if yes, please describe:

. . . .

. . . .

b. On a scale of 1–10, please mark the level of your physical disability (10 is your physical ability before illness):

●--●

   1   2   3   4   5   6   7   8   9   10

4. Current status

a. Are you currently doing any type of physical exercise? Yes ☐ No ☐;

if yes, please describe:. . . . .

How many times a week?. . . . .

b. Are you doing yogic practices? Yes ☐ No ☐; if yes, how many times a week? . . . .

c. Do you have any other diagnosed physical/mental condition? Yes ☐ No ☐; if yes, please describe . . . .

. . . .

d. Any particular instructions/recommendations given by your surgeon/doctor?

. . . .

e. Any contra-indications noted? Yes ☐ No ☐; if yes, please describe

. . . .

f. Have you seen a functional medical doctor, Ayurvedic or traditional Chinese medical practitioner? Yes ☐ No ☐; if yes, what advice were you given?

. . . .

g. What resources have been most useful throughout your care/treatment/ recovery (social, physical, mental/emotional, and spiritual)?

. . . .

h. What attitude would you say was most useful for you to have throughout your treatment and recovery?

....

5. Do you struggle with any emotional issues?

Yes ☐ No ☐; if yes, please describe:

....

....

....

6. Please describe the major events in the last 10 years that you think might have contributed to your health challenge

....

....

....

7. Please describe your typical daily routine (including mealtimes)

....

....

....

How regular is it? ....

8. If you were asked what belief about yourself or emotion contributed to your health challenge, what would your answer be?

....

....

....

So far, in the first part of this book, we have learned what yoga therapy is, and we have looked at its applications and modalities. We have presented the results of research on yoga and its proven effects on our wellbeing and health. We have also discussed spirituality as an inherent aspect of the healing journey, including the promise of spiritual, but not religious, transformation. Finally, we have presented the yogic way of assessing the status of a client's health, and outlined examples of assessments.

Throughout all these pages we have interwoven one aspect, yet it remains untouched and unnamed—what is needed to perform all of what we have talked about so far? Who has such knowledge to be able to assess with yogic modality the depth of a client's imbalances (dis-ease)? Who has the knowledge to understand a client's circadian rhythm imbalance and to interpret their nasal rhythm and what it means? Who can understand and assess breathing patterns? Who can build a close enough relationship with a client to be able to access their habitual thoughts and rigid belief system? Who can read the *pranic* and Ayurvedic pulse to assess imbalances in *doshas*? Who can assist or guide a client's spiritual transformation? Who knows all the modalities of yoga and is able to effectively match their application to their client's needs? And finally, what kind of skills and life experiences are needed to bring all of this knowledge together effectively, for the client's benefit? More importantly, who can do this?!

We attempt to answer these questions next, in our last chapter of this first part of the book, where we will discuss who yoga therapists are and what makes them "good." We make the case that in order to be yoga therapists we have to have our own continuous spiritual practice. We also offer ways of measuring and improving our skills as yoga therapists. Chapter 5 is based on the findings and practices described in the groundbreaking book by Richard Davidson and Sharon Begley, *The Emotional Life of Your Brain*.[13]

CHAPTER 5

What Makes a Good Yoga Therapist?

In this chapter we will cover what a yoga therapist is, what it means to be a "good" yoga therapist, and finally, how we can improve our skills as yoga therapists.

There seems to be quite a lot of confusion in the field as to the difference between a yoga teacher and a yoga therapist. This is no small matter considering that there are an estimated 36.7 million yoga practitioners and more than 100,000 teachers in the US alone,[1] with worldwide participation in yoga classes estimated to be 300 million students.[2]

In what follows we hope to clear up any confusion by providing an understanding of the profile of a yoga therapist as well as the nature of their relationship with their clients. The yoga teacher's goal is to teach a yoga class without causing harm, while the yoga therapist's goal is to assist in facilitating a client's healing. The training goal of yoga therapy is to prepare the trainee to engage in the process of empowering individuals to progress toward improved health and wellbeing through applying the teachings and practices of yoga.

What is a yoga therapist?

Yoga therapy as a profession has only emerged in the last three decades. While as yet the government has not regulated any of the yoga professions, there have been efforts for yoga therapists to self-regulate their standards in order to assure quality of skills across the board. In order to be accepted onto a yoga therapy course, you have to have finished at least 200 hours of course work, and be a certified yoga teacher. Yoga therapy training adds on 800 hours of additional training, both theoretical and practical.

The IAYT, founded in 1989, and other similar associations in Australia, India, Japan, and Korea, has a mission to establish yoga as a recognized and respected therapy worldwide. IAYT published its first yoga therapy school accreditation standards in 2012, and in an effort to make yoga therapy a broadly accepted professional association, introduced the therapist's certification standards in 2013. To ensure that therapists meet or exceed these standards, IAYT also introduced renewal and continuing education (CE) policies, which require therapists to renew their certification every three years by submitting at least 24 hours of CE credits.[3]

As of late 2017, IAYT has over 5600 members from over 50 countries and over 185 member schools. More than 3700 members (mid-2018) have passed their C-IAYT certification. This is all good news considering that in 2017, the Society for Integrative Oncology issued guidelines recommending the use of yoga for reducing anxiety, improving mood disturbances and depressive symptoms, and for improving breast cancer patients' quality of life.[4]

Many yoga therapists have been through some personal history of healing with the help of yoga, which then grants them a deeper understanding of the transformational healing process of yoga therapy. They tend to relinquish their current profession to move into yoga therapy as a professional calling. They therefore tend to be mature, have general life experience, and understand yoga and yoga therapy as a lifestyle.

Clients usually seek a yoga therapist for a completely different reason than a student seeking a yoga class—they usually have an unresolved health challenge. I often work with patients with an NCD in chronic form who have tried traditional medical treatments and have not found answers to their problems.

There are also a number of clients who, based on their own personal experience as well as those close to them, already know and believe in yoga as a possible answer to their health challenge. In other cases, clients may not want to know much about yoga but have heard that it may help them for their specific problem. Finally, in some situations there is a huge gap in medical care where yoga fits in perfectly, delivering solutions where there is no hope left. Such is the post-treatment situation for cancer patients where the medical treatment is finished and there is no support or information available to help them deal with the often-severe side effects of their disease.

The yoga therapist's relationship with the client

Being a yoga therapist itself indicates the need for building a very close relationship with the client, based on mutual trust, from the very beginning.

The relationship starts with an in-depth assessment during a one-to-one session, evaluating the client's physical, psychological, mental, lifestyle, and diet factors, and taking into consideration the client's goals. Based on such an in-depth evaluation, the therapist will then choose and recommend yogic practices, lifestyle changes, and perhaps diet changes. Both the client and therapist base the further relationship on constant evaluation of the effectiveness of their practice. At the core of the relationship is the continued evaluation and empowerment of the client. The therapist's goal is to facilitate the client's healing process. I often say that I am walking half a step behind the client, looking and waiting for the clues that they are ready to move forward in their healing journey.

Finally, unlike a yoga teacher who usually teaches *asanas* in the lineage they have been taught in, the yoga therapist will use a wide variety of yogic practices from many lineages, backed by scientific evidence. The therapist's loyalty lies with their client and their healing journey, and in addition to *asanas*, the therapist may use *yamas, niyamas, pranayama*, dietary and lifestyle changes, stress management, meditation techniques, mantra chanting, or *yoga nidra—* whatever they deem most effective for a particular client in the particular stage of healing of a particular disease.

To sum up, there is a great difference in the level of competencies between yoga teachers and yoga therapists. That difference is necessary in order to meet the very different goals in the minds of yoga teachers and yoga therapists. A yoga teacher's goal is to create a sequence of practices and effective delivery of yoga instructions to a group. A yoga therapist's goal is based on a close relationship with a client in a one-to-one or small group, where at the core is constant evaluation of the client's healing progress and the effectiveness of their practice. Those who come to a yoga class are looking to increase their flexibility and reduce their stress. Those who come to a yoga therapy class have specific health challenges and are looking for answers not perhaps found elsewhere. Their priority is to heal and they may not be interested in "studying" yoga.

Yoga is to be known through yoga

An important link in the chain of yoga seems to be missing in today's yoga therapy. This link is the therapist's own personal *sadhana*, or *practice of yoga*. By this we do not just mean the external practice of some techniques, but also the internalization of yogic principles as a consciously adopted yogic lifestyle. The strength of any chain depends on its weakest link. So, too, the strength of *yoga therapy* depends on the therapist's personal practice (*sadhana*), conscious yogic living, and on how clearly this 'spirit of yoga' is passed on to clients: "We do not think ourselves into new way of living, we live ourselves into new way of thinking" (Richard Rohr). Unless we ourselves know what to do, how to do it, why we do it, and what it feels like when it's done, how can we intelligently lead others? Indeed, isn't it against the very spirit of the moral-ethical foundations of yoga (*yama-niyama*) to recommend a practice without personal experience of the nature of the practice itself?

The above caveat also holds true for researchers studying the effects of yoga techniques. If they haven't a clue about the actual "yoga" involved in their investigations, what are they studying? Unless you have an experiential understanding of the technique, you cannot know the point at which you enter and become one with the practice. This being true, how can we know where the benefits of the practice manifest physically, mentally, emotionally, and spiritually? If we don't have the "experience" of the technique and its "state of being," what are we going to research, and what is the effect we are going to report?

A prominent contemporary mystic, Richard Rohr, said:

> Over the years, I met many…activists who were doing excellent work…but they were…still living out of their false self with the need to win, the need to look good—attached to a self-image.
>
> They might have the answer, but they are not themselves the answer. In fact, they are often part of the problem… For that very reason, I believe…great spiritual teachers first emphasize transformation of consciousness and soul. Without inner transformation, there is no grounded outside transformation.[5]

These words made us think of the situation we currently perceive among yoga community members. There seems to be a split of understanding in what yoga therapy is and what it is not, in addition to "reductionist" attitudes among some members of the yoga therapy community. The "reductionists" are usually working within the healthcare community (hospitals and medical clinics), which constrains therapists in two major ways. First, for those therapists existing within the medical system, this limits them to using medical diagnosis as their main assessment tool, with the exclusion of yogic assessment. Second, it limits the use of yogic tools to mainly *asanas*, some *pranayama*, and perhaps meditation, to deal mostly with symptoms of a medical assessment. This then tends to take yoga out of yoga therapy and creates "yogopathy," as described previously. Generally in such environments there is no permission or space to work with consciousness or spirituality, which is the essence of yoga, and provides the gateway to deeper inner healing work.

Such division, we believe, comes from the different approach people have to the whole field of yoga and yoga therapy. There seems to be much confusion about what yoga therapy is or is not. We have to remember that yoga is a two-pronged approach to life: it is an end goal (as the union of our consciousness with Universal Consciousness) and the means to achieve this goal—a multitude of yogic techniques and approaches to purify our body and to go beyond our mind. If we are to treat our clients with yoga therapy, we need to know these practices experientially and their effectiveness backed by evidence, in order to be effective in teaching: "Yoga is to be known through yoga. Yoga arises from yoga. One who is vigilant by means of yoga delights in yoga for a long time."[6] We need to understand these practices not through reading about them, but through experiencing and living them ourselves. Knowledge added to by experience results in wisdom of being and modeling the solution to our clients—we are then able to teach from the heart instead of the head.

Those who have had, for some time, their own established personal daily *sadhana* under the guidance of a teacher, were able to experience and understand the transformative power of yoga in their lives. Hence they tend to teach from their wisdom, from the "heart," from their own experience. Therefore they tend to teach yoga therapy, which treats the whole human as a being that functions on a multilevel system.

Those who do not have their own daily practice or who have not experienced transformation as yet, will usually teach from learned knowledge, from read research, or from that learned from books. In such cases yoga tends to be reduced to *asanas*, *pranayama*, and/or meditation to treat the disease and its symptoms, in accord with the approach of "a pill for every ill" or, to paraphrase, "a specific yoga technique for a particular symptom/disease." The *yamas* and *niyamas* seem to be forgotten. The teaching comes from the "head," becoming yogopathy that deals with symptoms. From that attitude the question often asked is, what yoga do you suggest for cancer patients?

During my six years in the Kaivalyadhama Yoga Institute in India I taught a "master class" for experienced yoga teachers (with over five years' teaching experience) who wanted to hone their skills further. Yoga teachers and sometimes trainers came from all over the world to study in this renowned institution. Sadly, the majority of them did not have their own daily practice. More than half of them were lacking in experience in *pranayama* and/or meditation.

Our own daily practice builds our own awareness, which is crucial to being effective in service to our clients. We need to know who we are as yoga therapists, why we are teaching our clients, and what we want to achieve while teaching. We need to realize that we can lead our client only as far as we have gone ourselves.

The well documented, but invisible, process of entrainment in a relationship plays a very important role in our practice. The vibrational frequency of two people in contact will frequently fall into sync. When the frequencies are the same, that is, both are happy, this is called "resonance." But when they are different, and a vibrational body of a stronger resonance influences another in its field, this is called "entrainment." Our bodies naturally entrain to external rhythms without us really noticing. Whether it is moon cycles or the vibrational strong presence of another person, we react to it without being aware of it. Try to sit next to someone who is angry, and in no time you will feel anger in yourself.

If we understand the power of entrainment and the effect it can have on our being and the being of our client, we can help our client to heal their physical, emotional, and spiritual body. But in order to have such a calming and healing effect on our client, we have to cultivate our own strong and high vibrational field through our own spiritual practice—*sadhana*. Our own progress allows us to teach more by the way of living than by doing, simply because yoga is primarily about being and not doing.

An important thing to remember is that there cannot really be any distinction between the professional and personal lives of a yoga therapist. Good yoga therapy is modeling how yoga should be lived regardless of the style or school of tradition from which the therapist comes. The quality of a yoga therapist's energy is the major factor in their yoga therapy success, and no amount of technical expertise will replace the projected energy.

Good yoga therapists will never impose their own will on a client. The process of facilitating healing must always be based on mutuality and agreement that, at the time, this is the best way to proceed. Yoga therapists meet clients where they are, and facilitate the process of healing by assessing and providing yogic tools best suited to a client's healing at the moment. Yoga therapists always walk half a step behind the client, always assessing and waiting for the client's signs of readiness for the next step.

We should never underestimate the impact a yoga therapist may have on a client's life. As the relationship of mutual trust develops with time, the therapist may become a lifeline for someone. Without realizing it, the yoga therapist may act in a similar capacity to a teacher, psychotherapist, physical therapist, priest, life coach, or even a parent.

How can yoga therapists improve their skills?

A fascinating book came out in 2012, *The Emotional Life of Your Brain*, by Richard Davidson and Sharon Begley, the culmination of neuropsychologist Davidson's 30-year research on the neuroscience of emotions. A meditator himself, Richardson has done groundbreaking research, working closely with the Dalai Lama and long-term meditators. He postulates that each of us is composed of six basic "emotional styles" where the "style" is defined as a consistent way of responding to the experience in our lives. Interestingly, each style is governed by specific, identifiable brain circuits, and can be measured by objective laboratory methods.

These styles and emotional states predict health problems. What is in the brain necessarily influences what is in the body. Moreover, the communication between these two is bi-directional, so that what is in the body influences what is in the brain. The brain circuits that underlie emotional styles have extensive two-way connections with the immune system, the endocrine system, and the autonomic nervous system.

Richardson suggests a way to measure oneself on the spectrum of each emotional style. His research in neuroplasticity has confirmed that purely mental activity—ranging from meditation to cognitive behavioral therapy— might increase or decrease activity in specific brain circuitry. Based on this, he then goes on to recommend ways to modify one's scores for each emotional style (and our health)—nothing short of a miracle made in a laboratory at the University of Wisconsin-Madison!

The emotional styles created by Richardson are as follows: social intuition, self-awareness, sensitivity to context, resilience, outlook, and attention. Each of these styles can be changed by yogic practices, if we desire, and three (social intuition, self-awareness, and sensitivity to context), suggests Richardson, are critical to being a good caretaker, therapist, or social worker. This also includes yoga therapist.[7]

Social intuition

Social intuition speaks to how adept one is in picking up social signals from the environment and the people around. The ability to "tune in" to another person is a hallmark of good yoga therapy. It is the ability to understand subtle non-verbal cues such as body language, vocal intonation, and the facial expression of others. It is a quality facilitating empathy and compassion—being able to decode the silent signals from clients means we can respond to them in an appropriate and effective manner.

Social intuition can be measured by answering the following questions, true or false:

1. When I talk with people I often notice subtle cues about their emotions—discomfort or anger—before they acknowledge these feelings in themselves.

2. I often find myself noticing facial expressions and body language.

3. I find it doesn't really matter if I talk with people on the phone or in person, since I rarely get any additional information from seeing whom I am speaking with.

4. I often feel that I know more about people's feeling than they do themselves.

5. I am often taken by surprise when someone I am talking with gets angry or upset at something I said, for no apparent reason.

6. At a restaurant I prefer to sit next to someone I'm speaking with so I don't have to see their full face.

7. I often find myself responding to another person's discomfort or distress on the basis of intuitive feel rather than explicit discussion.

8. When I am in public places with time to kill, I like to observe people around me.

9. I find it uncomfortable when someone I barely know looks directly into my eyes during a conversation.

10. I can often tell when something is bothering another person just by looking at them.

         1 ___ 2 ___ 3 ___ 4 ___ 5 ___ 6 ___ 7 ___ 8 ___ 9 ___10
         PUZZLED   INTUITIVE

SCORING

Give yourself one point for "True" in questions 1, 2, 4, 7, 8, and 10, and one point for "False" for questions 3, 5, 6, and 9. A total score above 8 means you are highly socially intuitive; a score below 3 means you are highly puzzled.

"Too puzzled" characterizes extreme insensitivity to the subtle signals of the surroundings. Such people, writes Richardson, are generally socially blind and deaf, with devastating personal and professional consequences.

If you are on the extreme mark of the socially intuitive scale, this may mean a tendency to forego your own needs and clues in order to meet others' needs and expectations.

WAYS TO INCREASE SOCIAL INTUITION

- Go out to a public place and begin observing people. Pay attention to eyes, body language, voice, posture, and emotional cues of strangers passing by. It is useful to choose one element per day such as, "Today it's about noticing different eye expressions." With time and a lot of practice you will gain sensitivity to the clues and start noticing differences. Practice, practice, practice observing and listening for cues.

- Mindfulness-Based Stress Reduction (MBSR) is the secular meditation technique developed by Dr Jon Kabat-Zinn. It is based on non-judgmental, moment-to-moment awareness, and is well researched and accepted in medical centers in the US and Europe. There are eight-week courses available everywhere that teach this technique. Alternatively you can get instructional CDs or DVDs that provide detailed guided instruction in mindful meditation. Of course the key is to practice, practice, practice.

Self-awareness

Self-awareness is the ability to self-introspect and to be aware and understand internal bodily cues. Self-awareness also implies a level of awareness of your inner emotions and thought processes. It is a critical factor for yoga therapists. In order to be able to "read" our clients and to be of service to them, we first need to be aware of what is in us and what our own trigger points or "buttons" are. We need to be aware if and how the reality we see outside of ourselves is skewed by our own inner world of emotions and beliefs. An ability to become a dispassionate witness to our own inner world comes only with awareness and acceptance of what is in it and prevents us from transference. Only then are we able to see the reality with empathy and to become non-judgmental and compassionate to others' suffering.

In our retreat many people come with little awareness of their negative feelings—the most common being anger, guilt, or depression. In the process of a cancer journey some people have trained themselves to numb their emotions and now have difficulties being aware of their feelings. The POMS test (see Chapter 11), which we do at the beginning of the retreat, measures tension, depression, and anger, among others. When we discuss the baseline results of these tests at the beginning of the retreat, many people have a hard time accepting how angry, depressed, or tense they are. Unless they become aware of their own internal state, they have no ability to change it! These people would qualify close to "self-opaque" on the scale.

However, a high score in self-awareness may also come with a cost. Those who have sensitive emotional antennas for their own feelings will feel another person's pain and suffering vividly, with consequences for their own body chemistry. They are likely to have a surge of stress hormone (cortisol) or elevated heart rate or blood pressure. Such extreme sensitivity is likely a factor in burnout of nurses, therapists, and social workers. It is therefore extremely important for yoga therapists to be self-aware, to maintain their own *sadhana*, and take the time for self-care.

Self-awareness can be assessed by answering the following questions, true or false:

1. Often, when someone asks me why I am so angry or sad, I respond (or think to myself) "But I am not!"

2. When those closest to me ask me why I treated someone brusquely or meanly, I often disagree that I did such a thing.

3. I frequently—more than a couple of times a month—find that my heart is racing or my pulse is pounding, and I have no idea why.

4. When I observe someone in pain, I feel the pain myself, both emotionally and physically.

5. I am usually sure enough how I am feeling that I can put my emotions into words.

6. I sometimes notice aches and pains and have no idea where they come from.

7. I like to spend time being quiet and relaxed, just feeling what is going on inside me.

8. I feel I very much inhabit my body and feel at home and comfortable with my body.

9. I am strongly oriented to the external world and rarely take note of what is happening in my body.

10. When I exercise, I am very sensitive to changes it produces in my body.

1 ___ 2 ___ 3 ___ 4 ___ 5 ___ 6 ___ 7 ___ 8 ___ 9 ___10

SELF-OPAQUE   SELF-AWARE

SCORING

Give yourself one point for "True" in questions 4, 5, 7, 8, and 10, and one point for "False" in questions 1, 2, 3, 6, and 9. A total score above 8 means you are highly self-aware; a score below 3 means a low level of self-awareness.

WAYS TO BALANCE SELF-AWARENESS

The way to move toward being more balanced is to practice:

- MBSR

- Breath awareness

- Body scan.

These practices have a regulating effect on the mind. If you lack self-awareness, it can help to make internal sensations more prominent and vivid. If you are hyper-aware—feeling and hearing your internal signals all too vividly—it can help to bring about internal equanimity so you are not bothered by internal noise; with time and practice the noise eventually dies down.

As with every emotional style, enduring change will come about through mental practice that shifts patterns in neural activity. But you can also rearrange the external environment to discourage or encourage self-awareness. To boost self-awareness, decrease the distractions and choose a quiet environment. To decrease self-awareness, do the opposite and focus on external stimuli.

Practice twice a day for four weeks, after which you may start noticing changes.

Sensitivity to context

Sensitivity to context expresses our ability to be attuned to our social environment. It means that we are able to choose to behave "the right way at the right place and time" according to roles, rules, and expectations. It is about our ability to understand the rules of social engagement. This is largely based on intuition and goes together with social intuition and self-awareness. Sensitivity to context allows for a greater ability to adapt to the environment. Failing to do so can lead to responses that are appropriate in one setting but not in another. It is like playing a card game in which we play by a different set of rules than everyone else, yet we do not know it.

People who are very tuned in to context tend to have strong connections from the hippocampus to areas in the prefrontal cortex that control executive function and hold long-term memories, writes Davidson. People who are tuned out tend to have a weaker connection. If you are too tuned in, you might be paying a personal cost of complying with expectations instead of meeting your own needs. If you are too tuned out, it may cause unconsciously offensive behavior.

Sensitivity to context can be assessed by answering the following questions, true or false:

1. I have been told by someone close to me that I am unusually sensitive to other people's feelings.

2. I have occasionally been told that my behavior is socially inappropriate, which surprised me.

3. I have sometimes suffered a setback at work or had a falling out with a friend because I was too chummy with a superior or too jovial when a good friend was distraught.

4. When I speak with people they sometimes move back to increase the distance between us.

5. I often find myself censoring what I was about to say because I sensed something in the situation that would make it inappropriate (e.g. "Honey, do these jeans make me look fat?").

6. When I am in a public setting like a restaurant, I am especially aware of modulating how loudly I speak.

7. I have frequently been reminded when in public to avoid mentioning the names of people who might be around.

8. I am almost always aware of whether I have been someplace before, even if it is a highway that I last drove on many years ago.

9. I notice when someone is acting in a way that seems out of place, such as behaving too casually at work.

10. I've been told by those close to me that I show good manners with strangers and in new situations.

1 ___ 2 ___ 3 ___ 4 ___ 5 ___ 6 ___ 7 ___ 8 ___ 9 ___ 10

TUNED OUT   TUNED IN

SCORING

Give yourself one point for "True" in questions 1, 5, 6, 8, 9, and 10, and one point for "False" in questions 2, 3, 4, and 7. A total score above 8 means you are highly tuned in; a score below 3 means you are highly tuned out.

WAYS TO INCREASE SENSITIVITY TO CONTEXT

To increase sensitivity to context, a practice of slow, deep breathing with the ratio of 1:1 exhale to inhale is helpful.

Another exercise Richardson recommends is as follows:

- In a safe setting bring to mind a situation that causes anxiety or discomfort. Spend some time making it as vivid in your mind as possible. Become aware of where the emotions of discomfort manifest in your body. After a few minutes start slow, deep breathing. Continue until the anxiety or discomfort lessens considerably.

All these exercises work through the mind to change the brain. Whether inspired by millennia-old contemplative traditions or 21st-century psychiatric techniques, they have the power to alter the neural systems that underlie every style. This gives us hope and the tools to become better yoga teachers or yoga therapists. As we do our own practice, hopefully under the guidance of a teacher, we are transforming ourselves. We are working out our own "stuff" and we are integrating the teaching into our life. We become yogis, living yoga on the mat, but more importantly, off the mat as well. Although the path of growth seems never-ending, such quiet yogis can be recognized by their demeanor—even, less reactive, they may be spontaneous but still radiate an inner peace. They seem to be somewhat quietly standing out from the crowd.

A great yoga therapist will teach from their true nature, from the place of unity and harmony, not from the ego. They will always be in service and have the client's interests in their heart. Their way of being will make the client feel welcome and will inspire them to want to practice yoga.

PART 2

CHRONIC DISEASE AND THE ROLE OF YOGA

In Part 1 we attempted to present the essence of yoga therapy, its tools and modalities, and finally, what lies at the core of yoga therapists' skills. In this part of the book we will present the general opportunities that yoga therapy brings to the field of healthcare.

As Sat Bir Khalsa pointed out at the Symposium on Yoga Therapy and Research (SYTAR) in 2017, NCDs are at an epidemic scale, and are the result of lifestyle and dysfunctional behaviors, including stress, diet, and sedentary habits, among others: "Our health care system, and the world as a whole, have made little investment in the area of NCD prevention…and treatment strategies have fallen short in trying to control NCDs. *And this is an area where yoga can be extremely helpful.*"[1] Matthew Taylor echoes this statement, saying, "*Yoga can effectively change these behaviors by providing tools to deal with stress, to increase client awareness and changes in life purpose and meaning. Yoga can alter spiritual perspective and it documents transcendence that practices bring.*"[2] This is the opportunity and the promise that yoga therapy brings to the world.

As the prevalence of NCDs is accelerating globally, advancing across each and every region of the world and pervading all socioeconomic classes, it is imperative that we, as yoga therapists, work with our clients to reduce their modifiable risk factors while promoting a healthy lifestyle.

This is even more necessary when we realize that the mortality, morbidity, and disability attributed to the major chronic diseases currently accounts for almost 60 percent of all deaths and 43 percent of the global burden of disease. The WHO estimates that by 2020 NCDs are expected to contribute to 73 percent of all deaths and 60 percent of the global burden of disease.[3] Data from 2016 is shown in the figure below.

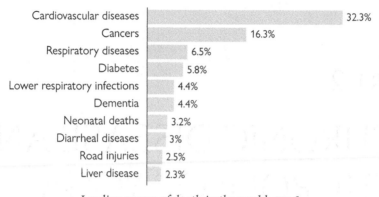

Leading causes of death in the world, 2016

Source: Institute for Health Metrics and Evaluation (IHME),
Global Burden of Disease (GBD), Our World in Data[4]

In this part of the book we will discuss in more detail the top four NCDs that are most relevant in today's world: chronic respiratory diseases, cardiovascular diseases, diabetes mellitus, and cancer. All are linked by many common and some preventable biological risk factors, notably high blood pressure, high blood cholesterol, and being overweight.

In each chapter we explain the disease in general terms, the risks, and aggravating factors. By now you will also understand that although the disease may be the same, each case and each client is different, and so don't be disappointed by the lack of recommended prescriptive methods. Instead, our aim is to help you to understand the client and what to watch for. We also discuss the role of yoga therapy in each disease.

NCDs and the role of yoga

As yoga therapists we often encounter clients suffering from various chronic diseases that today are the leading causes of death and disability worldwide. Many decades ago, infectious diseases were a threat to humankind, but with improved hygiene and the development of effective antibiotics, that challenge was managed for some time. In the last few decades, however, we have seen the emergence of NCDs caused by an unhealthy lifestyle and stress.

Poor lifestyle choices, such as smoking, over-use of alcohol, an unhealthy diet, lack of physical activity, and inadequate relief of chronic stress are key contributors in the development and progression of all chronic diseases, including obesity, type 2 diabetes mellitus, hypertension, cardiovascular disease, and several types of cancer. The issue is that even though many doctors encourage healthy behavior, clients are often either unwilling or inadequately prepared to transition to these appropriate, healthy lifestyle changes. There is a "gap" between the head and the hands as most clients understand the reasoning behind a healthy lifestyle but lack the behavioral skills and willpower to implement such transformative changes in their everyday life.

One of the positive aspects of the many research studies in this field is that we now have adequate empirical medical evidence to show that those who participate in comprehensive lifestyle modification programs experience rapid, significant, clinically meaningful, and sustainable improvements in biometric, laboratory, and psychosocial outcomes. This should be used to convince clients and create an appetite for healthy lifestyle changes. This is where a yoga therapist becomes a mentor and a guide as well as a friend on the client's path towards health, happiness, and wellbeing.

Important psychosocial aspects of chronic diseases

A chronic disease is normally understood to be a condition generally lasting for more than three months and often for the whole of a lifetime. It is often also considered to be one that cannot usually be prevented by vaccines or cured by medication. People with these diseases have a general misconception that they are free from the disease when there are no symptoms. It can never be stressed enough that a healthy diet, regular exercise, avoidance of negative habits, cultivating positive habits, and a healthy lifestyle can help us to prevent or postpone the onset of chronic diseases.

"DADA" is the acronym that explains the psychological turmoil that an individual and their family go through when diagnosed with a chronic ailment: denial, anger, depression, and acceptance. The technical terms and reports frighten them; fear and anxiety make them lose their innate sense of ease (*sukhasthanam*); and they end up in a state of dis-ease (*duhkha*).

- *Denial:* The person denies the condition—"It cannot be true, especially not for me." They check and double-check the reports and take umpteen opinions with many consultants. They start doing their own research, learning more about the disease. They end up overwhelmed by vast and sometimes conflicting information...

- *Anger:* When diagnosis is confirmed they get angry with everyone and even God has no escape from their wrath—"Why me?" "Why only me?"

- *Depression:* When the psychic clutter settles down, they subsequently begin to understand that there is no escape and sink into a state of depression followed by withdrawal from society and friends.

- *Acceptance:* When they finally decide to accept the problem and face it with courage, healing happens. (Acceptance is not in the form of passive resignation, but in the form of undertaking a dynamic resolute decision to progress and make the best efforts towards health.)

Stress and the role of yoga

The integrated approach of yoga in the prevention and management of chronic disorders works on cultivating appropriate and healthy attitudes towards every aspect of life. This is vital to reduce the stress that is more often an inner over-reaction than a response to any external stimuli. The adoption of a healthy, heart-friendly diet with adequate hydration and practicing the old adage, "Eat when hungry and only after the previous meal has been digested" is useful and very meaningful. All of the practices that work on breath–body movement coordination are to be advocated as they enhance mind–body harmony. Of course, modified versions of the various postures as per physical condition and other associated health problems of the individual should be used with a focus on simple "head-below-heart" postures that restore so many homeostatic reflex mechanisms. Self-healing may be encouraged by *pranayama*, and relaxation and simple hand gestures (*mudras*) can always be used, even by clients who are terminally ill. The head-rotating, breath-based practice of *brahma mudra* integrates slow, deep breathing with body movements, and adds on the vibration (*nada*) that reinvigorates the neck region through which both sensory and motor neuron pathways travel to and from the brain to the rest of the body.

Yoga is a boon to healthcare when we realize that it can play a role in all aspects of prevention, including primary, secondary, and tertiary prevention. It is also beneficial in health promotion, and may give the individual a sense of purpose (called *Ikigai in Japanese*[5] and *swadharma* in Indian[6]), helping them attain a sense of coherence that is essential for salutogenic wellbeing.[7]

This is why, we, as yoga therapists, must involve ourselves completely in helping our clients prevent and manage these major chronic diseases by showing them the way to reduce their stress levels, change their lifestyles, and thus control the key risk factors. As yoga works on the body, mind, and spirit, we truly have an unparalleled tool to help people at this crucial juncture of human history.

The modern human faces stress everywhere, caught in its claws in a vicious spiral, not knowing how to extradite themselves. For so many of us life has become a "rat race" and our body, emotions, and mind are all jangled by the physiological and psychological responses to the omnipresent stress at every stage of our existence.

As yoga therapists we need to help our clients understand that stress cannot be wished away and needs to be approached in a yogic manner if they are to deal with it effectively. If not, frequent stressful experiences lead to failure of the intrinsic homeostatic, self-regulating mechanisms, leading to disease, premature aging, and early or sudden death.

Hans Selye, the pioneering Hungarian-Canadian endocrinologist, postulated a model of stress and called this the "general adaptation syndrome" (GAS). It consists of three phases: the immediately reacting alarm reaction, the longer continual stage of resistance, that in turn finally leads to exhaustion after all resources are depleted:

- *Alarm reaction:* This is the immediate effect of stress where the individual responds to the perceived or real stress with the classic "fight or flight" response. Stress hormones such as adrenaline, noradrenaline, cortisol, glucagon, and aldosterone are secreted, and various physiological changes occur in the body to prepare us to respond to the stress. If the stress has been dealt with in an effective manner, everything returns to normal; if not, things go on to the next stage.

- *Resistance:* In this stage the body seems to return to normal but if the stress persists, the resources of the body keep getting depleted. Externally the problem is not visible and we end up thinking that all is well with our system. This is the stage where allostatic load starts to build up. The body keeps trying to help us "appear" normal but it is slowly and steadily using up resources from within.

- *Exhaustion:* Chronic stress places a constant load on the neuroendocrine adaptive mechanisms leading to distortion in the homeostatic mechanism, thus weakening the response of the organism to environmental challenges which, in turn, leads to ill health and disease. It is at this point that the system burns up, and fatigue and exhaustion manifest. All of the diseases associated with stress begin to manifest in this phase. We, as yoga therapists, need to be aware of this, as it is at this point that the proverbial "straw that broke the camel's back" happens, and the client may often only focus on the immediate cause and not give us details of the whole picture. We need to go deep into their history to find out the source of this chronic stress, as trying to repair just the "straw" part will not help much.

Chronic stress weakens our immune system and allows the innocuous agents to cause us trouble. Chronic inflammation and oxidative stress are part of the pathophysiology of virtually every chronic disease and need to be addressed through yoga. Much scientific research in recent times has shown that the physiological, psychological, and biochemical effects of yoga are of an anti-stress nature, and a large number of studies have described the beneficial effects of yoga, even endorsed by an Agency for Healthcare Research and Quality (AHRQ) report stating that "Yoga helped reduce stress."[8] This stated that reductions in perceived stress following yoga are as effective as therapies such as relaxation, cognitive behavioral therapy, and dance therapy.

Mechanisms postulated for these benefits include the restoration of autonomic balance as well as an improvement in the restorative, regenerative, and rehabilitative capacities of the individual. A healthy inner sense of wellbeing produced by a life of yoga percolates down through the different levels of our existence, from the higher to the lower, producing health and wellbeing of a holistic nature.

In this regard, the work of Chris Streeter and colleagues at the Boston University School of Medicine is pioneering, as in 2012 they proposed a theory to explain the benefits of yoga practice in diverse, frequently co-morbid, medical conditions.[9] This was based on the concept that such practices reduce allostatic load in stress response systems such that optimal homeostasis is restored.

They hypothesized that stress induces an:

- Imbalance of the autonomic nervous system with decreased parasympathetic and increased sympathetic activity

- Under-activity of the gamma-aminobutyric acid (GABA) system, the primary inhibitory neurotransmitter system, and

- Increased allostatic load.

They further hypothesized that yoga-based practices correct under-activity of the parasympathetic nervous system and GABA systems in part through stimulation of the vagus nerve, the main peripheral pathway of the parasympathetic nervous system, and in the overall picture, reduce allostatic load. For us as yoga therapists this is heartening, as we can have confidence in our efforts to support our clients in their struggle to effectively cope with stress. When an inefficient parasympathetic nervous system and GABA activity are corrected through yoga, amelioration of disease symptoms manifests, providing a holistic sense of enhanced wellbeing.

The WHO defines health as "The state of complete physical, mental and social wellbeing and not merely absence of disease or infirmity." The yogic way of living is a vital tool that helps attain that "state" of health. We must not forget that it is more important to have both a sense of "being" healthy as well as "feeling" healthy. Hence, the qualitative aspect of health, the spiritual nature of human life, is rightly considered more important in yoga and other Eastern systems of traditional medicine. The yogic principles useful in such disorders include psychological reconditioning and development of appropriate attitudes; stress management; normalization of metabolism; and relaxation, visualization, and contemplative practices.

We, as yoga therapists, must also never forget that yoga enhances our spiritual life and perspective beyond the physical body regardless of our particular religious, racial, social, cultural, or regional identity. When we use this approach we can enable our clients to attain and maintain a balance between exertion and relaxation, thus inducing a healthy and dynamic state of homeostatic equilibrium.

Dr W. Selvamurthy has given a beautiful summary of how yoga acts against stress: "We can think of it as a 3-in-1 action! Yoga enables and empowers individuals to modify their perceptions of the stressors, optimize their responses to them, and efficiently release the pent up stresses."[10]

CHAPTER 6

Chronic Respiratory Diseases

Swami Gitananda often described dyspnea (difficult or labored breathing) as an ancient condition as old as the medical history of humankind itself. Indeed, the problems of breathing begin as early as the "first breath of life" for many a human. Dyspnea not only robs the individual of their health, wealth, and happiness, but is also often a major challenge to doctors, medical researchers, and all health workers.[1]

As yoga therapists we often deal with clients suffering chronic respiratory diseases, and these are usually in the form of chronic obstructive pulmonary disease (COPD), asthma, occupational lung diseases, and pulmonary hypertension. According to the WHO, hundreds of millions of people suffer from chronic respiratory diseases, with 235 million having asthma, 64 million COPD, and millions allergic rhinitis and other often under-diagnosed conditions.[2]

Understanding the client and their presentation

In all of these conditions the major symptom is usually a shortness of breath resulting from obstruction to bronchial airflow. Excessive mucus secretion is a predominant symptom in those with asthma and bronchitis. In bronchial asthma, narrowing of the bronchial airway is common, but the major symptom is the severity and wide variation of the obstruction and the sudden onset of the attack. There is often spontaneous release of the obstruction when medication or yoga therapy is administered. Such a hypothesis is supported by Virendra Singh,[3] who postulated a non-specific broncho-protective or broncho-relaxing effect through yoga, while a study by M.K. Tandon[4] reported that subjects with chronic severe airway obstruction were able to exercise better after yoga, thus showing that a possible release of such an obstruction could be offered by yoga practices.

In emphysema, the air spaces beyond the terminal bronchiole become over-distended and the alveolar walls collapse, leading to the classic "pink puffer" appearance. On the other hand, in chronic bronchitis, the mucous membrane lining the inside of the bronchial tubes becomes inflamed and swollen, secreting excess, thick mucous into the lumen, thereby obstructing the airway passage. The classic description of the "blue bloater" is seen due to the cyanosis and peripheral edema that accompanies this condition. Both emphysema and chronic bronchitis are now classified under the term COPD. The most common symptoms of COPD are breathlessness or a "need for air," excessive sputum production, and a chronic cough. However, COPD is not just simply a "smoker's cough," but a major contributor to both morbidity and mortality, with the WHO predicting that it will become the third leading cause of death worldwide by 2030.

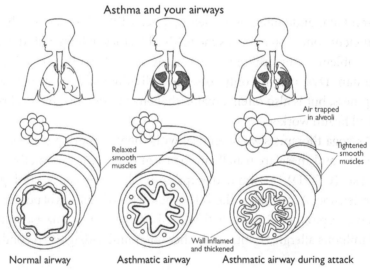

Asthma—a chronic disease in which your airway walls become sore and swollen, narrowing so that your lungs get less air

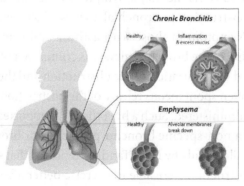

Chronic obstructive pulmonary disease (COPD)

In the case of bronchial asthma, the client usually reports a long-standing history of recurrent attacks of breathlessness and wheezing. This is usually set off by an allergy, and then due to its severity and frequency starts to take a great toll on the emotional and mental health of the individual. In the course of dyspnea or the common attack of labored breath, the bronchioles become so narrowed that the air can get into the lungs through active inspiration. Since the expiration is usually passive, the air is not expelled properly, resulting in the lungs being inflated beyond normal. As there is little space left in the already inflated lungs for more fresh air to get in, the client feels a sense of "being breathless." This is paradoxical as there is hyperinflation, but not enough air getting where it should. The statement "Water, water everywhere, nary a drop to drink" comes to mind in such cases.

In all cases the usual tendency of bronchiolar narrowing is increased by muscle spasms of the bronchiolar wall producing the common "bronchospasm," with accompanied swelling of the inner lining of the airways due to inflammation. This mucosal edema secretes thick mucus phlegm into the passages, complicating an already distressing condition.

As yoga therapists, we should guide our client and help them deal with this situation by using an explosive bellows-like breath through the mouth (*mukha bhastrika*), emptying the lungs as completely as possible.[5] This helps relieve the hyperinflation, and creates "space" for air to come in again. Of course this practice needs to be learned during a relatively "normal" time, and then used in times of need. Trying to teach it to someone in the middle of an attack is not advisable.

Understanding the aggravating factors

The main risk factors implicated in chronic respiratory conditions are tobacco smoking and air pollution along with occupational chemicals and dusts, as well as frequent lower respiratory infections during childhood.

Clients often express the aggravating role of air pollution from factories, heavy industries, or automobiles. We may help them to decide on moving to less polluted areas if possible, for any long-standing benefits. It does often seem counterproductive to teach anyone *pranayama* when they are living in a polluted environment, as we may be doing more harm than good.

Destructive personal habits (*viparita buddhi*), such as smoking cigarettes, chewing tobacco, inhaling snuff, and the use of certain street drugs, destroy the ciliary lining as well as dampen the body's response and immunity to infectious agents. We, as therapists, should gently bring to the client's attention the negative impacts of such habits, and then help them develop the inner strength to go beyond any cravings that are part of the vicious habitual cycles. Always be careful while teaching *pranayama* to those who are still active smokers—untouched areas of the lung tissue then become exposed to the noxious fumes.

Understanding the role of yoga therapy

The yoga life offers a holistic path to manage all of these conditions through its practical and philosophical aspects that deal with human existence at all levels. All aspects of yoga are useful, but *pranayama*, the yogic science of conscious expansion of *prana*, the life force, is the most valuable technique used to correct faulty breathing and chronic diseases associated with the nose, throat, and lungs. Even a moderate attempt at these breath controls will pay giant dividends to the sufferer. The client can quickly correct the faulty breathing habits that are the root cause of the disease, and then, by adhering to a proper diet and living a yogic life, may be freed from this malady to a great extent. The use of *pranayama* can enable the client to regain the normal physiological chest movement associated with good breathing, or to attain that condition if it has never been present. The essential principle of therapeutic *pranayama* is that the subject must learn to control the entire breathing mechanism in an aware manner. In the beginning this may be difficult for most people, but with time and with disciplined control, the client can learn to manage their breath while doing physical exercise, climbing stairs, and in other types of physical exertion. They can also lead to a control of the psychological and emotional factors that produce the rest and relaxation necessary to alleviate tensions that otherwise often cause an attack of breathlessness.

We need to detail the dietary aspects, as acid-forming and mucous-producing foods create phlegm and acid discharges that clog up airways. The inclusion of citrus fruits is wise, but these should be used as juices and with plenty of water to thin them down for quick and easy assimilation into the system. Oranges, lemons, pineapples, limes, and grapefruit are rich sources of vitamin C. Green leafy vegetables are a rich source of vitamin A, and help protect the respiratory mucous lining. Herbal teas may be included as they break up chronic mucous conditions. Teas made from an infusion of mint, barley, fenugreek, and other alkaline materials are useful, and herbal teas of tulsi are excellent for all respiratory complaints. Honey and natural jaggery may be used as natural sweeteners if required.

We also need to look into the client's emotional and psychological condition as an overly sensitive nature or a nature that is easily embarrassed will often be part of the causation. We must never forget that our emotions and breath are closely interrelated as the relationship of emotional volatility and asthma is well understood in psychosomatics. It is believed that asthma is connected strongly to the emotion of anger. Emotionality leads to the condition, which evokes an emotional response that further worsens the condition in a vicious cycle. Many breathing difficulties are just the surface manifestation of underlying emotional "hang ups." Unless the emotions are dealt with in a conscious manner, a long-lasting solution will not manifest.

Apart from diet and dietary restrictions, think in terms of doing regular *pranayama*, particularly out in the open air and sunshine in the early mornings and late afternoons. Short sunbaths are often of great help, but care should be taken not to get sunburnt. Sea baths aid in loosening congested mucous and a sunbath following a sea bath can have numerous added health benefits as well.

An evening or morning stroll while doing slow, deep breathing should be a daily routine for anyone with chronic breathing disorders. Sedentary city dwellers will find this an excellent daily constitutional, and although it may not permanently cure a condition by itself, the condition is, at times, greatly mitigated. The *sukha pranayama* (1:1 ratio for inhalation and exhalation), *savitri pranayama* (2:1:2:1 ratio for inhalation, held in, exhalation, and held out) or traditional (1:2 ratio for inhalation and exhalation) rhythm of breathing may be adopted while walking to deeply exercise the heart and lungs in a healthy manner.[6]

In recent times the scientific basis of using yoga as an adjunct therapy in chronic respiratory diseases is well established, with significant improvements in lung function, quality of life results, and bronchial provocation responses coupled with a decreased need for regular and rescue medicinal usage.[7] Dr R.L. Bijlani and his team gave evidence through a randomized controlled trial of the efficacy of a comprehensive lifestyle modification program based on yoga in the management of bronchial asthma.[8]

In India, cleansing practices are often advocated in managing respiratory disorders, and the team led by Dr Satyaprabha[9] showed that yogic cleaning techniques such as *dhauti kriya* (upper gastrointestinal cleansing with warm saline or a muslin cloth) and *neti kriya* (a warm boiled or distilled water with salt as nasal wash) remove excessive mucous secretions, decrease inflammation, reduce bronchial hypersensitivity, and increase the provocation threshold. They also reported that the dynamic forceful exhalations during *kapalbhati* improve the capacity to exhale against resistance.

Although we often think we need to do more complicated practices to get benefits, the works of Dr Luciano Bernardi and colleagues in Italy[10] have shown the immense benefits of simple deep breathing, six breaths per minute. They reported that slow and deep yogic breathing maintains better blood oxygenation without increasing minute ventilation, reduces sympathetic activation during altitude-induced hypoxia, and decreases chemoreflex sensitivity to hypoxia and hypercapnia. This enables clients who practice such techniques to have a better sense of "ease" that is so important for their "sense of wellbeing." This, in turn, influences the body and psychosomatic and somatopsychic mechanisms of health.

All of these findings help us to understand better how yoga brings about both objective and subjective improvements in the condition of clients, and this gives us the clarity and confidence to deal with them in an effective and competent manner. When discussing this with medical professionals we can also advocate the fact that yoga as a therapy is cost-effective, relatively simple, and carries minimal risk, and hence should be included as an adjunct, complementary therapy in an integrated system of medicine. The WHO is currently promoting such a system capable of producing health and wellbeing for all in the form of TCI (traditional, complementary, and integrative) medicine.

CHAPTER 7

Cardiovascular Diseases

In 2016 cardiovascular disease (CVD) was listed as the leading cause of death worldwide.[1] When we consider CVD, we are looking at a conglomeration of over 60 disorders affecting the heart and the vasculature. Millions all over the world (more than 25% in the US) have some form of CVD, with high blood pressure, heart disease, and stroke being the most common clinical presentations. In the developed world it accounts for nearly 40 percent of deaths each year. Yoga therapists are often asked to deal with clients with such issues, as more and more people are realizing the importance of a healthy lifestyle to prevent and manage CVD.

If we consider that CVD is basically a lifestyle disorder, the news for yoga is good, for the holistic science of yoga is the best lifestyle ever designed, with its preventive, possibly curative, as well as rehabilitative potential. This holistic action of yoga can be explained by ability to modulate autonomic functions and relieve stress by decreasing sympathetic (fight or flight) activity while concurrently enhancing vagal parasympathetic (rest and recuperate) activity. It has also been shown to improve all-round physiological functions, especially cardiorespiratory fitness, and developing a positive attitude helps improve quality of life. As is often said, "Yoga not only adds years to your life, but adds life to those years too."

Manifestations of CVD

Coronary artery disease (CAD) is a condition in which the arteries supplying the heart muscles harden with narrowing (atherosclerosis), thus reducing oxygen supply to the heart muscle. This may manifest as angina (temporary chest pain or discomfort) or a heart attack when a blood clot suddenly cuts off most or all of the blood supply to part of the heart. Heart muscle cells that do not receive enough oxygen-carrying blood die, leading to permanent damage. This, over time, can weaken the heart muscle and contribute to heart failure because the heart is not able to pump blood to the rest of the body effectively. Other issues such as arrhythmias or abnormalities in the normal heart rhythm may be very serious and life-threatening.

Although heart disease used to be known as a man's problem, it is now the number one killer of women in the US! Women are more likely to develop heart disease after menopause, as the production of estrogen drops. And women who have gone through an early menopause, either naturally or because of gynecological surgery, are twice as likely to develop heart disease as women of the same age who have not yet gone through menopause.

The symptoms narrated by clients usually include a combination such as chest or arm pain or discomfort (angina), shortness of breath, giddiness, a sense of the heart pounding in the chest, and extreme tiredness. There is also a "silent heart attack"—with no pain associated at the time.

Hypertension does not cause problems over days, weeks, or even months; rather, it causes problems over many years, and can affect the entire body. By adding strain to the blood vessel walls, hypertension makes them more likely to develop atherosclerosis, with a buildup of fat and cholesterol and the "hardening" of the arteries. This, in turn, puts extra strain on the heart as it pumps blood through the narrowed arteries. Over time, the strain this condition places on the heart and blood vessels can increase the risk of certain health problems, such as heart disease, stroke, heart attack, kidney, and eye damage. Most people do not have any hypertension symptoms. When they are noticeable, signs and symptoms may include blurred vision, dizziness, headache, or nausea. As it usually takes several years for problems from hypertension to become noticeable, by the time they manifest, serious damage may already have been done to body structures, such as the blood vessels, heart, eyes, brain, or kidneys.

Risk factors and CVD

As yoga therapists we need to focus on the factors that increase an individual's risk for such diseases. These are divided into non-modifiable risk factors that include age, family history of cardiovascular disease, ethnicity, and gender, and modifiable risk factors including deranged lipid levels, abnormal blood pressure, diabetes, atrial fibrillation, obesity, lack of physical activity, irregular circadian rhythm, and cigarette smoking. With this in mind it is essential that the management of CVD involves lifestyle changes including diet, exercise, attitude, and relaxation.

A large-scale study at the Harvard T.H. Chan School of Public Health in 2018 explored the effects of healthy habits on health and lifespan in a sample of women and men in the US.[2] Data from more than 78,000 women and 44,000 men who participated in two nationwide surveys—the Nurses' Health Study (NHS) and the Health Professionals Follow-up Study (HPFS)—was used along with data from the Centers for Disease Control and Prevention to estimate the distribution of lifestyle choices and death rates across the US population. They concluded that those who maintained five healthy lifestyle factors lived more than a decade longer than those who didn't maintain any of the five. These included maintaining a healthy eating pattern (getting the daily recommended amount of vegetables, fruit, nuts, whole grains, polyunsaturated fatty acids, and omega-3 fatty acids, further limiting red and processed meats, beverages with added sugar, trans fat, and sodium); not smoking; doing at least 3.5 hours of moderate to vigorous physical activity each week; drinking only moderate amounts of alcohol (one drink or less per day for women or two drinks or less per day for men); and maintaining a normal weight (BMI between 18.5 and 24.9).

Dr Kim E. Innes and her team conducted a series of comprehensive reviews[3] which suggested that yoga reduces a cardiovascular risk profile by decreasing activation of the sympathoadrenal system and hypothalamic-pituitary-adrenal (HPA) axis, and also by promoting a feeling of wellbeing along with direct enhancement of parasympathetic activity. They also suggested that yoga provides a positive source of social support that may also be one of the factors reducing risk for CVD.

The pioneering work of Dr Dean Ornish in the US is phenomenal with regard to reversing heart disease, as it was, in the 1990s, said to be irreversible.[4] Dr Ornish's four decades of research since have scientifically proven that the integrative lifestyle changes he recommends can: improve chronic conditions—such as heart disease, diabetes, and prostate cancer; change gene expression, turning on health-promoting genes and turning off disease-promoting genes; and lengthen telomeres—the ends of chromosomes—which begins to reverse aging on a cellular level.[5] The Ornish Lifestyle Medicine program claims to be the first that is scientifically proven to "undo" (reverse) heart disease by optimizing four important areas of life: what you eat, how you manage stress, how much you move, and how much love and support you have: "When you make comprehensive lifestyle choices, most people find that they feel much better, so quickly that it re-frames the reason for changing from fear of dying to joy of living." This work is summed up in his bestselling book, *UnDo It!*[6]

Understanding the role of yoga therapy ————————————

The yogic lifestyle is anti-atherogenic, and many researchers have proved that yoga practice increases HDL (good cholesterol) that is anti-atherogenic while decreasing LDL and VLDL (unhealthy or bad cholesterol). A comprehensive review by Dr Innes and colleagues reported that all 12 studies reviewed by them suggested that yoga improved lipid profile.[7]

Yoga is a vaccine against stress that is yet to manifest and the best antidote for stress, and along with a low fat–high fiber diet, provides proper exercise, thus improving circulation to all body parts. This, coupled with proper breathing and relaxation, induces the vagal, parasympathetic tone that is healing. Lifestyle modifications and a conscious cultivation of yogic attitudes towards life also aid in healing.

Yoga completely re-modulates our perception of stress itself. As Dr Bhavanani often says, "Nothing can stress you unless you let it do so!" By changing our perception and response to stressful stimuli, we subsequently reduce the negative manifestations of such stress in our whole system. When we don't perceive something as being stressful, we can short-circuit the whole stress response.

Normally stress manifests in us through the sympathoadrenal system that secretes adrenaline into the blood as well as the HPA axis that secretes cortisol, the stress hormone. At the same time, the vagal stimulation induces a healthier increase in heart rate variability (HRV), a sign that the heart and lungs are functioning together in a state of health. The aortic and carotid baroreceptor and their reflexes that modulate blood pressure are also brought into more harmony, in turn reducing heart rate and blood pressure. As a result of the balance between both of these limbs of the autonomic nervous system, many benefits are seen throughout the body. Inflammatory cytokines are reduced, insulin sensitivity increases, lipid profile is improved, and there is less fat accumulation in the body organs. All of this reduces the oxidative stress that is implicated in all chronic diseases and enhances the functioning of the inner endothelial layers of blood vessels, thus promoting a healthy circulation and reducing chances of atherosclerosis, stubborn blood clots, and their dangerous emboli. This cascade of positive changes reduces the risk for blockages in the blood vessels, premature blood clotting, hypertension, and CVD in the long run.

Yoga prescribes a *sattvic* diet with cereals, pulses, fruits, and raw vegetables to facilitate enhancement of *prana* through biogenic means. We advise regular and timely healthy meals that contain adequate amounts of green vegetables, salads, fresh fruit juices, and sprouts. We also advocate a fat-free or low-fat diet with minimal sugar and the lowest possible level of salt. Fruits are a good source of fiber and have potassium that help control blood pressure better. They are also excellent laxatives, and may help clear constipation. Maintaining an adequate level of hydration (a minimum of 2 liters of water per day) is necessary, as every cell needs to be hydrated if it is to function in a healthy manner. All of these changes will produce a healthy weight loss, which, in turn, reduces risk factors such as hypertension, breaks down insulin resistance, and reduces chronic inflammation.

Clients with heart disease are often found to have strong negative emotions and exaggerated stress responses. It is vital that we, as therapists, help them to develop yogic attitudes towards life. Adoption of the four-fold noble attitudes to places, people, and events (friendliness, compassion, etc.) as well as developing a contrary attitude (*pratipaksha bhavanam*) are often more important than any physical practices. We need to emphasize the cultivation of selfless action (*Karma Yoga*), higher intuition (*Raja Yoga*), and devotion (*Bhakti Yoga*) principles in daily life.

While doing *asanas*, we should focus on gentle practices that bring the head below the heart as these improve baroreflex sensitivity, an important aspect of cardiovascular regulation. Such postures when done in a non-stressful manner also attenuate the sympathetic nervous system and renin-angiotensin activity, thus resulting in better control of blood pressure.[8] Often the ego-based perspective plays a major role in stress and heart diseases, and hence, lowering the head in such practices plays a subtle role in reducing the ego-based stresses that are more often a creation of our mind than actual reality. All traditional cultures had head-below-heart postures embedded in their cultural aspects of worship, as submission to a higher power was always a way to reduce stresses and inner turmoil. When we realize that the Divine is within us and on our side, there is an automatic reduction in our tendency to worry unnecessarily.

The heart center (*anahata chakra*) and the subtle energy (*prana vayu*) of this region play a role in CVD, as emotional turmoil is known to precipitate and aggravate such conditions. When we consciously work on this area with love, compassion, and empathy, we develop a sense of gratitude to the universe. Giving and sharing is one of the best ways to "let go," and as we develop the ability to let go, so many of our perceived problems start to spontaneously fall away from our life. These changes in attitude come about over time with the practice of yoga.

Pranayama plays a vital role in enhancing the energies of this region, and slow, deep breathing (*sukha pranayama*),[9] as well as exclusive left nostril breathing (*chandra nadi pranayama*),[10] can improve blood pressure regulation as they enhance vagal activity and re-set baroreflex reactivity. They are actually very effective, even in a short-term immediate manner, and can be used as an effective antidote in stressful situations. *Pranava pranayama* utilizes deep breathing into all sections of the lungs in a sequential manner, and the audible chanting of "AAA" (*akara nada*), "UUU" (*ukara nada*), and "MMM" (*makara nada*) sounds on the prolonged exhalation has been found useful in both sitting[11] and supine positions.[12] Such simple and easy-to-use techniques can be suggested to our clients as they provide so much benefit with minimal stress and strain.

A middle-aged businessman from Pondicherry with multiple coronary blocks and breathlessness consulted Dr Bhavanani about his condition. He was given the practice of repeated chanting of the five-syllable chant (*panchakshara mantra japa*),[13] and advised to do this during the entire duration of his daily *puja*. After six months he came back overjoyed with his reports that showed the formation of numerous natural collaterals that were now keeping him hale and healthy. He asked for an explanation. "Well, whenever you chanted, you were prolonging the duration of your expiration phase," said Dr Bhavanani. Such a prolongation of the expiration in turn slows the heart rate down by enhancing the physiological phenomenon of sinus arrhythmia.[14] When the heart rate slows, there is more time for the diastole, the relaxatory phase of the cardiac cycle. It is during this relaxatory phase that the heart actually supplies blood to its own musculature. When practiced over many days and months, this enables the heart to start to take care of itself through the self-healing process by forming natural bypasses, the collaterals of circulation. This idea is supported by extensive research being done by Dr Bernardi and his team in Italy, who have highlighted the effects of chanting as well as a slow, deep breathing of six breaths per minute for cardiovascular health.[15, 16]

Cardiac rehabilitation, or cardiac rehab for short, is designed to help patients with heart disease recover faster and return to full and productive lives. They may be suffering from angina or have recently had open-heart surgery, angioplasty, a heart transplant, or a heart attack. The typical cardiac rehab team may include doctors, nurses, exercise specialists, physical therapists, or occupational therapists, dietitians and psychologists, or other behavioral therapists. Yoga can play a role in such programs as the practices improve cardiorespiratory health and musculoskeletal health, as well as general wellbeing. Breath–body movement coordination practices help to reconnect the mind–body complex and bring about a healthy psychosomatic state of being. Stress reduction programs using yoga can help develop a positive attitude and provide fortification against stressors while inculcating a positive attitude. Yoga provides better exercise tolerance and stress tolerability, as seen in numerous studies, and as the yogic lifestyle is anti-atherogenic, the vascular network can be regenerated in a healthy manner.

Relaxation is an essential prerequisite for healing to occur, and we cannot heal when we are stressed. Conscious relaxation facilitates self-healing, and this may well be yoga's greatest contribution to modern healthcare. It is all about inducing the "relaxation response." This, in turn, reduces peripheral resistance, enhances tissue perfusion, and facilitates the body system's harmony and holistic healing.

Swami Gitananda Giri postulated "four-fold relaxation" as a systematic and conscious adoption of attitudes resulting in deep experiential states of relaxation. This includes:

- "Letting go" of our prejudices and preconceived notions.

- "Giving up" our stresses in a positive, relaxing, and evolutionary process.

- "Giving in" and opening up to dictates of the inner mind.

- "Giving over" in an attitude of acceptance of the "Divine Will" in *ishwara pranidhana* and *Bhakti Yoga*.

With this in mind, we suggest that yogic protocols for cardiac health and rehab should always include elements of the following:

- Somatopsychic practices (*jathis*, *kriyas*, *mudras*, and *asanas*) to improve cardiorespiratory health, musculoskeletal health, and general wellbeing.

- Stress reduction programs to develop a positive attitude, with fortification against stressors and learning to "Do your best and leave the rest."

- *Pranayama* to revitalize the whole system and enhance cardiac function, healing, and healthy coronary circulation through the use of conscious and deep breathing in different ratios, with or without sound (*nada*).

- A *sattvic* yogic diet with less fat, more fiber, and adequate hydration. "Eat local, eat seasonal" is sane advice, whenever in doubt.

- Relaxation through practices such as visualization-based relaxation (*yoga nidra*), part-by-part relaxation (*marmanasthanam kriya*), alternate segmental tensing and relaxing (*spanda-nishpanda kriya*), dynamic relaxation (*kaya kriya*), and positive body image.

- Meditation techniques (*pratyahara*, *dharana*, and *dhyana*) as appropriate to induce reflective introspection and reduce sensory over-stimulation and hyper-reactivity.

- Enhancement of the personal worldview through lifestyle modification, inculcation of *Bhakti Yoga* principles, and adoption of *Karma Yoga* principles.

Prevention is always better!

It is often said that an ounce of prevention is worth a pound of cure, and this is very apt in CVD. We, as therapists, can help our clients lower their chances of developing CAD by enabling them to develop an understanding of the risk factors, and making healthy decisions. Important lifestyle changes for preventing CAD or controlling it include: becoming more active, maintaining a healthy weight, eating a well balanced, heart-healthy diet, as well as not smoking.

Often the whole process can be as simple as taking a brisk walk, eating wisely, and maintaining a healthy weight. What is most important is for us to reassure our clients that even making a few small and smart changes will pay rich dividends. We must motivate our clients to take a more active role in their own health and make changes to lead a healthier life. We can always remind them that the reward of a healthy heart and a better chance for a longer, more vigorous life is well worth the effort.

CHAPTER 8

Diabetes Mellitus

As diabetes has risen to pandemic proportions, it has become one of the most common health issues worldwide. According to the WHO,[1] the number of people with diabetes rose from 108 million in 1980 to 422 million in 2014, and the global prevalence of diabetes among adults over 18 years of age rose from 4.7 percent in 1980 to 8.5 percent in 2014. This really hits home when we look around at our own social circles, as all of us know one or more people who are trying to manage their diabetes. It is a chronic disease that opens up a plethora of complications, and hence it is dreaded for good reasons. While it is a major cause of blindness, kidney failure, heart attacks, stroke, and lower limb amputation, the WHO estimates that it was the seventh leading cause of death in 2016. The most frightening part of all of this is that it is a silent assassin, as more often than not it is missed until the individual gets a medical checkup done for some other issue.

The main pathology in diabetes is the inadequacy or insufficiency of insulin, where either the body doesn't make any insulin, doesn't make enough, or doesn't use it properly. In fact, the major issue today is of insulin resistance, where someone has the required levels of insulin in their bodies, but their cells are resistant to it, and so they cannot use it properly. Unless insulin attaches to its receptors on the cells, glucose, the essential fuel for cellular function, cannot get in and be processed. This is because insulin helps to "unlock" the cellular "door" that enables glucose to enter and fuel the cellular activity. In diabetes, lack of insulin or the resistance of the cells to insulin prevents the right amount of glucose from entering the cells. The unused glucose builds up in the blood, resulting in hyperglycemia, which is excess glucose in the blood.

Factors that lead to and aggravate the condition include heredity, obesity, mental and emotional stress and strain, prolonged anxiety and conflict, a sedentary lifestyle, lack of physical activity and exercise, as well as unhealthy eating habits.

There are primarily two types of diabetes:

- Type 1 diabetes, or insulin-dependent diabetes mellitus (IDDM), generally appears early in life (juvenile), and is an autoimmune disease where the individual's immune system turns on itself and destroys pancreatic beta cells that produce insulin. As there is no production of insulin by the pancreas, the individual requires lifelong supplementation of insulin through subcutaneous injections.

- Type 2 diabetes, the non-insulin-dependent diabetes mellitus (NIDDM), usually develops in middle age, and is due to relative deficiency of insulin, or most commonly, insulin resistance.

There are other forms such as gestational diabetes that develops during 2–5 percent of pregnancies as the body doesn't effectively use insulin because of metabolic changes caused by the hormones in pregnancy. It usually disappears after pregnancy, but more than half of such women eventually go on to have permanent type 2 diabetes.

When such clients come to us, common symptoms narrated include frequent urination (polyurea), extreme thirst (polydipsia), blurred vision, weight loss despite abnormal hunger and appetite (polyphagia), and fatigue. All of these are caused by persistent high levels of sugar in the circulating blood. Excess glucose in the blood increases water excretion in the urine, and the resultant dehydration creates extreme thirst. Although the blood has huge amounts of glucose, the lack of it being absorbed by the cells creates extreme hunger and lethargy. Clients may have a family history of diabetes and in the case of type 2 diabetes, are usually found to be overweight or obese. If the condition has been long-standing, they may narrate symptoms of complications affecting the nerves leading to an altered sensation in the extremities, loss of kidney function, visual loss, or cardiovascular complaints.

As yoga therapists, the most important thing we need to keep in mind is that the control of blood sugar is key to preventing and managing the short- and long-term complications of diabetes. Hence our effort should be focused on helping our clients to manage their life better through applying yogic principles and practices.

This is, of course, easier said than done, as most people are unwilling to change their lifestyle. This was reiterated to me in a recent conversation I happened to overhear between a diabetologist and his client.

Patient: Doc, how are my glucose numbers?

Doctor: Okay, but not great. You seem to have pre-diabetes, the stage before diabetes.

Patient: Ha… I knew it. My parents are diabetic. Okay… Give me some medications. I can only take one a day.

Doctor: I will give you a better deal. You need to take meds only zero times a day. Let's start lifestyle changes—diet, exercise, etc.

Patient: Why?

Doctor: So you can prevent diabetes and stop it in its tracks.

Patient: You mean to say that the best way to prevent diabetes is to live like I already have it?

Doctor: Err… Sort of…

Patient: Then why would I want to prevent diabetes? Let it come when it comes.

One of the hardest things to do is to motivate such people who prefer a "quick fix" with meds over doing something that would help them be healthy. In fact, I often used to tell the pharmaceutical reps visiting my office that they should tell their bosses to support yoga research. "Why should we do that? Aren't you a threat to us?" would be their incredulous question. "Well, human beings are so lazy that they will always prefer a drug they can take once/twice a day over making wholesome changes in their lifestyle. So, we will never be a threat to you." I used to also tell them, "Most clients stop medication for two reasons: one is the negative side effects of the drugs and the second is the high costs involved. Adjunct yoga therapy enables a reduction of the overall dosage, thus reducing negative side effects and cost. This, in turn, makes clients more compliant with the medical management. So it is a win, win." My last statement that would drive them away would be, "To top it all, if you guys support yoga research, you will also incur some merit in your karma account!" I must admit honestly that not many of them ever came back.

Understanding the role of yoga therapy in diabetes mellitus

Yoga is probably the best lifestyle ever designed, and as such can be safely advocated in stress-induced lifestyle disorders such as diabetes mellitus. Even small efforts are rewarded as the loss of a few pounds of body weight starts to show tremendous changes in indicators of the health status of clients with type 2 diabetes. Dr Bijlani and colleagues at the All India Institute of Medical Sciences (AIIMS), the premier medical institute at New Delhi in India, have also researched this.[2] Their results showed that a short lifestyle modification program based on yoga reduces risk factors for CVD and diabetes mellitus within a period of nine days.

The individualized yoga therapy protocol that we create for our client should aim at normalizing their body weight and reducing body fat. Such changes would, in turn, result in the normalization of blood pressure and blood sugar. These changes would also help correct lipid abnormalities and restore autonomic balance. A systematic review of 32 articles from 1980 to 2007 found yoga interventions to be effective in reducing body weight, normalizing blood pressure, reducing glucose levels, as well as reducing high cholesterol.[3]

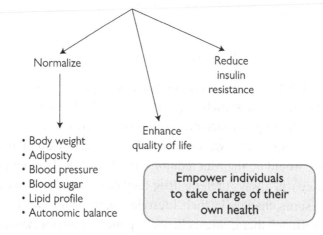

Aim of yoga therapy protocol

The role of sympathovagal balance in the pathophysiology of diabetes is well understood by researchers. Hence the use of yoga practices should be aimed at enhancing parasympathetic vagal activity and reducing sympathetic drive. Exclusive left nostril breathing (*chandra nadi*), left in and right out (*chandra bhedana*), and alternate nostril breathing (*anulom vilom, nadi shuddhi, nadi shodhana*) are very useful in this regard. Slow, deep breathing (at the rate of six breaths per minute) has been advocated as a means to bring about healthier sympathovagal balance, and the work of Dr Bernardi and colleagues[4] has even shown that it is useful in improving arterial function as well as enhancing baroreflex sensitivity in type 1 diabetes. This is an innovative finding as cardiac autonomic neuropathy is associated with increased morbidity and mortality rates in patients with type 1 diabetes. Such patients have been reported to have reduced baroreflex sensitivity. The fact that slow breathing, irrespective of disease duration, could balance baroreflex is great news for all of us.[5]

We must not look at these factors in isolation and remember that they are all interlinked. In this regard, it is worth going through the excellent comprehensive review by Dr Innes and H.K. Vincent,[6] where they reported beneficial changes in several risk factors, including glucose tolerance, insulin sensitivity, lipid profile, anthropometric characteristics, blood pressure, oxidative stress, coagulation profiles, sympathetic activation, and pulmonary function, as well as an improvement in specific clinical outcomes.

All of this can be achieved by an integrated yoga therapy module that takes into consideration basic yogic principles including:

- Psychological reconditioning and development of appropriate attitudes.

- Stress management through yogic practices.

- Enhancement of insulin sensitivity through physical practices including warming up and loosening techniques, postures, breath–body co-ordination and breath–energy harmonizing techniques (*pranayama*). Sun Salutation (*surya namaskar*) is also useful, and may need to be modified as per individual requirements and capacities.

- The use of relaxation, visualization, and contemplative practices to induce a sense of inner calmness and wellbeing.

Being relatively safe, simple, and cost-effective, yoga should be suggested as a beneficial adjuvant in diabetes mellitus when we communicate with healthcare providers. As suggested earlier in my dialog with medical representatives, adjunct yoga therapy may help obtain benefits at lower doses, reducing the side effects of medicines, enhancing metabolic control as well as patient compliance. For those skeptics who wish to always have confirmation from published works, you can always quote Innes and Vincent who concluded, "with no appreciable side effects and multiple collateral benefits, yoga is safe, simple to learn and can be practiced by even ill, elderly or disabled patients."[7]

For a long time, there was a general hypothesis that yoga, and especially the *asanas*, helped in managing diabetes mellitus by forcing a greater release of insulin, and that this was done by pressurizing the pancreas. It was suggested that the twisting postures and postures where the intra-abdominal contents were compressed would "squeeze" the pancreas, thus resulting in more insulin to control elevated sugar levels. It was only in 2005 that an excellent study by S. Manjunatha[8] and colleagues showed that serum insulin levels didn't increase after the performance of a series of *asanas* but rather, to the contrary, levels decreased! They also subjected their participants to a 75-gram oral glucose tolerance test (OGTT) after the *asanas*, where it was found that the serum insulin levels were higher than in the pre-study OGTT. Their findings confirmed that the performance of *asanas* leads to an increased sensitivity of the beta cells of the pancreas to a glucose signal. The breakdown of insulin resistance at the cellular level, and the simultaneous enhancement of insulin sensitivity, is now acknowledged as the mechanism of action for yoga practices in diabetes mellitus. Such an increased sensitivity can be attributed to a sustained change resulting from progressive long-term practice of the *asanas*. This is also now supported by studies showing that long-term yoga practice leads to enhanced insulin sensitivity as well as a healthy attenuation of the negative relationship between weight/waist circumference and insulin sensitivity.[9]

Diet is a vital component of yoga therapy in diabetes mellitus, and this must become part of the yoga therapy session. Processed food and junk foods in general must be avoided, while focusing on replacing such items with fiber-rich greens, vegetables, fruits, and salads. In India we often suggest the use of bitter gourd, fenugreek, and neem for clients as such bitter foods are highly effective in breaking down insulin resistance. We recommend the use of turmeric, an effective anti-inflammatory. We can never stress enough the need to maintain good hydration (a minimum of 2 liters per day of good quality water), as this is a major issue in diabetes mellitus. Small and frequent meals of complex carbohydrates, raw vegetables and fruits, and dietary fiber are useful to avoid unhealthy tsunami-like rises and falls of blood sugar that cause micro-vascular damage. We also suggest performing the heel sitting *vajrasana* (Thunderbolt Pose) after meals to aid in healthy digestion and assimilation of the meal.

Hypertension is often a co-morbidity, and hence we should advise avoidance or minimal use of salt, in both its direct and indirect forms. Additions of garlic and onion in the diet are useful to help keep blood pressure in its normal range.

We need to remind our clients that "You are what you eat. Eat healthy, be healthy!" Responsibility for client health always starts with the client and their own choices!

CHAPTER 9

Cancer

In this chapter we describe the disease, types, and stages of cancer, typical treatments, guidelines for yoga therapists, and finally, what to watch out for when working with cancer patients.

The WHO describes cancer as "a generic term for a large group of diseases characterized by the growth of abnormal cells beyond their usual boundaries that can then invade adjoining parts of the body and/or spread to other organs."[1] This means that the word "cancer" does not represent any particular disease; rather, it speaks to our own body's cells going haywire in an uncontrolled and often rapid growth in any part of the body. Other common terms used are malignant tumors and neoplasms.

According to the IHME and WHO,[2] cancer is the second leading cause of death globally, and is estimated to have accounted for 9.6 million deaths in 2018. In the US, lung, prostate, colorectal, stomach, and liver cancer are the most common types of cancer in men, while breast, colorectal, lung, cervical, and thyroid cancer are the most common among women. This also depends on the world's geographic region—in some parts of the world some cancers occur more often than in others, but in the Americas the WHO[3] lists cancer as the second leading cause of death. The lifetime probability of developing cancer is one in two for men and one in three for women.[4] For yoga therapists this means that most likely we are already dealing with people who have had cancer, or someone they love has had cancer.

Cancer is a collection of diseases that arise due to uncontrolled cell multiplication. In adults, cell multiplication is a highly controlled process that occurs mostly to replenish cells that die due to normal wear and tear or damage from external factors (called cell apoptosis). If the processes that control normal cell multiplication and lifespan go awry, cells start mutating and then multiplying uncontrollably, ultimately failing to die when they should. These accumulating cells form masses called tumors in body organs and tissues. When it happens in the blood or bone marrow, the mutated cell growth simply crowds out normal cells. Over time, by entering the bloodstream or lymphatic network, some cancer cells invade local and then distant tissues, a process called metastasis, and form secondary tumors at remote sites. Most deaths from cancer are due to metastasis.

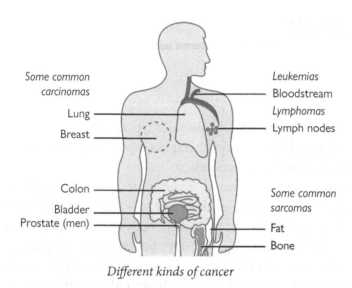

Some common carcinomas

Lung

Breast

Colon

Bladder

Prostate (men)

Leukemias
Bloodstream

Lymphomas
Lymph nodes

Some common sarcomas

Fat

Bone

Different kinds of cancer

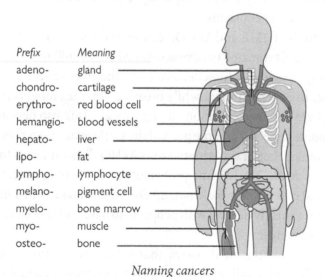

Prefix	Meaning
adeno-	gland
chondro-	cartilage
erythro-	red blood cell
hemangio-	blood vessels
hepato-	liver
lipo-	fat
lympho-	lymphocyte
melano-	pigment cell
myelo-	bone marrow
myo-	muscle
osteo-	bone

Naming cancers

Diagnosis

Cancer diagnosis may be done by several means, although only a few are conclusive. There are blood tests for markers CA-19-9, CA-125, and PSA. Usually, elevated levels of the markers in the blood are of concern and lead to further testing. Often imaging is used in the form of X-rays, ultrasound, CT or PET scans, and/or an MRI to find the exact location and size of the cancer.

The most conclusive test, however, is a pathology-based test such as a local biopsy, bone marrow biopsy, or lumbar puncture. During a biopsy tissue is retrieved from the cancer site and then tested in a laboratory. This invasive procedure gives fairly accurate results and we get to know if the cancer is aggressive or benign.

Recent studies have shown that it is possible to use a blood sample, also called a liquid biopsy, instead of the invasive traditional tissue biopsy, to obtain material that can be analyzed to provide information about a patient's cancer.[5] Liquid biopsies have the potential to transform early detection, diagnosis, treatment, and surveillance of cancer by identifying markers of disease, therapeutic response, resistance, and recurrence.

Once a diagnosis has been made, details of how advanced the disease is are then determined and measured in stages. The stages of cancer are determined by detailed pathological examination of the tumor's tissue, which is usually obtained during surgery. The lab report is based on different factors of the sample, such as:

- Appearance—irregularity in shape of dividing cells

- Large, variably shaped nuclei

- Variation in cell size and shape

- Loss of normal specialized cell features

- Poorly defined tumor boundary.

Categories:

- Grade—differentiation

- Tumor markers

- Level of invasion (lymphatics and blood vessels)

- Gene mutation.

To determine all these factors the lab performs specialized tests on the tumor tissue sample, which may typically take one to two weeks for the results to come back. This multitude of factors indicates the stage of the cancer and the level of its aggressiveness.

Cancer stages

In general, cancer advancement is divided into four stages, which are then additionally also sub-graded by letters. We only consider general stages here, as such sub-grading goes beyond the broad scope of this book.

Stage 1 is the earliest stage marked by local involvement and usually a small size of tumor. This is the stage where for some cancers chemotherapy may not be recommended and in many cases surgery may be enough.

Stage 2 means that the cancer is locally advanced and the tumor is larger than in stage 1. Cancer might also have spread to some nearby lymph nodes.

Stage 3 involves cancerous tumors locally advanced and spread to more lymph nodes. Its margins may have extended into tissue surrounding the tumor.

Stage 4 involves the spread of primary cancer to distant areas of the body. This is called metastasis. For instance, breast cancer in its advanced stage typically spreads to the lungs, brain, or bones. We then say that the primary breast cancer has metastasized to the lungs, brain, or bones. This is as opposed to lung cancer or bone cancer, which, when primary, are completely different kinds of cancer. Stage 4 is usually regarded by the medical world as a terminal cancer.

Surgery

Depending on the tumor and its location, different types of surgery may be applicable. The most common type of surgery for tumors is the most invasive one, which involves full anesthesia and many hours on the operating table. Fortunately, with new discoveries being made all the time, more alternative surgeries are now available that are less invasive and may only involve local anesthesia.

There can be *laparoscopic* surgery, during which the operation is performed far from the location of the cancer. This involves a small incision (1.5 cm) elsewhere on the body through which the surgeon can reach the tumor.

Cryotherapy uses a very low temperature to freeze the tumor locally.

In *radiofrequency ablation,* a small needle is inserted into the tumor and destroys it by applying a high frequency electrical signal.

Or the tumor can be burnt with a laser beam.

For the purposes of our discussion in yoga therapy we simply need to know how invasive the surgery was. We also need to know where and how big the incision was (if any), and to what degree it is healed. We should also assess if the incision site limits any movements of the body.

Chemotherapy

Chemotherapy is a systemic anti-cancer therapy in the form of infusion or pills. Also called chemo, it may typically come in different stages for different cancers. For lymphoma and leukemia, chemo comes right after diagnosis, as no surgery is involved.

For cancers that involve tumors—carcinomas and sarcomas—chemo typically comes after surgery, as a preventive measure. In cases where the tumor may be too big to operate on, chemo may be recommended before surgery to shrink it. Depending on the stage of the cancer, chemo may not be recommended at all.

In the traditional medical model there are several different systemic chemotherapies depending on the type of cancer.

Traditional chemo hits the whole body indiscriminately, and kills healthy and unhealthy cells equally. It has most severe side effects because it acts indiscriminately all over the body, and especially targets rapidly proliferating cells such as the hair, skin, and stomach lining. Hormonal chemotherapy is used for those cancers that are hormone-dependent (most commonly breast and prostate). Biologically targeted chemotherapy, such as HER2 or VEGF inhibitors, can be used. All of these different types have their side effects, which we will discuss in what follows.

The Cancer Immunology Program at Johns Hopkins University School of Medicine is leading the rapidly growing field of immunotherapy. Immunotherapy involves engineering or enhancing the immune cells of the cancer patient to wipe out their cancer cells.

According to a recently published editorial in the prestigious *Lancet Oncology*,[6] "the prices of cancer drugs continue to increase uncontrollably, sometimes doubling within 5 years, with an average return of US$15–50 on every $1 spent on research and development." A recent WHO report[7] reiterates that the problem is now even more rampant, and drastic measures are needed to tackle what seems to be gross profiteering by the pharmaceutical industry. "This burden," proposes *The Lancet Oncology*, "will only be reduced by addressing prevention and profit in parallel—and, if profit margins continue to remain out of reach, one of the most effective ways will be to reduce the reliance on these medicines altogether."

Fortunately, due to the availability of information in the last few years, other therapies may be complementary or even alternative to the conventional medical model. Some of these therapies are offered by specializing naturopathic doctors or other functional medical practitioners:

- *Detoxification:* A 2005 study found 287 industrial chemicals in the umbilical cords of newborns.[8] Over half of these chemicals are known to cause cancer. Naturopathic or functional doctors can provide advice on detoxifying protocols. There are other natural methods to purify the body such as coffee enemas, fasting, and intermittent fasting or infrared saunas.

- *Diet:* Elimination of the source of toxins by eating non-processed foods, organic, and anti-inflammatory foods (such as turmeric), and many other diets that claim anti-cancer properties.

- *Gerson therapy:* Developed in the 1930s, this is a natural treatment that may activate the body's extraordinary ability to heal itself through an organic, plant-based diet, raw juices, coffee enemas, and natural supplements. With its whole-body approach to healing, it naturally reactivates the body's ability to heal itself, with no damaging side effects.

- *Vitamin C* is proven to be highly effective in the treatment of colorectal cancer, which claims the lives of some 50,000 people annually. It is particularly effective in the treatment of colorectal cancers bearing both KRAS and BRAF gene mutations, which happen to respond quite poorly to conventional therapies, including chemotherapy. Naturopathic doctors in other types of cancer treatment also commonly use it as a complementary support.

- *Antineoplastons* are chemical compounds normally found in the blood and urine. They are made up of amino acids and peptides. In the 1970s, Dr Stanislaw Burzynski developed antineoplaston therapy.[9] However, the Food and Drug Administration (FDA) has been fighting the Burzynski Clinic for years, and so he is limiting his services to the state of Texas.

- *Ozone therapy*[10] used in oral and other cancers. In Asia doctors commonly use ozone therapy to treat infected tissue. Although it is a common therapy in much of the Eastern world, it is not widely used in the US.

- *Mistletoe extract,* used since 1917, directly prevents cancer cell growth while stimulating the immune system to fight the cancer cells. Studies[11] show that mistletoe improves symptoms as well as quality of life and general wellbeing in patients afflicted with multiple types of cancer. Simultaneously, it reduces the side effects of conventional cancer treatments, and may help patients survive the harsh side effects of chemo and radiation.

- *Hyperthermia*[12] can be used as both a primary treatment and an adjunct treatment, because it weakens cells and makes them less resistant to other treatment therapies. Local hyperthermia concentrates very high temperatures in targeted locations to weaken and destroy cancer cells. Full body hyperthermia uses less intense heat (around 38–39°C or 101–102°F) to create what is essentially an artificial fever. This activates the immune system to combat disease. Full body hyperthermia also eliminates toxins through sweat.

- *Cannabis*[13] has been cultivated in Asia for millennia and has been documented in traditional Chinese medicine for approximately 1800 years. Many doctors in Asia use cannabis successfully to treat cancer. Cannabis has a wide array of benefits, including tumor reduction. Studies have indicated that cannabis can help induce apoptosis, stopping the spread of cancer and encouraging programmed cell death.

- *Microbiome*—in other words, our gut health—research abounds linking the development of cancer to a compromised microbiome. The systemic failures that are the results of microbiota out of harmony can lead to tumors, and even full-blown cancer. A 2015 paper[14] revealed that epidemiological studies indicate damage to the microbiome as a major risk factor in cancer development.

An excellent website providing comprehensive and trustworthy information is Beyond Conventional Cancer Therapy.[15] Designed for patients, families and friends, and health professionals, it provides therapy summaries and evidence-based cancer-specific reports. These include diets and metabolic therapies, biologic treatments, energy therapies, mind–body, spiritual, and consciousness-changing approaches, exercise and movement therapies, approaches using heat, sound, light, and other cutting-edge therapies. I have found it an excellent resource for all those who have been touched directly or indirectly by cancer.

We may also hopefully be witness to a rapid paradigm change, with two Nobel Prize[16] winners in 2018 (James P. Allison and Tasuku Honjo) for their work on human immune cells isolating and killing cancer. It may take some time before it comes out of the lab into the clinical stage (it's said that the lab-to-clinic time takes around 15 years!), but perhaps these are the first steps to outdate the conventional treatment of chemotherapy and its terrible side effects.

The dispensation of conventional chemotherapy can be by infusion or oral administration. It can be daily, every three weeks, or perhaps once a month. The length of treatment may also vary, from weeks to years. This is important to yoga therapists—usually the days of chemo and post chemo are very difficult for patients.

It often causes multiple side effects such as fatigue, depression, and cognitive impairments. The severity of these symptoms depends on the type and duration of chemotherapy, on the type of cancer, and on the individual person. Most often these side effects manifest in tandem. We cover these side effects in Chapter 10, "Coping with Cancer."

The typical treatment course involves diagnosis followed by surgery, which establishes the pathology of the cancer. Based on the pathology results, usually chemotherapy and then radiation is recommended. However, chemo and/or radiation may come before surgery depending on several factors, such as the size and location of the tumor.

Prevention

In the US eliminating risk factors can prevent 4 out of 10 cancer cases and almost 50 percent of deaths.[17] Unfortunately, the multiplicity of factors causing cancer is still not understood completely by medical science, but research points to the following key risk factors:[18]

- Tobacco use

- Alcohol abuse

- Unhealthy diet

- Lifestyle

- Physical inactivity.

There are also other factors involved in cancer formation, such as environmental toxicity. According to the WHO, environmental risk factors account for nearly 20 percent of all cancers globally, most of which occur in low- and middle-income countries. Other risk factors include:

- Infections (viral and bacterial)

- Compromised immune system

- Chronic sub-clinical inflammation

- Chronic stress

- Gut microbiome imbalances

- Genetic inheritance

- Emotional, mental, and spiritual distress

- Other unknown reasons.

Many cancer risk factors are also risk factors for other chronic diseases, such as CVD, respiratory diseases, and diabetes.

Although 5–10 percent of cancer-causing mutations can be inherited, most are acquired over an individual's lifetime due to the factors mentioned above, or coexisting health conditions that fuel chronic inflammation. Based on this, each person's cancer is unique, in part because it is influenced by the patient's biological characteristics and lifestyle factors.

However, yoga therapy can play a major role in cancer prevention and at any stage of the cancer journey, for that matter. Yogic lifestyle, diet, and attitudes, as well as many yoga therapy techniques, match exactly the requirements in lifestyle and attitudinal changes for creating health in our clients. A wonderful description of such lifestyle changes and their results is outlined in a new bestseller by Anne Ornish and Dean Ornish in *UnDo It!* (January 2019),[19] where yoga therapy is highly recommended. In fact, Dean Ornish worked extensively with Swami Satchchidananda of Mysore, and Nischala Devi, on creating his famous Dean Ornish Lifestyle Medicine program. The happy news is that the Lifestyle Medicine program is now covered by insurance. My hope is that yoga therapy, with time and growing evidence, will also be covered by insurance.

Yoga therapy can additionally address a critical issue hindering improvements in public health by effectively communicating the current knowledge on avoidable cancer risk factors and suggesting interventions to minimize these risks. In fact, according to a recent report, most adults in the US are still unaware of the significant cancer risks associated with obesity and alcohol use.[20] In 2014, overweight- and obesity-related cancers accounted for 40 percent of all cancer cases in the US.[21]

The subject of the side effects of conventional cancer treatments will be covered in detail in the following pages of this book. We will also look at objective measures in using techniques such as *asanas*, *pranayama*, meditation, chanting, *mudras*, and *yoga nidra*. For those who are lucky enough not to have to walk this path, we also describe the cancer journey from a survivor's subjective point of view. For now, we present a few general guidelines to help our clients deal with the different stages of the cancer journey.

Guidelines for yoga therapists ─────────────────────

During the assessment process we get a glimpse of our client's physical abilities, mental attitudes, and psychological state. We also find out where on the cancer journey the person is. The stages of the journey are:

- Diagnosis

- Pre-surgery

- Surgery

- Post-surgery

- Chemotherapy

- Radiation

- Post-treatment.

Each of the stages presents its own distinctive challenges for the client, but there are also factors that weave throughout the complete journey (described in detail in Chapter 10, "Coping with Cancer"). We need to take all of this into account when working with our client and choosing the appropriate tools to meet their goals. Our guidelines here are rather general as, of course, each client is different and we need to understand that what works for one may not work for another. We realize that there is a tendency to look for the tools you would use working with cancer patients, but we must keep in mind that yoga therapy must not be prescriptive in nature. Therefore we need to shift our paradigm into working with the individual, the wholesome being in front of us, and not get entangled by focusing solely on the disease.

We must also remember that the evaluation process never really ends throughout the time we work with the client. Since our approach is helping to heal people on all levels, we need to be constantly on watch to see if what we recommend really works for the client. At the same time, however, we need to keep in mind that yogic practices require time to produce effects, and we may have to wait for even four weeks or more before we will see any results.

There are no easy and simple answers. Yoga is not prescriptive science. It takes time to get to know the client and their most inner territory. Our initial assessment is rather superficial, and as we build a relationship with the client, we get to appreciate more their level of awareness and the deeper cause of imbalances. It takes time to match the sequence of practices to a particular client, and we may have to adjust what we initially recommended several times as the client progresses.

In my experience with the Beyond Cancer retreats, the majority of patients have either never done yoga or practiced it way back in their youth. Most of them have done very little physical movement, although in recent years we have seen a 300 percent increase in attendance in yoga classes in the older population.[22]

Although cancer touches a very diverse population, most of the clients we have worked with were mature people, usually in their 50s or 60s (although more and more often we see clients in their 40s), and not familiar with yogic practices. Therefore the following guidelines are geared towards the beginners' population. We also need to keep in mind that recommended practices should always be checked with and modified for the specific condition, limitations, and needs of a particular client.

Typically our work may occur only once or twice a week, yet it is so important for the client to work these practices every day—and then the desired results will come much more quickly. So, making guiding materials available in audio recordings or video clips will make it easy for clients to follow the practices.

Diagnosis and pre-surgery stages

Cancer diagnosis and the pre-op (pre-surgery) stage is the time of the great "unknown," leading to high levels of anxiety, confusion, fear, and generally an immensely stressful time. Therefore our task, as yoga therapists, is to help our clients to effectively cope with these states.

PRANAYAMA

The first and perhaps quickest way to make our clients aware of their state is by turning attention to the breath. We find that 99 percent of the clients we work with have a very short and quick breath (16+ breaths per minute), engaging only the upper part of the lungs, so they hyperventilate.

The most common aberrations in breathing to watch for (while doing *asanas*) are:

- Interrupted breathing

- Shallow breathing

- Long inhale—very short exhale

- Reversed breathing—belly in on the inhale (which happens when the client only breathes with the upper part of their lung)

- Fits-and-starts breathing—inhalation with breaks.

We recommend spending a fair amount of time making the client aware of how they breathe. Since we work with the adult population, we spend time explaining the mechanism of breathing, showing a short video so that clients can visualize the working of the diaphragm while practicing its engagement later on. For some clients, conscious engaging of the diaphragm is extremely difficult, and in rare cases we have to manually assist them in releasing it, by pushing their stomach in during exhale. The following inhale usually results in a "bulging belly," which means full engagement of the diaphragm and all parts of the lungs. For many this is the first time they have consciously taken a full deep breath in many years.

We then proceed to explain the interdependency between the body, the mind, and the breath, and ask them to practice "proper" slow and deep breathing several times an hour throughout the day. This is the first thing we follow up on during subsequent sessions.

If they practice at home, clients tend to grow in their awareness of their body and mental states. They also usually become self-motivated, seeing how effectively this modulates stress in their daily living.

If there are no contraindications for a specific cancer, we recommend all-around *pranayama* practice with the inclusion of alternate nostril breathing (*nadi shuddhi*), *surya bhedana*, *sitali*, *chandra bhedana*, *ujjayi*, and *bhramari*.

What is important to note here is that *pranayama* is an extremely powerful tool. If done incorrectly, it may create more problems rather than healing. Therefore, before we recommend that the client practices it at home, we need to make sure that they have learned the practices properly. For the same reason we do not describe the practices here—you know them if you practice them. If you do not practice them, you should not teach them.

Note that *sitali* is listed in the *Hatha Yoga Pradipika* as an effective *pranayama* for tumors and inflammations in the body. Hence it has become a very important *pranayama* for all patients with cancer and chronic diseases.

Finally, since for most of the clients this will be an introduction to *pranayama*, which they have never done before, we recommend a 1:2 ratio without *kumbhaka*. We teach 1:2 ratio breathing *before* the client starts *pranayama*. The ratio is important, and we find that learning the ability to control the breath ratio is best done with normal, two-nostril breathing.

Many clients begin to develop sleeping difficulties at this stage of the cancer journey. We recommend 10–15 minutes of silent meditation or *kirtan kriya*,[23] followed by 20 rounds of *bhramari pranayama* just before going to bed.

Asanas

The pre-surgery period is also a good time for *asana* practices, which will help the client to effectively release psychosomatic stress and tension from the body. It can be done as an individual class or in a beginners' group. The general recommended practice here is based on gentle *Hatha Yoga* and includes simple *asanas* assuming a beginner's level of ability, with emphasis on spine flexibility.

The more important factor, perhaps, is how it is done. The recommendation is to move into an *asana* slowly with the client's full awareness in the body as well as a long and deep breath throughout the process. Hold the *asana* without changing the rhythm of the breath and keep the awareness on the emotional and mental field. Then slowly release the posture with full awareness of body changes. Finally, relax the full body for 15–30 seconds before moving on to the next *asana*.

At the beginning, many clients may have great difficulty controlling their mind, and most of them have rather stiff and stressed bodies; however, we can help them to become aware of their breath and teach them to use slow and deep breathing during an *asana* class. When they slow down the breath, the mind will relax, and the body's self-healing mechanism will be activated.

This way the *asana* class becomes not so much about the correct posture and muscles, as it is usually used in the West, but about deepening awareness of the inner world of the mind and emotions, and reconnecting with the body. It is also a way to encourage "being in *asana*" or "relaxing into *asana*" rather than "doing *asana*."

Meditation[24]

Many of our clients may have never meditated. And many novices have preconceived ideas that you only meditate when the thought process ceases. So they struggle with "not having" thoughts, and end up being convinced that they cannot meditate.

In such cases, we recommend simple guided meditation, with the emphasis on the posture of witnessing the thoughts. The task, then, is to simply observe the thoughts coming in and out of awareness. We have found that guided meditation works very well in such cases, especially for those who have a strong mind. We recommend pre-recording the meditation and offering it to be practiced daily at home.

Meditating with awareness on the breath and using the "so hum" mantra works well for beginners. It sometimes has quite unexpected results:

> During my stay, I had a pancreatic crisis which is very painful and for which none of the painkillers are effective. Desperate, I decided to practice meditation.

> Then, miraculously, the feeling of pain disappeared. I could not believe it but it was really happening. The pain was gone. It came back 8 hours later and then I did again a longer meditation and again the pain was gone forever. (Colette Casmir)

After some time of practicing a "so hum" meditation we introduce a "forgiveness" meditation, which helps clients deal with unresolved emotional issues and relationships. In the words of a Beyond Cancer retreat participant:

> Another tool I found very powerful was the guided forgiveness meditation. Thanks to this type of meditation, I had been able to make some "cleaning" in my life in order to reach a level of serenity which I never have had before in my life. (Colette Casmir)

We often introduce clients to *kirtan kriya*, a *Kundalini Yoga* meditation, which is known to increase telomerese by 43 percent if done daily for eight weeks.[25] This 12-minute active meditation includes mantra chanting with *mudras*, leaving beginners with very little time for thinking of anything else. It has a very calming effect and is also a great tool for increasing blood flow to the brain to recover from "chemo brain" in the post-treatment stage.

Post-surgery stage

Anxiety and fear are now added to by pain after surgery. It usually takes four to six weeks to heal wounds, and at this time *asanas* are not recommended. However, gentle *pranayama*, *kirtan kriya*, and meditation may be very helpful.

At this point we also recommend introducing *yoga nidra* (see Chapter 13 and Appendix 2) with healing visualization. The text can be recorded and used daily after setting a short, positive affirmation for speeding up the post-surgery healing. It is a very powerful technique and many clients use it with great effect.

Chemotherapy or radiation stages

During chemotherapy and radiation treatments the client's energy levels may greatly fluctuate from one class to another. The closer to the end of the treatment, the more severe the side effects—physical and mental.

This is a good time to reintroduce a few gentle *asanas* if the client's condition allows for it. Needless to say, all the practices, especially the *asanas*, should be modified and adapted to the type of cancer and the patient's physical limitation in the moment. There may initially be some resistance to such practice because of possible high levels of fatigue, but a recent review of 24 studies "supports the recommendation of yoga as a supportive intervention for improving health-related quality of life and reducing fatigue and sleep disturbances when compared with no therapy, as well as for reducing depression, anxiety and fatigue."[26]

Another study[27] at the University of Rochester found that exercise reduced chemotherapy-induced peripheral neuropathy. Our experience during Beyond Cancer retreats confirms these findings—typically, by the end of the three-week retreat, our clients report complete regression in their neuropathy symptoms.

Remember, given this stage of the cancer journey, typically our client is dealing with:

- Long-term inactivity

- Possible breath irregularities

- Lack of connection with the body.

Hence we can use *asanas* as a way to deal with these issues with appropriate cues. More importantly we can take this opportunity to use an *asana* class to introduce awareness of inner sensations and develop the posture of an "observer" of the inner world. With practice this will develop mental stillness and emotional calm in our clients.

It is possible, however, that because of high levels of fatigue as treatments progress, the *asana* class may not be feasible. Staying with *pranayama*, *kirtan kriya*, *yoga nidra*, and meditation—which can all be prerecorded for clients—is a good solution for daily practice. This way we recommend a daily routine for the client, encouraging them to do daily individual work at home until such time when they are ready for gentle *asanas*.

Post-treatment stage

We describe in great detail post-treatment in Part 3 and in the appendices outlining our retreat protocols.

Hands-on/off approach

In the following we discuss precautions in teaching *asanas* and *pranayama* to specifically a cancer population. Before we do so, however, I would like to discuss the hands-on/off approach—that is, should we, or should we not, touch the client while teaching a yoga class?

There is an ongoing discussion whether we should or should not touch clients in order to help them achieve the correct posture. I understand that it mainly depends on teacher/therapist preference and, of course, the population they are working with. What is appropriate for one may not be comfortable for someone else. Also, touching may be a quick and easy way for the therapist to correct a client.

But I want to stress that when we are applying yoga therapy, the concept of "correct posture" changes from the book picture to what is safe and correct for a particular client. There is no "box" that we need to fit our client into.

However, the question remains, what is the client's or therapist's goal in the class? What is more important to the client? I have worked with people who have lost touch with their body—the cancer treatment or chronic diseases created great discomfort or pain in the body. For the majority of my clients the easiest way to deal with this was to disassociate from the body and live from the neck up. If attaining the perfect position in an *asana* is the client's or therapist's aim, then touching or not really depends on the client's and therapist's preference. If the aim is *also* regaining contact with the body, understanding and feeling the limits of the body when going into *asana*, than touching can be counterproductive. In such cases we should allow our clients to find their own way into *asana* or *pranayama* with just our verbal or visual cues.

In our experience, the best approach lies in proper verbal explanation and/or demonstration, and then checking with the client, to teach them to reconnect with the body. When we corrected the posture by touching or moving the client's body, we found that our action would encourage a rather passive attitude in the client. In some cases, the client even waited for us to manually help them into the *asana* without trying on their own.

Such a situation was counter-productive as it encouraged passivity rather than independence and responsibility for the client's own action. In our experience, non-touching encourages and teaches clients to reconnect with their body. It may make the therapist's job a little harder, but in our opinion every touch is a lost opportunity to direct the client into self-awareness.

In addition, if we want to lead trauma-informed sessions, we need to be sensitive to the fact that manual adjustment can be perceived as invasive, intrusive, or even triggering. Finally, it is much safer to have a "non-touching" attitude, thus avoiding the danger of the therapist injuring a client. According to Matthew Remski,[28] his "interviews [with yoga students] and research show that a surprising number of senior Ashtanga and Iyengar teachers who adjust students, have caused injuries, sometimes life-altering."

Our job as therapists is to teach our clients practices that will be effective for their condition, and encourage them to continue the practice daily at home by themselves, where they will have no one to adjust them. In order to prevent possible injuries it is important for us to teach clients awareness of the body's messages and its limits.

Taking all this into account, we much prefer to have a "no touching" rule in our classes, although we realize that there are many situations that require manual adjustments at the beginning. So the only golden rule we can think of is to meet the client where they are, and start from there, always erring on the cautious but safe side.

Precautions in teaching *asanas* and *pranayama*

Chemotherapy and radiation causes side effects that greatly influence a client's ability to manage the body, their fragility, sense of balance, and energy levels. The scars after surgery may limit their movements, and clients may have surgically implanted medical devices that are used to administer drugs.

The first rule of thumb is safety. Make sure you know where the client is in their cancer journey and be aware of their limitations ahead of time. *Never* push clients to exceed their limits. Instead, turn their awareness to their body's limits, and once they reach the limit, ask them to back off a little. We never encourage clients to go into pain; instead, we encourage them to be aware of their pain threshold and to back off from it.

We now look at how fatigue, recent surgery, chemo brain, balance and coordination, and medical devices affect the teaching of asanas and pranayama.

Fatigue

It is therefore imperative for us to know our client and their history, and to be sensitive during each session as their conditions may fluctuate—their energy levels and fatigue especially may change from session to session. Depending on where the client is in their treatment, their energy levels may even change during a session.

Levels of fatigue tend to increase the closer the client is to the end of traditional medical treatment. Unfortunately, such fatigue, caused by either chemotherapy or radiation, does not depend on how much they rest. They can be as fatigued after a full night's sleep as after a mild activity.

At the beginning of a Beyond Cancer retreat we have often found that we needed to encourage people to do gentle *asanas* despite their feeling of fatigue. Interestingly, by the end of the retreat, after three weeks of daily intense yogic practices, their levels of fatigue generally were substantially diminished, and their vitality significantly increased.[29]

We need to be very aware of the client's psychological state and how far we can "push" through the feeling of fatigue. Some people are "fighters" and respond well to a challenge. Others are more passive, and presenting a challenge to them may have an adverse effect. Keep this in mind in your assessment of the client, and moderate your approach accordingly.

Recent surgery

We do not recommend *asanas* until the client's wound is completely healed, so it is important to know which area is affected by surgery. With breast cancer, the axillary nodes are often taken out and the scar is not only on the breast but also under the arm. At the beginning this typically limits the movement of the arm to some degree and may cause lymphedema.

For surgeries in the abdomen or pelvic areas, the outer scars can be of different sizes, depending on the type of surgery. Abdominal laparoscopy involves only a small outer incision (usually near the belly button) to remove the fallopian tubes and/or ovaries in women. Although the outer incision may be very small, be very cautious and give time for the healing of the inner body.

The rule of thumb is to avoid stretching or putting pressure on the surgery area within one month or until the incision is completely healed. With tumors in the breast, limit the movement of the hand on the side of the operation, for which modification must be offered. With abdominal and pelvic operations, be very cautious with twists of the torso and leg movements in the supine position.

Any limited range of motion caused by scar tissue will have to be treated individually as the tolerance for stretching will depend on the client. One of my clients couldn't lift her left hand more than 30 degrees in a supine position. Within three weeks of daily *asanas* and without pushing, she was able to regain the full motion of this hand. For others, however, it may take more time.

Chemo brain

The hippocampus is responsible for our memory, and in particular, for the capacity and quality of memory as well as our spatial memory. It is also responsible for our mood and emotions. Formerly thought of as unchanging, we know today that our brain and hippocampus constantly transform through neurogenesis. In fact, Jonas Friesen of the Karolinska Institute in Stockholm estimates that on average we produce 700 new neurons a day in our hippocampus.[30] It doesn't seem that much, but by the time we are 50, we will have completely replaced the entire brain we were born with.

Our ability to create new neurons is modulated by diet, our lifestyle, and environmental factors such as heavy metals (like lead) in our body. Some of the chemotherapies used today to treat cancers are also known to stop neurogenesis. This creates impaired cognitive function and is known as chemo brain or brain fog. In practical terms this means that our client typically has an impaired short memory and speed of mental processing, which usually manifests in:

- Forgetfulness

- Confusion

- Inability to understand or follow up on what is being said

- Feeling of hopelessness

- Anxiety and depression

- Fear

- Confusion

- Struggle to find the right word

- Lack of focus

- Difficulty in multitasking.

In practical terms it means that in order to effectively reach our client we need to adjust our teaching methods accordingly. Patience, understanding, and compassion are key to this process. We also need to know if our client learns visually, orally, or kinesthetically. Then we need to make sure to deliver simple and clear instructions with a demonstration, always checking that the client understands what we are conveying.

Do not be surprised if the client forgets what you have just told them. It took me a couple of years to stop being frustrated with myself and ashamed that I immediately forget what had been said to me. It took me a couple of years before I learned to joke about it and say, "Oh, you know, that's the chemo brain in me!"

Especially embarrassing were moments when I was introducing two good friends of mine who were just meeting each other for the first time. I introduced one by name and as I came to the second one, I would forget their name! It felt like the word was at the back of my head but it didn't want to come out...

It is especially humiliating when such a feeling of "going blank" happens during a lecture. This still happens to me today—my mind goes blank and I am stuck! Forgetting a word or getting stuck is a typical symptom of chemo brain. Give the client space to come back from such a blackout.

If we discuss the next appointment, we help the client record it in their calendar. In our case record (see Chapter 4), which clients fill in prior to attending a retreat, we use pictures and scales instead of descriptions for the client's ease to indicate where the pain is and its level. All these little hints are to help the client deal with very frustrating and often frightening symptoms of cognitive impairment.

Balance and coordination

There are several factors in cancer treatments that may cause a fall. One of them is simply the age of the client, who, with time in treatment, is less stable on their feet.

During chemotherapy the platelets may become very low, and this may lead to bruising or bleeding on even insignificant traumas. In such cases it is recommended that "head-below-heart" positions be avoided as we do not want to risk intracranial bleeds. Caution during an *asana* class in preventing falls is also very important as falling may lead to excessive bruising.

Traditional medical treatment may often lead to osteopenia or even osteoporosis. In such cases any fall may end up in broken bones. If our client has a bone metastasis or advanced osteoporosis, excessive weight bearing or twisting may result in broken bones. We usually consult with the client's doctor and keep their spine and neck in a safe neutral position.

If our client has had radiation, we make sure we know exactly where the radiation was applied. Local radiation tends to lead to local osteoporosis. I found this out myself when I fell on the radiated side of my body and broke two ribs—a total surprise to me. As a rule of thumb, avoid *asanas* that threaten the area of concern, and make it as safe as possible to hold an *asana*. If there is metastasis to the bones or suspicion of such, communicate with the client's doctor for their weight-bearing status.

A side effect of chemotherapy is peripheral neuropathy. This means lack of feeling or changes in sensations in the feet, legs, or hands, resulting in poor balance issues. In such cases use props to make sure that the client is secure in any *asana* that bears weight on the hand or leg affected by neuropathy. For instance, use a chair or wall for modified Tree Pose (*vrkrasana*), have the client do Plank Pose (*kumbhakasana*) on their elbows instead of their hands, etc. Once again, in our intensive yogic retreats, most of the participants recovered from neuropathy within three weeks.

Lymphedema is a swelling of the hand, leg, or torso due to poor lymph circulation. It often happens after the lymph nodes are taken out during surgery, and thus the circulation of the lymph is greatly impaired locally. It may also produce a feeling of tightness or heaviness, aching or discomfort. It often results in a restricted range of motion if it affects the extremities.

In such cases encourage the client to wear a leg or hand compression sock during a yoga session. Avoid prolonged sitting or standing poses. Avoid poses that may cut off circulation and return of the lymphatic fluid to the affected area. The hand or leg should not be put in a dependent position for too long. Change positions frequently.

Medical devices

Devices such as a portacath, drain, or oxygen supply may create some movement restrictions. They may not in themselves introduce restrictions, but we need to know that the client has a portacath installed, for example, to avoid certain positions that may exert pressure on this area. The same applies to drains inserted after surgery.

Pranayama

Although there are no major research studies on contradiction of any *pranayama* technique, we can take our cue from the *Hatha Yoga Pradipika* as to the effects of some breathing techniques on the body, our energy, and our mind.

Bhastrika

> ...cures diseases of *vata*, *pitta* and *kapha* and increases the gastric heat. (*Hatha Yoga Pradipika* II:65)

We want to err on the cautious side and do not recommend the use of *bhastrika* for abdominal and head cancers or diseases, so we do not increase the heat in these areas. (*Bhastrika* is also considered by yogis to infuse vigor and stamina, alertness and memory, while removing depression.)

Suryabhedana

This removes from the throat diseases caused by phlegm and increases the gastric fire. (*Hatha Yoga Pradipika* II:52)

The same precaution applies as above, and we do not recommend it for any abdominal cancers.

Kapalbhati

Kapalbhati is mentioned in *Hatha Yoga Pradipika* as a cleansing *kriya*, not a *pranayama* (*Hatha Yoga Pradipika* II:36). This is why we do not recommend using it (or any other cleansing practices) during chemotherapy. Since this *kriya* stimulates second, third, and sixth chakras (energy centers in the areas of the pelvis, solar plexus, and between the eyebrows) we err on the cautious side and do not recommend its use for brain cancers, high blood pressure, heart disease, brain tumors, stroke, vertigo, stomach or intestinal ulcers, gastroesophageal reflux disease (GERD), gastritis, glaucoma, diarrhea, systemic inflammation, and hyperventilation.

Some respected yogis of recent times, however, regard *kapalbhati* as a *pranayama* and offer it as a remedy for poor blood circulation, slow peristaltic movement, and poor digestion.

Contraindications for other diseases

An excellent resource offered by Dr Loren Fishman is a website listing contraindications for every *asana* in the context of a particular disease.[31] Another excellent resource is "Understanding and preventing yoga injuries"[32] published in the *International Journal of Yoga Therapy*.

Finally, at the time of writing this book (2019), a new smartphone app was introduced called Yoga Therapeutics Pro. It is an app created by (and for) yoga and healthcare professionals to help keep clients and students safe in their practice. The user-friendly app helps to quickly discern which yogic practices to potentially avoid (and which might be beneficial) when a client presents with a health challenge or injury. It provides quick access to the cautions, benefits, therapeutic applications, and modification considerations with accompanying photography, including chair restorative yoga.

Pulmonary capacity

In the case of a pleural infusion diagnosis there should be no forced deep breathing. In asthma or shortness of breath, proceed with caution depending on the client's capacity.

Cardiovascular status

For congestive heart failure, high blood pressure, and untreated CAD, use very gentle *asanas* and no strenuous activity. No *kapalbhati* or *bhastrika*.

Deep vein thrombosis (DVT)

If there is swelling on one leg only and calf pain, no *asanas*, and advise seeing a doctor.

CHAPTER 10

Coping with Cancer–
A Personal Journey

I dedicate this chapter to all those who are dealing with cancer, their caregivers and families, as well as yoga teachers and therapists. There is extensive literature on traditional cancer treatments and on what is available, but so far, I have not found anything that would describe what a patient goes through internally during a cancer journey.

Those who are just at the beginning of such a journey or even in the middle of it will find it essential to know and embrace all the possible tools to help make their journey easier. It is critical for caregivers and families to understand what our loved ones are going through internally. It is also important for yoga teachers and yoga therapists to know what our clients are dealing with over a long period of time, and to facilitate the relief that yoga can provide.

And so, in these pages I give a bird's-eye view of a typical cancer treatment and then focus on the cancer journey from a patient's perspective. I then point to the yogic tools that may be useful in dealing with the challenges along the way. Finally, I explain what yoga therapy is and the difference between a yoga therapist and a yoga teacher.

When I say "cancer journey," I mean the time from when we first learn that there might be a problem through to post-treatment. This takes a long time, and it is important to understand this journey from the patient's point of view.

Of course, there is a problem in assuming a "typical" journey as such, because each journey is highly individual. How we experience it depends on many individual factors such as age, level of awareness, mental resilience, belief systems, determination, energy, and psychological flexibility, not to mention the type and stage of cancer and type of allopathic treatments.

However, even with this diversity of individual factors, there are things we have to deal with that are common to everyone, and these include the stages of a cancer journey. In these pages I cover the stages of a typical journey from the patient's perspective, and consider how yoga science could be helpful in each case. I hope that cancer patients as well as yoga therapists and teachers, luckily never touched by cancer, will find it helpful.

I cover diagnosis, surgery, post-surgery, chemotherapy, radiation and post-treatment. I write from my own experience and include the experiences that my clients have shared with me. In this way, I hope to make it more "typical."

I invite your comments, thoughts, and perhaps your own experiences, which may differ from those I write about.[1]

Diagnosis

Diagnosis is the first stage of the cancer journey. We live somewhat balanced lives, with long- and short-term plans, and think that we know where we are going! However, a phone call from our doctor can destroy this balance with the news that "there may be a problem and we have to do more tests." So, we now enter a new world where time stops, where all is suspended, and we start living from one test result to another.

None of the tests are usually conclusive, so the shadow of cancer grows with every step, and this brings high levels of stress and anxiety. We must now deal with an unknown tomorrow and plans need to be suspended until we receive the test results and know the next steps.

We must also deal with our environment and with friends and family: what to tell them, and, if so, how to tell them about the dreaded challenge growing on our horizon.

During the first session of our healing yoga retreat, clients share how they learned about the possibility of cancer and their reaction. Often, we hear comments like, "My life has stopped in this moment...and now what?" A feeling of fear and hopelessness sets in. Much also depends on how the news is delivered—around 30 percent of cancer patients suffer from post-traumatic stress disorder (PTSD), something we do not hear about.

We also have to understand that social and cultural factors may be at play and may often determine how we deal with the emerging challenge. In most Western countries, cancer patients are surrounded by loving care and the understanding that they are experiencing exceptionally difficult times.

I remember losing my hair when going through chemo and choosing not to wear a wig. Seeing my bald head, strangers would smile tenderly and "knowingly" at me, and some would even ask how long I had been in treatment. We would have a warm exchange and I would be left feeling supported and uplifted, that I was not alone.

However, in some countries, cancer carries the stigma of shame. It is believed that the patient did something terrible in their past life and must now suffer punishment through cancer. Unfortunately, this results in people hiding their condition before their family and so the diagnosis usually comes at a late stage of the disease. So levels of anxiety, tension, confusion, and fear are elevated even further by the social environment.

When conducting our Beyond Cancer retreat[2] in India for the first time, we had a dedicated yoga studio where all the classes were taking place. Curiosity would get the better of some of the staff members at the clinic, who would come to peek into the room to see the "cancer people." And when our group entered the dining hall for the first time, there was suddenly a dead silence, as all eyes focused on us.

On another occasion, a 27-year-old male shared that he had been engaged to a lovely girl whose father, after hearing of his diagnosis, decided to terminate the relationship, leaving both of them heartbroken. I can only imagine that such stigma makes this client's cancer journey so much more difficult.

After an agonizing time of waiting, we are finally asked to do a biopsy (in the case of a tumor). This is the only test that gives 100 percent certainty, but it is also the most expensive one. As we leave the doctor's office afterwards, the dreaded words "It is cancer!" still ring in our ears. But many people hear something different—they hear "Death is coming for you *now!*"

Dealing with reality

Now comes the time when we have to tell our friends and family that all plans are off, that we have a bigger challenge to deal with. Friends and family have different reactions to our news. In some cases, they do not really know how to deal with it. They would like to help but do not know how, so they withdraw. Some are shaken and offer not only their condolences, but also wonderful ongoing support. But some situations become very difficult.

At one of the workshops for cancer patients I heard the following:

> I have stage 4 colon cancer but so far I feel okay. The doctors told me they cannot do anything for me, but I do not feel sick, and apart from few symptoms my life would be normal. Life would be as before if I didn't have to deal with people around me. My family and friends treat me as if I was going to die tomorrow.

Friends invite me to parties or dinners where they talk openly about farewells and say, "Perhaps this is the last time we will meet." Or they call and talk to me as if there was no tomorrow. "Have you planned your funeral? Have you made a will?" With family members I have to deal with their emotions and their fear of losing me! It feels like in addition to taking care of my kids I have to take care of everyone around and their emotions. I am really tired of that!

I think the subject of how a diagnosis impacts a patient's social circle might be good material for another blog or a book. Living with someone or taking care of someone who has stage 4 cancer (regarded as terminal) is challenging and brings many difficult emotions and situations. This short chapter, however, is limited to the patient's perspective.

Coming back to the subject of diagnosis, the dread becomes reality, and many people deal with it by denial. Such was my case. Luckily, I only had to wait for a week for the diagnosis, so I was spared a long time of anxiety. When my diagnosis was confirmed, I felt myself facing a huge challenge and tremendous energy rushing through me with the thought—okay, let's see who wins! At the same time, I had already planned six months of my life with trips to Europe and Trinidad, and nothing was going to stop me! I felt invincible…

How little did I know…

The time between "suspicion of…" and final diagnosis is one of the most difficult during the cancer journey. Our so far normal life is disrupted by the unexpected possibility of "what if…?" As we go from test to test, the anxiety grows exponentially.

This uncertainty may last a week or several weeks. We usually cope with this sudden stress by going into denial, "not thinking about it; not worrying about it." But even then, the voice in the back of our head saying, "what if…?" gets louder and louder. And these few weeks feel like years—time moves so painfully slowly.

Yoga therapy

This is where yoga therapy shines and can be a great help for anyone dealing with emotional tension, fear, often anger, and high levels of stress brought on by the prolonged process of diagnosis and uncertain future prospects.

A skillfully conducted *asana* class can also become a meditative practice. It will bring relief to the tensed body and frightened, busy mind.

Connecting to your breath and slowing it down will also slow thoughts running here and there.[3] It may help with sleep patterns, which are often disrupted at such times.

There are *pranayama* (breathing) techniques, which are distinctively for activating our parasympathetic nervous system (relaxation of all body systems) and calming down the sympathetic nervous system (fight or flight mode). The ability to manage our autonomic nervous system to a certain degree is perhaps one of the most important gifts that yoga therapy can give to us. According to traditional medicine, this is something we have no control over. And yet, a body of research[4, 5, 6] confirms that by using yogic techniques skillfully on a daily basis, we are actually able to influence the balance of our autonomic nervous system.

Techniques like guided meditation, *yoga nidra*, and chanting have a deep healing impact on all levels of human existence. Research[7, 8, 9] shows that by using yogic techniques over time, we can change our brains on physical and functional levels. We can become calm and collected while standing in the eye of the storm.

A few sessions with a yoga therapist will hopefully result in building a daily yoga practice geared specifically to help us deal with the great challenges we meet at the beginning of the journey.

We often need to make decisions with very little information. These decisions are difficult to make in the first place, and a lot of conflicting pressures from family, friends, and doctors only adds to stress levels.

But throughout the diagnosis process we can use yoga therapy tools to bring us internally to the place from where we can act in a rational and calm way to choose the best option possible, despite our anxiety, fear, and confusion.

Surgery

The next step after diagnosis, for those of us who are dealing with tumors (carcinomas or some sarcomas) is surgery. Now the dreaded world that we call "the cancer journey" has opened to us, but the reality is that we do not know what is in store for us—we just know that everyone dreads it. So now we anxiously wait for the day of the operation.

When we show up at the hospital, this is perhaps our first experience of being treated by a multidisciplinary team. For me, personally, it was an eye-opener. I was told to arrive very early in the morning, that my procedure was only a one-day event, and that if everything went okay, I would be released from hospital late in the afternoon.

On the day of the operation, after being admitted by admin at 7am, I was led to an open cubicle on the surgical floor. Once I was there, a nurse did an intake interview, took my vital signs, and then told me to wait. After some time, I was asked to go to another cubicle with a chair and again told to wait. A nurse said, "The doctor will come in a minute." He did come after some time and he marked the location on my body where the operation was to take place; he then confirmed with me that this was the correct spot. Another nurse then came and moved me to yet another cubicle. This one had a chair and a stretcher, and I was again told to wait. This cubicle was supposed to be the last one—the final wait before surgery.

As I waited, I looked around. I could see a large open hall with two rows of six to seven semi-open cubicles, with a lot of patients being moved by nurses from one cubicle to another, just like myself. I realized this place was obviously the prep room, right before the operating theaters.

There was something strange about this environment: it felt very sterile, like we were objects or perhaps numbers being moved from one cubicle to the next, like on a production conveyor belt. The nurses were politely impersonal, efficiently going about their tasks. They were very scarce with words, and their most often used phrase was "Sit here and please wait." There was no time for any questions.

And so I waited. This last cubicle had a stretcher, and since it was early morning, I lay down and started to meditate. I switched off the external noise and went into my own center. I was calm; I felt supported by my many friends who were meditating for me at the same time. I didn't think of the surgery—instead, I managed to stay in the present moment and felt completely at peace with the world and with myself. A gift from my years of yoga practice!

Suddenly, I was abruptly brought back to reality. A nurse had just rushed into my cubicle and demanded that I immediately get up... "I need this stretcher!" she exclaimed, with urgency. A little disoriented, I got up slowly. She noticed my confused reaction and offered a short explanation—"We are short of stretchers and I need it for a patient waiting for spine surgery"—she then left in a hurry, taking the stretcher with her.

After about an hour of being moved from one cubicle to another and being told to "Sit here and please wait," a nurse came and said, "Follow me please." I got up and we walked into the operating theater. I laid down on the table and was then put to sleep. The next thing I knew I woke up on a stretcher in another big room that was full of stretchers with people lying on them.

In hindsight

When I look back at this experience 12 years ago, there is only one thing that stands out in my memory: that everyone in the hospital was efficient and coldly polite. I was given no opportunity to talk to anyone or ask any questions—all the nurses were busy and spent only the necessary time with me to accomplish what they needed me to do. I felt as if I were an object that needed to be directed and told what to do and where to go. I was not entitled to have an opinion or any questions for that matter, and my cooperation was limited to doing exactly what I was told to do. I cannot imagine a more disempowering environment than this.

For those who have lost parts of their body during surgery, this unfriendly environment is even worse. I know of women with breast cancer who have undergone a mastectomy. Losing a breast or even both breasts is a very traumatic experience for many women, so I cannot imagine how traumatic it can feel to be treated in such an impersonal, cold way, as if one were merely an object.

Thank God for yoga! It allowed me to keep my inner peace and calm despite the rather unsettling environment. I cannot imagine how difficult this experience might be for someone who does not have the tools of yoga, tools to help manage thoughts and emotions while they are in such an unfriendly environment, with growing anxiety and fear just before surgery.

Post-surgery

The first few days after surgery passed in a fog—I was heavily sedated but comfortable at home. I was surrounded by love and friendship, and took my time to heal the wound and recover from complete anesthesia.

Post-surgery time is marred with dealing with pain and more anxious waiting. We are told that the full pathology will be available after a few weeks, and only then will we know exactly the kind and stage of cancer. We still do not know the next steps of the journey. "*What now?*" That drilling question is still active in our minds.

After a couple of weeks we will go to our surgeon for a follow-up appointment. Hopefully, the surgery was a success and we will finally know what type of cancer we are challenged with.

This will be the first opportunity to discuss what's next. "You will discuss this with your oncologist, but most likely you will have to have chemotherapy and radiation," my surgeon said. "Such treatment will take some time."

Well, I wasn't having any of it. I still clung to my original plans to travel through Europe and to Trinidad. I said, "No way. I don't have the time for chemo. I need to be in London for Christmas and then on to do lectures in different locations in Europe!" My lovely doctor smiled kindly and said simply, "You'll talk this over with your oncologist."

As I was discussing the next appointment with his secretary before leaving the office, she asked, "So you do not want to do the chemo treatments?" I explained to her that I had my plans set and wanted to stick to them. She looked at me with compassion and said, "Oh Lee, but you are so young; much too young to die."

I left the office speechless, her words still ringing in my ears. Does it really mean that if I do not do chemo, I will die tomorrow? What did she mean? She said it with such compassionate conviction...

Today, I realize how many conscious and unconscious scare tactics the industry uses to have us do what they think we should do.

What to do?

The time I call "post-surgery" is the time for healing after surgery. Depending on the individual and the seriousness of the operation, it may take four to six weeks to recover. Recovery in this case means the time before going to the next step of the recommended treatment.

Increasing levels of anxiety, fear of the unknown, and physical pain mark this four- to six-week period. Friends and family advising us what we should do surround us. So many well-wishers tell us about what they have heard from others.

So many directions we can take: "We can go on this wonderful diet someone applied and cured herself from cancer!" "We can look for an alternative therapy someone took and won the battle with cancer!" Friends and family usually "know for sure" that theirs is the best option to follow. We also check the internet and do our own research! All of this results in loads of unverified information flying around us. This information overload and the pressure we feel from our well-wishers leaves us confused. What to do?

Finally, I went to my first appointment with the oncologist. Now we enter into another stage of the cancer journey—dealing with long-term treatments. In my case, it was a prestigious hospital in Toronto, Canada, that somehow evoked deep respect for the opinion I was about to hear. After the initial intake I was told that the cancer was aggressive and needed to be treated aggressively with eight sessions of chemotherapy, plus 28 days of radiation and 12 months of another adjuvant chemotherapy.

I asked my oncologist how he had come to this conclusion. He said, "I have a computer program where I enter the data from your pathology and it tells me what is the best treatment." I did not comment. We left, and the family member accompanying me, who happened to be a nurse, commented, "Oh boy, they really make you feel completely disempowered!"

That's exactly how I felt—disempowered, confused, anxious, and tired of this ordeal. So now what to do? The time of decision came and yet I wasn't clear on the right thing to do and felt pressure from every direction.

Making a decision

Yoga became my refuge over these four to six weeks. I meditated at least three times a day for 30 minutes, to reset my mind.

I chanted for 45 minutes first thing in the morning to set my day right. I couldn't do *asanas*, but I could maintain my *pranayama* practice. I also slowed down and became aware of my own body and what was happening to it. I slowly started to live in a more relaxed state. As time passed, I was regaining the connection to my own center. The access to peace of mind became easier and stayed longer.

Although my confusion decreased, I still didn't know what to do or which therapy to choose. However, each time I accessed my center in meditation, I felt an idea growing to do the traditional allopathic cancer treatment.

I didn't know where it was coming from and why it felt important to work with the oncologist on my healing, but my practice of yoga helped me to find my way. Despite the feeling of confusion, I was able to connect to my inner center, and I decided to follow it and do the traditional cancer treatment.

Today, I feel grateful for my yoga practice and for that decision. I didn't exactly know at the time why it was important, but I followed my intuition anyway. Now I understand why. I would not have been able to stand in my power and help others now had I not followed my inner voice then.

This is what yoga therapy can do—through meditation, help patients to slow down and speed up the healing. Through *asanas*, rebuild the connection with the body. Through *pranayama*, decrease the fear, anxiety, and stress of having to make a decision. It helps to find our own center to deal with our immediate surroundings and to understand that our friends and family are much impacted by our journey and mean well, despite adding to our confusion.

Finding my body...

I didn't realize how big of an impact complete anesthesia can have on a person. I was healing very quickly, so about three weeks after surgery I felt well enough for my husband to take me skiing. We both loved it, and it was a great relief from the gloom and doom of the "C" word.

But as I was putting on the skis my body felt weird, as if it wasn't mine. We went to the ski lift and suddenly I had the feeling that I didn't know my body. To my dismay, the lift was slowly approaching, and I didn't know if I would be able to maneuver my body in accordance with the movement of the ski lift. Somehow, however, I managed to sit on the lift. What a feeling of great accomplishment and relief!

As we were coming up the hill I realized that I had no idea of how to get off the lift and start skiing. I am a fairly good skier, and in the past getting on and off the lift was never a problem. This feeling was completely new. I lost all confidence in managing my body's movements. It felt as if I was completely disconnected from it.

When we reached the top I stood up from the lift and skied down the little hill, with my legs feeling like stilts and not knowing how to turn for fear of falling. After three or four times of coming down the hill I slowly regained and remembered the connection to the body and the skill came back, so I could enjoy the rest of the wonderful day.

It was an illuminating experience. For the first time, as I was trying to use my body, I witnessed with awareness the process of rebuilding my connection with it. It was much more than remembering a once-acquired skill. It felt literally as if I was sending signals down to my legs or hands and then slowly rebuilding the nerve connection back to my brain with each downhill pass. My surgeon confirmed that it usually takes about 30 days after full anesthesia to reconnect completely with the body.

Chemotherapy

Depending on what type and stage of cancer you have, your oncologist will recommend the appropriate treatment—chemotherapy, or perhaps, if you are lucky, they will recommend skipping it.

During one recent yoga therapy class at an oncology clinic I listened to a breast cancer patient talking about her experience of chemo. She said she was surprised how little effect the usually dreaded chemotherapy had on her. She said she felt just fine even right after treatment and that no one would know she was in treatment if it wasn't for her lack of hair. "I hope you realize how lucky you are," one of the other students said.

Indeed, the side effects vary depending on the drug, on the person, and on the stage of the cancer. For most of the patients I talked to, however, the experience was quite different from that of this student who had shared in class, and closer to my own.

In my case the chemotherapy involved two different drugs, with four intravenous sessions of each, every three weeks. First I had the dreaded Adriamycin with Cytoxan, and then Taxol followed by Herceptin, then called a "wonder drug."

Prior to starting the treatment I received an information package from my doctor's office containing the list of possible side effects from the chemo. It included:

- Hair loss

- Vomiting

- Sores in the mouth

- Loss of appetite

- Signs of fever, chills, and cough

- Tiredness

- Mental confusion.

Nevertheless, full of pep I went for my first session thinking, "I can beat this!" But nothing prepared me for the ordeal that spread over the next 18 months.

The first session didn't go too badly. I sat there, for 4 hours in a La-Z-Boy, reading a book, talking to other neighboring patients in the room close to me. The nurses were lovely—it was quite a different experience from my surgery time. I was a human being here; the nurses conversed with me rather than just talking at me.

There was a feeling of camaraderie and community I suddenly belonged to— the same thing tormented us and we suffered the same way and all was going to pass, eventually. We just had to endure it. There was even a bell you could ring at the end of your chemo treatment.

After 4 hours in the La-Z-Boy I got up and thought, I am okay, not too much damage done! The next couple of days were rather difficult but I was able to do *pranayama* and some *asanas* as well. By the seventh day I was back to normal, actively participating in normal life.

The next seven months were punctuated by this three-week ordeal. My visits to hospital for chemotherapy were the main excitement, which I began to dread as time went by. After the second session I decided to shave my head, as I would wake up in the morning with my pillow covered in my hair. I didn't mind losing my hair—actually, I quite enjoyed being bald. It was convenient during shower times, and everyone complemented me on the shape of my head.

After the third chemo session, I got off the La-Z-Boy feeling as if a truck had run me over. Every bone and every muscle in my body was hurting. I could barely walk and I felt disoriented. It wasn't a piece of cake anymore.

As time went by, every session became a bigger disaster in my life. By the third month of chemo treatment I would spend the three first days lying in a stupor in my bed, unable to function. Than I needed the next four days to come out of zombie mode, to show an interest in anything, to get off my bed and look out of the window and somehow slowly function during the day.

And so a pattern emerged in my treatment. The first week after treatment was a total waste. I couldn't meditate, I couldn't read, I couldn't even watch TV. The second week I would slowly recover, perhaps go for a walk outside if the weather permitted, show some interest in life.

But I couldn't do *asanas* anymore. I wasn't able to even meditate—when I sat to go within I heard every cell in my body literally screaming at me, "WHAT ARE YOU DOING TO US! DO YOU WANT TO KILLS US ALL??!!" The only yogic tool left for me was slow and deep breathing…

The swing of week 1—totally wasted, week 2—slow recovery, and week 3—functioning more or less went on for over six months. What the doctor's pamphlets didn't say was that each recovery after treatment would never reach my previous energy levels. I would recover somewhat physically, but never to the extent I had felt prior to treatment. The side effects would increase with time as the drugs poisoning my body had cumulative effects. Consequently, slowly but imperceptibly to me, I grew weaker, more fatigued, and more sluggish.

What they don't say…

Since chemotherapy also hits the immune system, patients are usually advised to avoid social gatherings for fear of becoming infected with a cold or flu. I was advised that if I woke up with a fever I should immediately go to emergency, as I had no immune system left to fight any infection.

My social life went to pits and I communicated with friends only by phone or email. This, in turn, created in me a feeling of social isolation as everyone went on with their lives and I was sitting at home trying to recover from the previous chemo treatment before going to the dreaded next one.

What the doctor's pamphlet also didn't mention was that my physical state would be reflected by my mental state. At the time I didn't realize, but I was slowly succumbing to depression. The fatigue, which was just the same as before and after the rest, took away any joy of life.

I was watching comedies but it was really difficult to find something that would make me laugh. I bought a whole series of Victor Borge DVDs—I have always loved music comedians—and he was the only one who made me forget my ordeal.

Loss of hair makes it even more difficult for some women. Losing what is regarded as the very essence of womanhood diminishes self-worth as a partner. Some women are embarrassed, some angry, some feel ashamed, some even feel naked without hair. Fortunately for me, I actually enjoyed being bald.

Living with the thought of the next treatment looming, I hit the lows a couple of times. My mental state was even worse when I realized towards the second part of treatment that I was unable to hold focus long enough to read an article or a book. I was growing more and more passive. I thought, *if this is what my life will be about, I would rather check out.*

Loving care...

What kept me going was the love I was surrounded by. One of my friends kept mailing me a new set of outrageously long earrings and matching lipsticks before each chemo session so that I could wear it for my next session. She claimed that I needed to look my best in a room full of sick and bald people. I still have some of these earrings as a reminder of the love that would lift me in difficult times.

Other friends divided each day of the week between them and I would get a phone call every day asking if I needed shopping done or whether they could bring me lunch or dinner they had just made for me. These expressions of care and love would lift me in my despair.

Often I would also get this "knowing" look from someone in an elevator or store line up, and would be asked how long still to go in my treatment. We would then have a nice conversation, which would leave me feeling somewhat lifted, "I am not alone" and "I am special."

In these times yoga therapy has a very limited possibility of helping. The overwhelming fatigue and usual depression makes it very difficult for patients to practice any form of yoga on their own. It is difficult enough to get up in the morning let alone maintain any discipline, unless we have one-on-one sessions with a therapist. Also in such cases most likely the practices would be limited to non-physical techniques like *pranayama*, chanting, *yoga nidra*, or perhaps meditation.

Chemo brain

At the end of the seven months of chemo, I was in a poor state—mentally and physically fatigued, severely depressed, with a lack of focus, no short-term memory, unable to express myself, and often not understanding what I was being told. This created embarrassing situations—such as inviting friends for lunch and not remembering they were coming. I am a fairly good driver, but my car during those seven months ended up scratched and bumped on all sides.

I remember going to a big store in my neighborhood that I used to frequent. I asked for assistance from the attendant who took me to the desired shelf and left. When I picked up my item and turned to leave, I felt completely lost and couldn't find the exit. Then I would lose my way driving back home, in my own neighborhood!

I used to be able to multitask efficiently, but that also "went out the window." I could barely muster the focus to finish one task. When someone talked to me too fast my brain would switch off and their speech became a cacophony of unrecognizable noise. I really didn't know what was going on with me.

The doctor's pamphlet mentioned confusion, but what I was experiencing felt much worse. Only later, after I had finished treatment, did I stumble on the expression "chemo brain" or "brain fog."

Where is my brain?

Little research has yet been done on the phenomenon of mental impairment caused by decreased oxygen supply to the brain and impairment of neurogenesis in the hippocampus. Apparently, scientists do not know yet why some react more strongly than others, and how long the mental impairment may last.

Typical side effects of chemo brain include:

- Depression

- Tension

- Feelings of hopelessness

- Difficulty multitasking

- Confusion over dates and appointments

- Misplacing objects

- Forgetting the details of recent events or conversations

- Struggling for the right word

- Slower mental processing

- Difficulty focusing on one task

- Feeling mentally slower than before.

Some may say, "I do that too!" But the distinctive feature here is the scale of impairment. Functioning with a completely blank brain that cannot focus, understand incoming information, or think straight *all the time* is not something

I would wish on anyone. It is like living behind a veil separating you not only from the world outside but also from your own self.

No one knows

Perhaps the most difficult part of chemo brain is that it is invisible. It creeps up on us gradually, mostly unnoticed as we progress in treatment, incrementally disabling our capacity. We notice it only in extreme times, when we do something "really stupid" and out of the ordinary. But most of my clients who come to Beyond Cancer retreats do not realize the advanced side effects they have, simply because the changes happen slowly.

Chemo brain is invisible, so our environment does not see it either. At the end of the chemo treatments everyone—family, friends, and co-workers—seems to think that we are now cured, we are okay. And yet, many of us feel that we are at the lowest point in our lives. My assessment of my abilities was that my capacities were only 30 percent of what I was before my treatment. It is a lonely place to be. Lack of information on how long these symptoms will last or what we can do to change them makes the situation even more difficult.

Yet there is also some good news. The brain has its own plasticity and we can work actively on improving our mental functions. This plasticity is based on neurogenesis—the brain's capacity to generate new neurons by itself. We can impact and enhance our brain's ability to grow new neurons through diet, lifestyle, and some activities. Below is a table listing factors that modulate our ability to generate new neurons.

Increased neurogenesis	Decreased neurogenesis
• Learning new languages	• Stress
• Exercise	• Lack of proper sleep
• Reducing normal calorie intake by 20%	• Getting older
• Intermittent fasting (minimum 18 hours)	• Ruminating thoughts
• Consumption of flavonoids	• Persistent negative emotions
• Sex	• Saturated fats
• Laughter	• Alcohol
• Activity that increases oxygen flow to the brain	• Street drugs
• Supplements—omega-3, folic acid, zinc, curcumin	• High sugar
• Crunchy food	• Depression
	• Processed foods
	• Vitamins E, B, and A deficiency
	• Soft foods

Software games are also available for those who specifically want to improve their cognitive functions. I use www.brainHQ.com, a website created by Dr Merzenich,[10] a neurosurgeon, for his clients to use after a brain operation. It involves playing certain games that train the brain in several aspects. Another similar website is www.lumocity.com

There are also other side effects of chemotherapy that are perhaps not as frequent as the ones mentioned previously.

Hypersensitive reactions can be inconvenient. I remember my cousin wearing gloves throughout the day, because touching cold or hot things felt painful for her. Eating meals or drinking was possible only when the food was at room temperature. Although she craved it very much, eating ice cream was out of the question.

Peripheral neuropathy, a result of damage to the peripheral nerves, often causes weakness, numbness, and pain, usually in the hands and feet. Walking may not be problematic but difficult when the feet feel completely numb. Handling food or a simple activity like handwriting can be tricky if we do not feel objects in our hand. Many patients attending Beyond Cancer retreats come with neuropathy in the feet or hands. Most start rebuilding these nerve connections in three weeks of intensive yoga training. From the point of view of yoga therapy it is important for us to understand when a patient has neuropathy. The ability to maintain balance during *asanas* may be compromised, and clients may be prone to fall and hurt themselves.

All kinds of infections may be happening as a result of a weakened immune system. As mentioned earlier, I was advised to go to emergency as soon as I discovered I had a fever. In some cases the body's self-defense mechanism is unable to deal with even the smallest attacks from viruses or bacteria. One of my clients had to stop coming to classes as she couldn't get rid of the flu. And so I had to visit her until she became well again.

There is also the portacath, an implanted venous access device for patients who need frequent or continuous administration of chemotherapy. Drugs used for chemotherapy are often toxic and can damage skin, muscle tissue, and veins. This can also cause discomfort in a number of *asanas*, so we always need to ask our clients if they have had an implant.

Long-term implications

And there are also the long-term side effects of treatment. During the 12 months of receiving Herceptin I had heart tests every three months, as this medication can cause heart problems. At one point during my checkup the assistant to my oncologist was alarmed by the results. However, it turned out that the oncologist ignored the warning signs and recommended continuing with the treatment. As a result, even now, 10 years after my treatments, I am still short of breath while walking at a normal pace and talking with a friend. And my legs keep swelling.

In some cases of breast cancer, women undergo induced menopause. It seems to be acceptable for women who have children and do not plan to have any more, but this is a different experience for someone who would like to have children and now will not be able to. More and more young women in their 30s and early 40s are being diagnosed with cancer. Inducing menopause and taking away the possibility of becoming a birth mother can be traumatic.

Finally, and this is something that rarely gets talked about, some chemotherapies and radiation can directly cause secondary cancers. A large study in the UK published in the well-respected *Lancet*[11] revealed that in some hospitals many cancer patients died because of chemotherapy treatment and not because of cancer. It was painful to watch my cousin vanishing before my eyes as she was being treated with chemotherapy. She and her family firmly believed in traditional treatment and there was no room for any discussion. She finally died a few days after chemo treatment.

I find it very difficult to accept the fact that we are not informed about the risk possibility when we are presented with treatment recommendations. At a training session for yoga teachers I asked the oncologist, "Why is radiation and some chemo drugs recommended despite the fact that they themselves cause cancer?" He replied that the research shows that these treatments prolong survival rates.

There is also another side effect that is so far not talked about. I remember my initial discussion with the oncologist about the recommended treatment. After he explained the process of chemotherapy, I asked, "Is there anything I can do to increase the effectiveness of treatment?" His reply left me speechless: "Don't you worry your head about it, we will take care of everything." I am sure he meant well, but this took all my power away!

Being immersed for a long time in a traditional healthcare system encourages us to invest all the power in our doctors. There are very few doctors who will leave ownership of the body to the patient and advise about different treatment options. Most doctors will "know better" and claim the right to decisions over our body and health. This leaves us powerless and encourages an attitude of victimhood. Unfortunately, as patients we usually readily accept that position as it relieves us from being responsible for our own health.

The problem with being a victim is really serious as it costs us our own health. The pay-off for the victim is lack of responsibility, but the cost of such an attitude is lack of possibility of changing anything. Cancer or disease happens to us and we feel helpless, we cannot do anything about it, we are not responsible for it. So we listen to the doctor who tells us what, when, how, and where.

Once the treatment is done, we do not actually change anything in our lives. This means we keep on doing what was partially responsible for us getting cancer in the first place.

Taking your power back

If we want to be empowered, *we* need to take a part in being responsible for *our own health* and educate ourselves as to our condition. We need to understand what in our life contributed to us getting cancer. We need to learn all carcinogenic factors under our control, and change them. Cancer is a "last call" to corrective action on our part.

The statistics cited previously do not tell us much if we do not experience any of these afflictions ourselves. But try to imagine how it would feel if, on top of chemo treatments, you suffered with insomnia. You are fatigued and in pain and on top of this, not having proper rest every night, instead, tossing and turning through the night. After a while you go on dreading another evening followed by a sleepless night. That would make anyone crazy!

Here is one of my client's accounts of what this meant for her:

> From January 2018 I experienced chronic insomnia and anxiety. I didn't want to use sleeping pills but I was getting desperate!
>
> Lee suggested certain breathing exercises just before bed. By the fourth night I was sleeping through the night! I feel I now have the tools to help myself without any side effects. (R.C.)

Yoga science is uniquely poised to provide all these tools. In our three-week intensive retreat, Beyond Cancer, we teach people a yogic approach to life. We teach them *yamas* and *niyamas*—a yogic ethical guide to living a healthy, balanced life. We teach people *mitahara*—a yogic approach to food, drink, balanced diet, and consumption habits, and its effect on our body and mind. We teach people yogic tools to manage their emotions and thought processes, especially negative ones. We teach them to be aware at all times and to choose from the variety of yogic practices the best one for the moment.

The results are astounding every time we finish the retreat. People transform their lives in almost a magical way. No longer victims, they transform helplessness into empowerment. Their attitudes to life change and they become partners with their doctors in the quest for long-term health. Amazingly, this works no matter what kind of cancer and stage. Their eyes become sparkling and their steps gain a spring.

One of our patients summed this up perfectly. Coming from France to India, he signed up for a course three months before the start of retreat. He had stage 4 colon cancer. Nevertheless, he gave 100 percent to working with the program. On the last day, when leaving, he said:

> When I signed up for this retreat I was trying to survive long enough to be able to travel to India. Now, after three weeks, I am going back to a new life!

Indeed, yoga therapy has the capacity to completely transform lives if the patient is ready...

Radiation

As the chemotherapy ends, to our relief, we are usually in a pretty precarious position. Usually life energy is low, fatigue levels are high, and we are often depressed and isolated socially. But at least we have this nightmare of the every-three-weeks ordeal behind us.

I remember my initial visit with the radiologist. First she asked me a few questions and then she kept talking to me... She probably wanted to infuse me with the maximum amount of information in the little time she had, because she talked so fast that my chemo brain simply switched off. I stopped registering what she was saying. Instead, I had a feeling that I was sitting in front of a machine gun spitting words at me—noises that I wasn't able to connect into sensible sentences. So I sat there, just looking at her, and didn't even try to break this cacophony of noise. I am sure she didn't realize that my chemo brain was not efficient enough to register all she wanted to convey to me.

I was to have 28 radiation sessions, which became a different challenge. From now on, for the duration of radiation (usually 20-odd days), I was to visit hospital on a daily basis. The treatment itself is short and painless, but the trips to the hospital and waiting in line became more and more difficult.

Managing radiation

We may not have a family member able to drive us every day, so either we rely on public transport or, if we are lucky, the local cancer society provides volunteers to drive us from and to home. This means more waiting, as usually several patients are carpooling and we have to wait for them to finish treatment. This way, at least half of the day was spent in hospital, day after day, coming back home exhausted.

Once again, almost unnoticeably, extreme fatigue creeps into our lives as we proceed. In a few days we dread having to spend another half a day in hospital, waiting before and after a few minutes of treatment. And somehow it feels like the life energy is being sucked out of us. I remember at the end of treatment not being able to walk 50 meters, not to mention one flight of stairs.

Extreme exhaustion marches hand in hand with mental weariness. You really feel like a victim, and the treatment from the doctors usually doesn't help at all. I remember my radiologist (the same machine gun) insisting on seeing me every week. Spending extra time in the hospital waiting for the doctor's appointment was simply too much for me. By mid-point of radiation, for 1 hour of activity I had to rest for 2 hours. Since I had no other side effects of radiation, no burned or inflamed skin, I explained to her that there was no need for her to see me every week. She would have none of it—"I will make an appointment for you anyway," she said "I must see you every week."

HUH?!

Finally, the end of traditional treatment came and I found myself in front of my oncologist. I was depressed, exhausted, and barely able to function with my brain hiding somewhere behind a thick fog. I was hoping that I would hear something uplifting.

"The treatments went well," I heard, "and we did everything we could. Now you can go and live your life!" I heard.

I sat there looking at my doctor thinking, "Life? What life?! This is not a life, not even existence!" I felt totally abandoned and discarded. The life I had lived in the last 18 months had been based on pure survival in the name of killing the "C." This ordeal, caused by my doctors, had left me almost completely mentally and physically incapacitated. All I heard was, "Go and live your life," as if my present condition could be completely ignored.

When patients undergo open-heart surgery they have access to long rehabilitation programs helping them to heal quickly. The oncology health system, once treatments are finished, does not suggest any next steps and nor does it provide any aftercare.

No information is offered on how to deal with side effects and what would be useful to speed up recovery. Consequently, in most cases, patients are left to their own devices at a time when they are most vulnerable and need support the most.

This is where yoga therapy picks up and shines. It deals with every person individually. With a skillful yoga therapist, the patient is empowered with self-care yogic tools. Now they are able to influence the way they feel.

Using *asanas* (body postures), breath and awareness, yoga therapy moves the body out of long-term inactivity. It establishes a close connection between mind and body. Life then becomes fuller and is experienced on deeper levels. Fatigue decreases.[12]

Other yogic tools like meditation, *yoga nidra*,[13] and chanting[14] help to develop mental stillness and emotional calm. The depression, anxiety, and anger lift, and the outlook on life changes. With time, the spring in the step and spark in the eye return.

Most importantly, through skillful yoga, the therapist will choose and modify yogic practices to the patient's physical and mental limitations, also taking into account the type and stage of cancer. This makes the therapy highly individualized and most effective for every patient.

Post-treatment

I came back home from my last visit to the oncologist disappointed with his reaction but at the same time elated that my ordeal was done. Finally finished! So now what?

I sat and pondered my situation. During the treatment I had felt somehow special. I was a "protected species" as someone undergoing extremely difficult times. People all around me were sympathetic and made me feel special.

I remember speeding through the streets of Toronto, driving back from the chemo treatment and wanting to get home ASAP. A policewoman stopped me and asked for my driver's license. "Why are you speeding?!" she asked. I didn't know I was speeding but I said, "I just finished chemo treatment, there was no driver available and so I had to drive myself. I want to get home to bed ASAP." She looked at me with compassion and gave me back my driver's license saying, "Go ahead, but slow down!"

But this aura of being special, now that the treatment was finished, was gone—I became normal, just like everyone else. I had finished my treatment and was pronounced cancer free by the doctor. Hurray!

My family and friends were celebrating and encouraging me to share in the joy. My workplace wanted me back ASAP now that I was back to normal.

Yet...

It seemed to me that the adverse symptoms of treatment were now in full force. The treatments that lasted almost two years had resulted in cumulative side effects, which I now felt unequivocally. Of course, the side effects will be different and specific to each type of cancer and treatment. Also, the level of adverse effects will be different for different people. However, below I have listed the most common side effects for all patients undergoing chemotherapy and/or radiation. These symptoms tend to occur in tandem:[15]

- Physical symptoms:

  - Pain 96%

  - Fatigue 90%

  - Anorexia 92%

  - Shortness of breath 70%

  - Insomnia 69%

  - Nausea 68%

- Psychological concerns:

  - Depression 77%

  - Anxiety 79%

  - Anger

  - Grief

  - Frustration

  - Fear

- Spiritual distress:

  - Existential concerns

  - Loss of meaning

  - Feeling of hopelessness.

Other research[16] mentions fatigue as a predominant side effect, which affects 80–90 percent of patients. It is not relieved by rest or sleep, and has both physical and cognitive components. Although my friends wanted to celebrate the end of treatment with me, my level of fatigue was such that I didn't have enough energy to go outside of my home.

I was confused. I knew my memory was not what it had been before, and all I wanted to do was to sleep. I didn't realize how depressed I was, but I felt that my life was the pits. I felt terrible, I felt isolated and extremely lonely, and yet nobody seemed to notice that. I knew I wasn't as efficient as before, but I had no idea how long this state would last or what I could do to improve things.

I found it very frustrating to deal with all the people around me. They perceived me as cured and yet I felt worse than I had done during the treatment.

My co-workers expected me to be like before—on top of my work—yet I sat there not really knowing what I should do. Life felt scary and hopeless, and I felt helpless not knowing what to do.

When I heard my oncologist say at the end of treatment, "We did everything for you. Now you can go and live your life," I thought to myself, *if this is supposed to be life, I would rather check out!*

Where is the light?

The most difficult part of my condition was that there seemed to be no light at the end of the tunnel. I was constantly exhausted and my mind was behind a veil. The world seemed different and I felt very lonely...

But life had a way of showing me the way and bringing me back, although at that moment I didn't realize it. About three months after finishing treatments I was scheduled to travel to Poland with a friend. It was the home of her ancestors and her first trip there. She is a naturopathic doctor specializing in breast cancer, and I thought it would be nice to organize some lectures for her in Warsaw. We had all the slides ready and we were set to have two workshops for the Cancer Society over the weekends.

About three weeks before our takeoff she had to cancel her trip. And I was left with pre-sold workshops, which now I had to do on my own. I had this idea that since I would be doing the talking I might just as well do it in Polish. This meant, of course, that I had to translate the slides from English to Polish. All 120 of them in three weeks!

I opened the file and started with the first slide. It had five points and I thought, no problem. I read the first point and then switched to the blank screen to translate...but my brain somehow forgot what the point to translate was. So I went back to the English slide, read the point again, went back to the blank slide...and my mind was blank again! It wasn't a joke—my mind had no memory!

That day it took me 3 hours to translate five points of the slide, and at the end of the process I felt completely exhausted. It was terrifying—I now realized how badly my mind was impaired. I looked at the 120 slides to be translated and I had three weeks to do it! This meant about six slides per day!

Nevertheless, I kept at it, and as I was proceeding, the process became easier and easier. Sometimes it felt almost like I was forcing a neuron connection to happen, and when it did, the right word would appear. It was interesting to watch this process—there was this sense that my mind was very slowly coming back from behind the veil and it was waking up!

I also noticed about three-quarters of the way into the work that my mind started to work in a different way. Instead of trying to translate word for word, I would read the point and go into inner silence, from which a corresponding phrase in Polish would come out. Often it was a much better translation than trying to match word for word.

In the end I managed to translate all the slides. In this progression I found that my mind had great plasticity and had improved quite a lot. Moreover, I felt that this whole exercise had managed to activate parts of my mind I had never accessed before. Today, 12 years later, I can see how differently my mind functions. I have lost the ability to "multifunction" and "multitask" but instead I have gained a laser-like ability to focus on what is in front of me, although I am far from where I used to be. I still keep working on exercising my mind by using, for example, the www.brainhq.com program.

As I progressed with the translation, the levels of mental fatigue lifted, but I was still physically exhausted. Walking 100 meters was an effort, and climbing a flight of stairs seemed an impossible challenge. At the time I was living by Lake Ontario near a big park. It was summer and I made a point of walking every day and challenging myself to achieve longer and longer distances. I would then sit by the water and simply be with nature. This was very nurturing—both physically and mentally. Slowly, week by week, I felt I was improving.

As I was progressing my depression also lifted. I became busy and productive—this gave me a mental lift. I went back to daily disciplines—doing asanas, pranayama, and meditation. I felt I was succeeding in recovering, and this gave me hope that I might one day reach the levels of functioning I had had before the cancer.

Today, 12 years later, I realize that this is not possible. In the two years between diagnosis and the end of the treatment, I aged about 20 years—physically and mentally. I still function pretty well, but in different ways. My body is not capable of doing what it used to do before. My mind is not the same, but I like the way it functions better now—I can achieve great focus, which was not possible before, and I can be mindful in the moment. I also know now that I can still change and improve as I keep working with it.

The end of treatment was by far the most difficult part of my cancer journey... I couldn't see the way out of the terrible state I felt I was in. And there was neither recognition nor any help forthcoming from my environment. But as I worked on my recovery using yoga and other tools, the light in the tunnel slowly started to flicker...

To finally shine with full force!

PART 3

APPLICATION OF YOGA THERAPY

In Part 2 of the book we discussed the four major NCDs that are expected to contribute to 73 percent of all deaths worldwide by 2020. We also attempted to point to the possibility yoga therapy may have of alleviating human suffering and decreasing these statistics. "Yoga can effectively change these behaviors by providing tools to deal with stress, to increase client awareness and changes in life purpose and meaning," [1] writes Matthew Taylor.

We see exactly these results in our clients after they complete three weeks of our residential retreats—Beyond Cancer and Chronic Solutions. In a way these retreats replicate intensive training in yogic ashrams, where students are subjected to long daily practices. In many cases these practices result in personality, spiritual, and health transformation. Such retreats are needed and effective in helping people rebound from cancer treatments or from a chronic NCD. The spark in the eye and spring in the step come back, and the hope for a better life returns in only three weeks of intensive yogic retreat.

In this part of the book we describe these three-week intensive yogic retreats that we have been running since 2013. We begin with a general description followed by a detailed protocol, including yogic practices and yogic tools. We have found such retreats to be of great help for people suffering from NCDs and who are going through or have completed traditional cancer treatment.

I believe that part of the effectiveness and dramatic results we describe at the end of retreats is due to the intensity of the yogic practices over the longer period of time. Doing yoga twice or three times a week for an hour or two is one thing, but doing yoga for 6 hours a day, day in, day out, for a full three weeks results in dramatic transformations and deep healing in patients not seen in normal weekly sessions.

The retreats were sparked by my personal experience of the cancer journey. There is a huge gap in cancer medical care. Typically, after surgery, cancer patients undergo chemotherapy and radiation, which may last from four weeks to a few years. Often such intensive treatments result in severe side effects, both mental and physical.

We started with Beyond Cancer retreats but very soon we expanded the offering to other NCD patients and saw equal transformation and healing in them that we recorded with objective measures. To my understanding there are a few other programs available of a much shorter duration—a weekend or a week. I am not aware of any retreat offering that is longer in duration. I find this unfortunate given that we noted such wonderful healings happening in the third week. Therefore my intention is to present as much detail as possible in the hope that some day someone else will pick up this concept and, after appropriate training, start offering it to those in need.

CHAPTER 11

The Healing Process

My body is a house, I build for me,
Myself the architect shall be;
I cannot accept the stubborn fact
That I am fashioned by every act
Which I must determine with my own will,
And there I live, for good or ill.

(Author unknown)

Introduction

I designed a three-week residential retreat for cancer patients (Beyond Cancer) in Kaivalyadhama Yoga Institute, India, in 2013. My intention was to fill in the gap in healthcare for cancer patients in need, just like I was in the past. This meant retreats were to be offered to *all* cancer patients in *all* stages of cancer. Because there is such a wide variety of cancer cases, and because yoga therapy lends itself to a highly individual approach, the number of participants in a given retreat is limited to a maximum of eight at a time, with three facilitators running the retreats. Two facilitators are certified C-IAYT and are fully trained to run the program. They conduct group classes, as well as facilitating discussions, and offer individual yogic counseling sessions. A third person, ideally a psychologist or social worker and simultaneously a yoga teacher, has a more supportive role. They respond to the everyday needs of the participants and support the two main facilitators throughout the three weeks of the program. Support for the participants' needs is very important—they have generally come from a medical environment, which is usually disempowering and unfriendly. A warm and empathic personality coupled with an understanding of how to handle human suffering is very much welcomed and appreciated by participants.

A three-week comprehensive protocol was designed, with six days per week of progressive yogic practices, including the following each day:

- 1 hour of gentle *asanas*

- 1 hour of *pranayama* (breath management techniques)

- 1 hour of meditation

- 1 hour of *yoga nidra* (deep relaxation)

- 45 minutes of chanting and meditation

- 1.5 hours of lecture or group work

- 30 minutes of yogic counseling on request.

Providing participants can move about independently, those with all cancers at all stages are accepted. Most come within 12 months of finishing treatment. Most also come with the severe side effects of chemotherapy and radiation—high levels of tension, depression, anger, fatigue, anxiety, and chemo brain. Most also have a "victim" attitude, well entrenched by the healthcare system. All of this creates the need for a high level of individual support. As the retreat is residential, participants stay and work together for three weeks in the same small group, which in itself becomes a therapeutic tool.

Yoga classes offered for cancer patients are usually free of charge, conducted by wonderful yoga teachers who have a lot of good will. These classes are typically limited to gentle *asanas* and some *pranayama*, offered once or twice a week. These are very helpful, but the effect is limited, especially if the tools used are limited to *asanas*.

Our programs differ in many ways. First of all, acceptance of a participant into the retreat begins with the client filling in a case record, a three-page assessment questionnaire (see Chapter 4). This gives us a picture of the physical state the participant is in, and what their expectation is of the retreat. Based on this, we determine if the participant would be able to attend and enjoy the benefits of the retreat.

The retreat has a very comprehensive protocol, which uses all elements of yoga, and not just *asanas*. It takes clients from Day 1 to Day 21 in a systematic way. Yogic techniques are used to work not only on the body, but also more importantly, we work on emotions and the mind. We want to address the causes of the diseases, not just the symptoms.[1] We help participants to recognize carcinogenic thought processes and give them the tools to learn to change their thought patterns and manage their minds. We help to resolve or release negative emotions, which also contribute to the disease and are stored somewhere deep down.

This emphasis, coupled with the intensity of the protocol and length of the retreat, creates a deep spiritual transformation in many. But most importantly, I believe these retreats move people—in 21 days—from victimhood to empowerment, helping them to feel "in charge" of their lives. This, in itself, is a tremendous change in life attitude. As one participant stated:

> I am so glad I found this course and was able to come. It's exactly what I needed at this point in my cancer recovery. I came into this course feeling depressed, hopeless, fatigued, and disconnected from my body. I am now leaving three weeks later with a sense of hope for a meaningful and rich life, a feeling of joy returning and with greater energy and belief in my body. (N.O.)

We also spend a lot of time educating participants on carcinogenic factors in their diet, lifestyle, and environment. Finally, we help them to examine their old belief systems and to create a new, healthier one. I believe that there isn't any program like ours at the moment. I am hopeful that this book may spread the word around, and as a result, more programs like this will become available, as there is a great need for them.

Our Beyond Cancer retreats have been so effective that we have created a sister program called Chronic Solutions for Chronic Diseases (also called NCDs). The Chronic Solutions retreat is based on the same principles using the same tools as Beyond Cancer. The difference lies only in some lectures that are more relevant for NCDs and that are not cancer-specific.

We found that the Chronic Solutions retreat is very effective in helping patients with CVD, diabetes, psoriasis, anxiety, depression, and many other diseases caused by stress and a destructive lifestyle. We have been conducting Chronic Solutions retreats since 2014 with equal success—by addressing the core causes of the problem, which then reduces symptoms.[2]

The classes are small, with no more than eight participants and no fewer than three. There is great value in being a part of a group, which, with time, becomes a powerful support tool for each participant.[3] Therefore, the program has a designated room in which all group classes take place: yoga, lectures, film projections, etc. And there is also a private space to provide individual yogic counseling for participants upon request.

The food provided is mostly organic, and the participants have three vegetarian meals daily, including a cold pressed juice in the morning, before breakfast.

Usually, while assessing participants, we detect stumbling blocks in *manomaya* or *pranamaya koshas* in the form of a rigidity of core beliefs, attitudes, emotions, convictions, or some kind of mental weaknesses. Disturbances in breathing or a short and shallow breath point to disturbances on mental or emotional levels. The program helps to move participants over the three weeks from their established patterns and to create new ones. We encourage them to keep a detailed diary from Day 1. This can help them to become aware of their own progress as well as to build their self-awareness. As one of our participants wrote in their three-month review:

> The retreat has further propelled me on path of self-discovery. I understand my body, my feelings, and my needs in a much better way now… There are days when I can't even close my eyes because I am scared. There are days when I cry. I started a diary again where I write every day…it has enabled me to mirror myself and look at myself and accept all my emotions with love and appreciation. (J.S.)

Perhaps the most important thing in this process is to help our participants, no matter the nature of their problem, move from victimhood to owning their part in the problem. Victim posturing is the most common predicament. Typically our clients have gone through a long and traumatic process, which has rendered them powerless, where the medical doctors appeared to be all-mighty and all-knowing. This encourages our participants to feel victims to a disease or sometimes identify with the disease, that is, "I am diabetic." If you are settled in such an attitude, you cannot do anything to improve your life. Victimhood can be a very comforting place to be—it relieves us from personal responsibility for our thoughts, emotions, and actions—but when we are victims, we cannot change anything because nothing depends on us.

Moving into an empowering position might be very challenging and scary, and requires people to own their contribution to creating the problem; not everyone wants to take that responsibility. For many it may be too difficult to accept the discrepancy between their image of themselves and who they truly are. However, victimhood means disempowerment, and so no changes can be made. Healing can only begin when the client moves into personal responsibility for their own health.

Here is one of the more dramatic accounts of taking health into your own hands:

> During my stay, I faced an unexpected significant health issue. I had a pancreatic crisis which is very painful and for which no painkillers are efficient. Desperate, I decided to practice meditation. Then, miraculously, the feeling of pain disappeared. I could not believe it but it was really happening. The pain was gone. It came back eight hours later and then I did again a longer meditation

and again the pain was gone forever. From that point, my level of motivation skyrocketed and ever since I have been practicing meditation regularly. (Colette Casmir)

In the following pages we describe in detail the principle of the retreats and the tools used. But first we look at the stages of healing that our patients generally go through during the three-week retreat.

Stages of healing

As mentioned above, we have noticed certain trends in our participants' healing and transformation during the 21 days of the retreats. These can be divided into three stages.

Stage one

Typically, we spend the first week helping patients settle into the routine of the day in the new-for-them environment. By the end of the first week or the beginning of the second, depending on the participant's earnestness, we see them going through some kind of crisis. The yogic practices start working, and their pain connected to disease or any major incident in life is coming out. Their long-held negative emotions are coming out. Their rigid attitudes are challenged. Yoga practices force them out of their established comfort zones to vulnerability, where they have to face themselves and their own inner issues.

We help participants meet their internal challenges by teaching them appropriate yogic practices and by supporting them with yogic counseling sessions. We hold the space for them, so that they can feel supported in meeting their inner challenges. We help them to reconnect with their bodies. We teach them yogic tools to deal with their strong negative emotions. We help them to become aware of their routine negative thought processes and teach them how to change them.

Here is another participant's recollection:

On a third day [of the retreat] during meditation after chanting mantra for 30 min I, an avid atheist, I had a vivid vision of Christ and light entering through top of my head. I was shaken, moved to tears and deeply feeling the truth of the experience.

I asked for [a] counseling session during which I discovered my life long struggle. My mother became pregnant at 45 and was crying through pregnancy in fear of being too old to bring her daughter up. Since my birth, I was trying to make as little trouble to my parents as possible. I never had a period of rebellion when growing up. Denying my own truth since childhood for the sake of pleasing others seemed to have been my life long struggle. I found this discovery to be very helpful and very freeing. (A.R.)

This first week is also a time during which we work on building a sense of community within the group by encouraging dialog, sharing our stories, and general interactions during classes. Thus the group becomes an added support and important factor in the participants' healing over the three weeks.

Who we need to be

This is the time when the participants need a lot of care and support. We usually have a dedicated person on the facilitation team, a "care taker" who does just that. They make the participants feel that there are people who are genuinely concerned with their wellbeing, ready to help them to solve any and all of their problems, and answer any questions they may have.

By the second day we have the results of the participants' tests (described in detail in the following) and we know their levels of anger, anxiety, depression, tension, fatigue, and energy. We observe and get to know their strengths and weaknesses and address them in an indirect way. For us, as yoga therapists, it is a time of increased sensitivity, reading covert and overt signs from our participants, even if they are only expressed by body language. Based on this feedback, we adjust the details of the program according to the needs of the group. So, for example, if we have someone in the group with a high level of anger, we may choose a guided meditation dealing with forgiveness or heart opening. The sharing in the circle after the practices usually reveals the effectiveness (or lack thereof) of our adjustments.

Right after we calculate the results of the first day's tests we sit down with each participant individually and discuss the results. This is a time for building a rapport between the facilitators and participant. Often people are not aware of their negative emotional states and this initial discussion may reveal many more details. Based on this initial discussion, we may also recognize a need and offer individual yogic counseling with any of the qualified facilitators. The offering needs to come out as a general open-ended proposal for the participant to act upon. In most cases the yogic counseling works only if and when people are willingly going through the process.

We also watch for the participant's attitude towards each person on the facilitating team. As the days pass each participant will connect to a greater or lesser degree with each facilitator and will have their favorite. This person will be the one to do the most effective yogic counseling. We always need to keep in mind that in our relationship with the participant we risk the possibility of their transference, that is, redirection of emotions that were originally felt in childhood, onto the facilitator. And so for them we become an archetype of a loving or cruel mother or father, a worst enemy, or greatest friend, etc....

As one of the participants said:

> The second week seems to be the week when "the stuff rises" so to speak, and in my case this was most certainly the case. It took the form of finding myself almost uncontrollably angry at our course leader...poor Lee. This exploded one day and I attacked her verbally, an assault in the face of which she stood calmly firm and looked at me with increased attention. We subsequently had a chat about it and I realized I was projecting an old hatred born of fear onto her, and having seen it, as is the way with these things...it collapsed and I was free of it! (N.P.)

Our role, then, as facilitators is to accept the participant's anger or love with equanimity and to remain a composed and compassionate listener, holding the space for them. If we see a need, we may suggest additional yogic practices.

Stage two

In stage two relationships within the group and with the facilitators are somewhat established. The six days of intensive yoga training brings into the light the "stuff" which, in the past, was pushed into the unconscious mind, or brings to the surface issues that are in the consciousness but remain unresolved. Thus a time of crisis arrives.

The second week is also the week of intense spiritual work, and inching from victimhood to empowerment. As all the classes are held in a group setting for the three weeks, the participants also watch each other going through this process, knowing that they are not alone! They can observe others progressing through the second week's tribulations, and the group becomes a very strong support and encouragement system for everyone. People open up, and their deepest desires and pains are shared freely in the group. In such a supportive environment the true healing happens.

The manifestation of the crisis is, of course, very varied depending on the person, their history, issues, and attitudes. Over the years of running the retreat programs we have experienced everything, including simple negativity creeping into the client's judgment of people and situations, people resisting opening to their own feelings until the end of the program, people resigning from the program "because it's not for me," bouts of overt anger at someone or something, and we also had full-fledged panic attacks.

Here is an account of one of the participants:

Her first incident of anxiety attack happened six days into the program. The group planned to go shopping to a city that is 2 hours' drive from here on a Sunday. On that day, she came to one of the facilitator's rooms at 5:30 in the morning, complaining about fainting spells with some strong discomfort in the abdomen (where the cancer had been). She was shaking and it was apparent that she had a strong anxiety. We started with a long, deep yogic breathing for 10 minutes, followed by *nadi shuddhi* for another 15 minutes. Then we chanted "*omkar*" for quite a while. As we proceeded, her anxiety level decreased and her discomfort and fainting spells lost intensity. However, she was convinced that her state was purely physical.

The medical doctor came and checked her blood pressure and pulse, and as they were normal, he suggested that she attend class as usual. She, however, found it very difficult to believe that her reaction was purely psychosomatic. [Her previous experience with allopathic doctors made her very distrustful of the correctness of any diagnosis.] She attended morning yoga and the rest of the day went relatively well. The group decided to postpone the shopping trip to the next week.

The following Sunday [end of the second week], Lee met our participant early in the morning by the tea spot. The patient said that she had an anxiety attack again and that she didn't sleep the whole night. However, this time she didn't give in to panic. She said: "Throughout the night I sat on my bed and used *pranayama* (*nadi shuddhi*, *sitali*) and chanted '*omkar*' and was able to manage my level of anxiety on my own. And we are going shopping!" she exclaimed, with a smile at the end. (A.R.)

This is where the value of an intensive residential program comes in. I suspect that if people are not confined to a space and only come for a day program, in times of crisis they may stop coming altogether. Facing oneself is sometimes very difficult and can be a very painful process. If the program is residential, the participant has nowhere to go, and they have other members of the group encouraging them to continue. But we did have participants who, although they stayed in the program until the end, refused to honestly work on themselves and simply sailed through the three weeks. Needless to say, they failed to reap the effects of the program in their lives.

WHO WE NEED TO BE

Most of the time people do not realize that what they are going through is simply "their own stuff" manifesting in life. This is, in a way, a critical moment; our challenge and opportunity is to turn the participant's eyes from looking outside for the blame to actually realizing that the "button" lies within them. You cannot perceive outside yourself that which you are not, or cannot feel, within yourself. Once we can help them realize that their reaction is a projection of their own issues onto others, then an outside reality is seen only as a trigger, allowing them to own and become conscious of the blocks in their individual inner world.

This is a great challenge to us as facilitators—we need to adjust our approach to the level of awareness of our participant. This requires sensitivity, spiritual maturity, knowledge of yogic assessment, and understanding of where our client is coming from and what will work for them. It also requires a good understanding of which yogic tools will be most effective in this particular case. But most of all, it requires from us spiritual maturity and an ability to be aware of our own triggers so that we can rise above them and not allow them to contaminate our relationship with the participant.

Needless to say, this is also a time when the participant will choose who they would like to confide in and who they would like to have for private yogic therapy sessions. We have to have at least two, preferably three, able facilitators to give our participants a choice. There is no possible way for one person to be able to fill the demanding role of a yoga therapist for all participants. In case of a strong negative transference onto one facilitator, another one can play the role of the "good guy" and do effective yogic counseling.

Yoga has a very important role to play in this healing, as it provides a great number of very effective tools allowing us to facilitate and speed up the process of the participant becoming more aware of their own issues. It also provides very effective methods of successfully dealing with and resolving them, as illustrated above. Here is a statement from one of the participants speaking to this issue:

> I didn't have a belief in myself to make the decisions as to the next step of my cancer journey. And now I do! I have to say that that is a miracle in itself—to feel empowered moving forward to make my own decisions. I found the guidance from within and I now know that I can find the answers within myself. I feel connected to myself and I feel strong. I am very grateful for that to this program. *Yoga nidra* had perhaps the biggest impact on me from all the yogic tools we practiced. I felt most resistance to it at the beginning. But at the end I gained the most from the experiences I had during *yoga nidra* sessions. (J.)

Stage three

In week two the participant recognized the surfacing issue to be dealt with and tried yogic tools, which began to improve the situation. Stage three is about continuing and refining what has been suggested in week two. For some it may be specific *asanas*, for some *pranayama*, for some additional meditations, for some it may be reframing through yogic counseling, and for others it may be chanting. The focus now is to use with awareness whatever modality of the program works for the participant and to be aware of any changes.

The third week is usually marked by considerable change in the participant's attitude and mood. The emotional, mental, and spiritual work they did in the second week, as painful and difficult as it was, now makes them feel empowered and strong. They now feel that their health depends on *them*, and not on their doctors. Their enthusiasm for life replaces their former hopelessness, depression, and anxiety. Their energy levels are rising, and the hope and acceptance of their lot is apparent. They begin to feel powerful and motivated to continue with yogic practices after going back home. Their minds are now focused on boldly looking forward and planning how to change their lives to live healthier and longer.

Upon completion of the retreat, patients are usually able to take full responsibility for their health and the choices they make in everyday life. That gives them tremendous energy to look forward to a new life. As one of our recent participants said:

> Several of my friends have said how much more positive I have been since returning from [retreat in] Poland and I certainly feel so much calmer, in charge of my life and ability to do what I enjoy doing. The retreat gave me lots to think about and I am so pleased that I was privileged to be able to experience all it had to offer. (M.G.)

Since the program is fairly intensive, the changes and improvements happen quite quickly and are often dramatic. Such spiritual transformation motivates participants to work even more to continue practices at home. Perhaps this is the most important part of the program, the realization by the participant that their wellbeing depends on them rather than a doctor and medication. Such a feeling of empowerment becomes a very powerful motivator to continue using yoga long after they finish the program and return home. Perhaps this is the reason why we get such good results in our tests after the three-month follow-up.

Here is another participant during their three-month follow-up interview:

> I no longer suffer nausea, anemia, fatigue, difficulty in focusing on one task, and I don't feel mentally slower than before anymore. I have no anxiety attacks like before

and my sleep is great. My colon is clean as a whistle but I have been diagnosed now with irritable bowel syndrome. The doctor gave me Sulpirod [a psychotropic med], and I took it for two weeks but I stopped it. I just rely on my yoga to keep me well. Looking back the main benefit of the retreat for me is twofold. First, it empowered me, gave me self-confidence and belief in myself. It gave me tools to deal with my life and health. It also gave me focus and discipline to maintain my daily program, which makes me feel good and healthy. (A.R.)

WHO WE NEED TO BE

Our role now becomes much easier. We become a friend and true supporter in the work our participants are doing and the results they are getting. Our focus is on the improvements we see in the participants, and we are quick to point them out. We are now free to explain the process they went through, point out the positive changes in them, encourage them to continue, and invite the group to discuss it.

During this week participants spend two to three days working on a life mandala. This is, for many, a time of setting new goals, reviewing old thought patterns and belief structures, and creating new ones. By now we know each participant well enough to tailor our approach in helping them to create a meaningful document that becomes their new roadmap for when they return home. Again, this is a very important role in that we may encourage our participants to "dig a little deeper" into their own inner world in order to create a more meaningful plan for the future. We do so by asking probing questions and not letting them "off the hook." If the group is homogeneous and time allows for it, sharing or reviewing individual mandalas and experiences can become a very powerful tool.

Another participant notes:

Amazing what a difference this yoga makes. I feel more confident, balanced, and look more positively into the future. I have a very clear idea of how I will implement positive changes into my daily life when I get home. (N.W.)

For the last two days of this week participants practice yoga on their own. We prepare for each participant an individualized list of practices, which they perform during normal scheduled hours on their own. The therapists are available for any questions or corrections. The idea is to have each person feel comfortable and confident that they are doing all the practices in a proper and safe way, on their own. This will help them to feel confident when they do yoga in their home environment. We also encourage them to use whatever they have learned at the retreat in their daily life. Here is one account:

> In 2017, two days before an annual general meeting of *about* 300 people, I learn that I have to replace the hospitalized president, run the meeting, and give a speech. But I am away from the office professional in 200 km [meaning that she was 200 km away from the office]. I leave my work at 4.30pm to be at 7pm at the place of the meeting. I have a spare moment of 30 minutes; I take advantage of it, by isolating myself and make 15 minutes of *asanas* by ending by *sirsana* that I just hold for 5 minutes. And miracle, in spite of the full working day, the drive, and the stress to speak in public, I felt as rested and calm mentally. And, of course, the meeting went very well... (B.M.)

One day before the last we also have participants submit the same tests they did at the beginning. We then prepare the scores for the outgoing interview. This usually happens on the last day, with each participant individually. This is the time for privately summarizing their stay here, reviewing test scores and achievements, and for setting the yogic routines to be continued at home daily. We use the "Home Plan" document (see Appendix 4) with individual notes so that participants are left with written and clear instructions. We also give them electronic files for guided mediations and for *yoga nidra* sessions.

In the words of one participant:

> As I arrived back at Heathrow my partner commented that the old me had returned home. The world had been lifted from my shoulders, I felt happy again and more peaceful than I have ever felt. I now had some direction, I had taken back some control and most importantly I had the tools to keep myself well.
>
> After a month of being home it became quite clear that incorporating all these practices into a regular busy lifestyle was not going to be easy. It takes effort and time to get into a routine and results are not always seen immediately. The shifts at first are quite subtle but there is no doubt that over time the impact it can have on your life is immeasurable and worth every effort. (Z.A.)

Testing

We started to test our clients from the very first retreat to have some kind of objective indication of the effectiveness of the retreat. We chose three standard psychological tools, due to the lack of availability of yogic assessments at the time, and continued gathering data for years to come. These tools were suggested as standard tests, which would indicate to us the effectiveness of the retreats in the best way, yet would not overburden the client with too many complicated tests. We used the abbreviated WHO Quality of Life (WHOQOL-)BREF questionnaire,[4] developed by 15 international WHO field centers to reflect the cross-cultural application. We felt it was exceptionally suited for our purpose since we had clients attending from all over the world.

The WHOQOL-BREF expressed assessment in four categories—Physical health, Psychological health, Social relationship, and Environment. The figures below show the psychological means for two groups of participants (six cancer survivors from a Beyond Cancer retreat and seven NCD patients from a Chronic Solutions retreat). The data was gathered on the first day of the retreat (D1), 20 days of the retreat (D20), after three months (3M), after six months (6M), and after 12 months (12M). As you can see, significant improvement is shown on the D20 point, with little deviation over time.

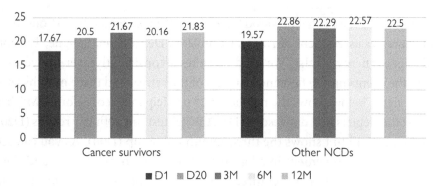

Long-term psychological means of the two groups

Another tool we use is the Hospital Anxiety and Depression test, which has 14 questions and is very simple to use. It expresses the levels of depression and anxiety, since these two most often go together and are one of the main side effects of the cancer journey. The same two groups' median (see the two figures below for anxiety and depression) show significant improvements, which hold over 12 months, none coming back to the baseline.

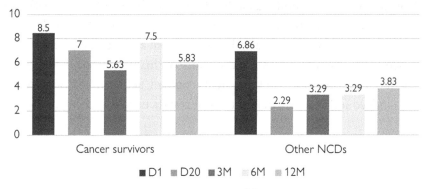

Long-term anxiety means of the two groups

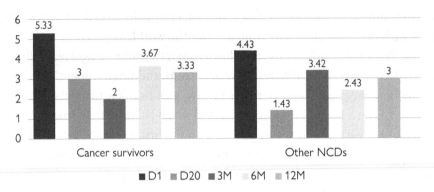

Long-term depression means of the two groups

Finally, we use the Profile of Mood States (POMS) test, which has 65 questions and expresses assessment of Anger, Confusion, Depression, Fatigue, Tension, and Vigor (energy levels). We used these tests consistently over the years to assess the clients on the first and last days of the retreat and three months later.

The figure below shows the median of 27 participants' scores for POMS. The darkest tint depicts first day results (D1), the lightest tint 20th day results (D20), and the medium tint shows the three-month follow-up (D90). As you can see, there is great improvement in all aspects of the score over 21 days, and these levels do not change much after three months—so improvements hold and none of the factors come back to the baseline of the first day of the retreats. These results are in synch with many research projects done on the effectiveness of yoga, including the recent "Review of yoga therapy during cancer treatment."[5]

Since the test results of POMS list the levels of six factors, we discuss with each client individually every test result. We do this for two reasons—first, to assess their own awareness of their inner emotional state. The summary of tests is often quite illuminating for them as they are normally not aware of their mood states. Levels of depression, tension, and anger in particular are habitually underestimated. The second reason for discussing these test results with clients is to bring their attention to their inner states throughout the 21 days of the retreat—they know we will do another assessment at the end of the retreat, and this encourages them to become more aware of their emotions throughout the retreat. It is also good to see that the clients confirm, at the end of the retreat, that they do indeed feel much better, as the test results usually indicate.

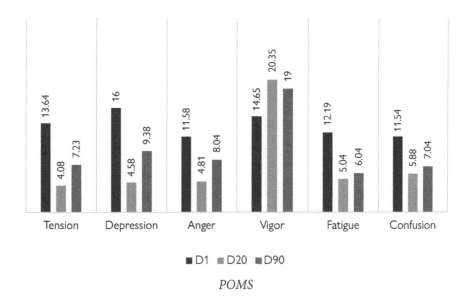

POMS

Over the years we gathered data, testing our participants in both retreats—Beyond Cancer and Chronic Solutions—on the first and last days of the retreat and following up three months later. Based on that data, we published a paper in a research journal[6] in 2014 and wrote an article[7] in 2016. In addition, we are currently at the end of gathering data from a longitudinal research study where we followed up on our clients for 12 months, with more thorough testing. The results will be published at the end of 2020.

CHAPTER 12

Yogic Practices

In this chapter we describe in detail the yogic practices we use during our retreats. We also explain why we use them. Most of our participants are over 50 years old, with very little experience of yoga. With this in mind, the practices we choose are meant to move the body out of long-term inactivity, with the participants re-establishing a close connection with the body.

Move the body out of long-term inactivity

During treatments many of the participants lead a sedentary lifestyle due to lack of energy and the side effects of the treatments. Even regular gym-goers tend to slack on their discipline due to constant visits to the hospital and the tendency to avoid public places due to a low immune system. Consequently, many have been fairly inactive compared with the time before their diagnosis and treatments.

Some participants may initially show resistance to physical exercises due to neuropathy and/or high levels of fatigue. A multicenter, randomized controlled trial, however, showed that gentle body movement and resistance training was effective in reducing chemotherapy-induced neuropathy and fatigue in 355 patients.[1]

In rare cases we may encounter a strong resistance from a client to trying something new. Here is the note I made in my diary about a 37-year-old client who had breast cancer and who had never tried yoga before:

> She negotiates every *asana*, every *pranayama* with questions "How do I know it will work?" "Will it work if I do not believe in it?" "How much do I have to do?"
>
> Additionally there was a great resistance in her to take responsibility for her own actions and behavior.

Re-establish a close connection with the body

The clients coming to the program may have different levels of awareness of their own body. Some lose that awareness during chemotherapy—the side effects may be severe and they simply distract themselves in order to not think of and feel the side effects in their bodies. Over a period of time this may lead to losing touch with their body.

For us, as yoga therapists, this means that our participants may push themselves to do yoga practice beyond their capacity, causing them to suffer injuries. We therefore need to be very cautious and observant in making sure that we do not allow over-exertion. "Gentle, slow, and easy" is the name of the game.

We introduce our participants to and develop awareness of the inner landscape, encouraging the posture of "observer" over the three-week program. We all live with our awareness and senses directed to the outside world. When we concentrate on the outside, what is going on inside is unnoticed. We are often not aware of the pain until we sit and calm down. Sometimes we are not aware of our emotions, especially those that are unwanted—until we cannot contain them anymore and we burst out, surprising ourselves and every one else.

All yogic practices are designed to develop awareness of our inner life, awareness of the body, of our emotions, and of our thought processes. And so we teach all yogic practices in such a way as to redirect a client's awareness from "outside into inside."

This is extremely important for the NCD population. Before participants come to the program they will have lived their lives for an extended period of time typically in high levels of anxiety, fear, depression, and other mental disturbances. Using appropriate commands and reminders, we help them to develop mental stillness, focus, and emotional calm by promoting the "witnessing" stance during all our classes.

More importantly, perhaps, we also want them to become aware of how each practice affects them. In order to do that, we start and finish each class with a moment of awareness. At the beginning, in sitting position, with closed eyes, we direct their attention to:

- Their physical body—how does it feel?

- Their emotional body—what are the feelings and emotions in the moment?

- The quality of their thoughts in the moment.

At the end of the class we do the same by asking them:

- Is there any difference in the way your physical body feels now, compared with the beginning of the class?

- Is there any difference in your feelings and emotions now, compared with the beginning of the class?

- Is there any difference in the quality of your thoughts now, compared with the beginning of the class?

We empower participants with self-care yogic tools and gently move them from victimhood to empowerment. Through yogic counseling we help them "to be with" an emotion or a thought without judgment and to deal with whatever comes up by using yogic practices. This way they experience self-empowerment and are able to control their inner states with newfound tools.

The ability to recognize and self-manage their own inner disturbances, as well as mental and bodily states, becomes a very powerful motivator to continue practicing yoga at home after the program is finished. They feel empowered and not as dependent on the doctors and medicines as before.

We encourage our clients from Day 1 to keep written diaries in which they record their experiences right after the practices and at the end of each day. We help them by asking them to answer two basic questions:

- "Please elaborate on your experiences, feelings, difficulties, if any, after each yoga practice."

- "Describe any significant changes in your feelings and/or perceptions today."

Keeping notes after each practice and at the end of the day helps to keep clients introspective and to track changes and their own progress.

In what follows you will find a detailed description of yogic techniques and practices with detailed instructions on how to run each class throughout the three weeks. But before this, we must stress the need for intelligent flexibility.

The participants are coming from all walks of life and their knowledge of yoga, their psychological predisposition, and their physical flexibility may differ greatly. There may be a yoga instructor in the class sitting next to someone who has never heard about yoga. Each group of participants will be different, with different dynamics and at different levels of physical flexibility. So the facilitators' adaptability in their approach and the methods within a given framework are key to successfully leading participants towards health.

It is also very important to note that we, as yoga therapists, do not heal the participants. We use our skills to constantly assess them, and when they are ready, we offer suggestions for the next steps. We always wait for them to show a sign that they are ready to proceed to the next stage. This way we "walk half a pace" behind them, facilitating their own healing.

Throughout the day they do all the practices, but it is important to recognize which yogic practices they respond to favorably. For some people, *asanas* are the most beneficial, some people respond very well to *pranayama*, others to meditation or chanting. As we proceed we need to recognize, as soon as possible, individual preferences so that we can recommend individual practices for particular participants as we help them to move through a possible crisis if or when it comes in the second week.

The importance of finding the meaning of the disease or the suffering that participants have been through for their healing process has been documented by many researchers. This "meaning-making" empowers them and accelerates recovery. Many studies of meaning in life have shown that finding such meaning is related to higher levels of psychological wellbeing and also to some dimensions of physical health, including a health-related quality of life.[2]

It helps participants to see the sense and reason for their suffering. Often after recovering they use their own experiences to assists others, which helps them to have a sense of a purposeful and happy life. They transform their suffering into their strength. We introduce life mandalas, which participants do in the third and last week, for exactly such a purpose, to move them from weakness to finding their own strength within.

CHAPTER 13

Yogic Protocol

In this chapter we describe yogic tools we use and how and why we use them. We start with *asanas*, go through *pranayama*, meditation, *kirtan kriya, mantras, mudras, yoga nidra*, and chanting.

Our typical daily schedule, Monday to Saturday, is as follows:

Time	Activity
6:45–7:45	*Asana* class
7:45–8:15	*Pranayama*
8:30–9:30	Breakfast
9:30–11:00	Lecture/group work
11:00–11:30	*Pranayama*
11:30–12:00	Meditation
12:30–1:30	Lunch
1:30–3:00	Break
3:00–3:15	*Kirtan kriya*
3:20–4:50	*Mudras* with meditation
5:00–6:00	*Yoga nidra*
6:30–7:30	Dinner
8:00–8:45	Chanting and meditation
9:00	Lights out

According to *pancha kosha*, disturbance usually starts in *vijnamaya kosha* or *manomaya kosha*, and if not corrected, it steps down to *pranamaya*, and will then finally manifest itself in *annamaya kosha*. The yogic tools we use during each day of the retreats are chosen to deal with all of these levels. In the morning we start with 1 hour of *asanas*, which predominantly move the organs of the physical body. However, even our *asana* classes are conducted with an emphasis on mind management by keeping awareness of the body during the *asanas* and maintaining slow and deep breaths. This way the participants work simultaneously with *pranamaya* and *manomaya koshas*. The 60 minutes of meditation and 1 hour of *yoga nidra* daily may have a direct impact on *manomaya kosha* and *vijnamaya kosha*. *Kirtan kriya*, as you will see, has a direct impact on the cellular level and at the same time is a great tool in healing brain fog. We end the day with chanting, which spreads its impact across all four of the lower *koshas*.

Asanas

The morning class consists of 60-minute easy *asanas* based on the *Hatha Yoga* tradition. *Asanas*, or yogic postures, differ from normal stretching exercises in the way they are performed. Therefore, it is very important for us, as yoga therapists, to lead participants in an *asana* class in the proper way with an understanding of what we want to achieve.

Our first aim is to relax, reduce the feeling of stress, and connect participants to their body and emotions. We do this by first explaining the interconnectedness between the mind, the body, and the breath.

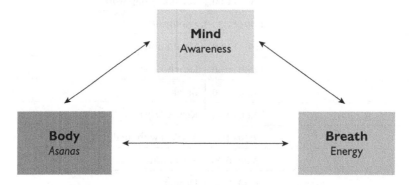

Interdependence of mind–body–breath rate

There is interdependence between mind–body–breath. When we have disturbing thoughts, the breath quickens and the body's biology changes in response to mental stress. When we willfully change our thoughts into those that are more agreeable and peaceful, the breath automatically slows down and the body relaxes. The same interdependence happens between the body and the other two factors. When we slowly stretch our body in *asanas*, the mind quiets down and breath becomes steady. Finally, when we start controlling our breath, willfully making it deep and slow, both the body and the mind relax and slow down.

At the beginning, most of our participants cannot control their mind (see side effects of treatment in Chapter 10) and most have rather stiff and stressed bodies; however, we can help them to become aware of their breath and teach them slow and deep breathing to use during an *asana* class. When they slow down the breath to as low as six breaths per minute, the mind will relax and the body's self-healing mechanism will be activated.[1] The breath also becomes a bridge between body and mind—that is, between the *asana* and awareness. This way an *asana* class becomes not so much about the body and muscles, as it is usually used in the West, but rather about deepening one's awareness of the inner world of mind, emotions, and body.

The *asana* is taught in three stages that are explained to the participants before the beginning of the class:

- Dynamic stage: From a relaxed posture, participants are led to move slowly and smoothly into the final posture, where they find their limit and back off a little.

- Static stage: As they hold the *asana*, they are led to find a comfort zone and relax into it. The whole static stage of *asana* is about teaching them the feeling of "being" in *asana*, rather than "doing" *asana*. This is achieved by slow and deep breathing combined with body awareness while comfortably holding the posture.

  This is the stage where their inner work starts. The participants are led to become aware of their body, which muscles are contracted, and which can be relaxed as they hold the posture. If they feel slight muscle tightness or stress in the body, we ask them to direct their breath and attention to that point, breathing in and out of that point of the body. We remind them to continue slow and deep breathing so they can relax into the *asana* even more. We also remind them to be aware of their mental and emotional states. We gently increase the length of holding the *asana* as they gain strength during the three weeks of the program.

- Dynamic stage: We lead them into releasing the *asana* to a relaxation posture in a slow and smooth way. At the end of the *asana* we make them aware of the experience they have just had and of any changes in the body due to the *asana* they have just performed.

As we lead participants into *asanas* we emphasize what is most important in each. For instance, in *paschimootasana* (Sitting Forward Fold) we teach our participants to elongate their spine on the inhale and to hinge from the hip joint on the exhale without overcompensating by lumbar or thoracic spine flexion.

Asanas are always interwoven with short periods (15–20 seconds) of total relaxation. We prepare participants to come out of them by connecting them to the breath and stressing the need to keep an unchanged rhythm of the breath throughout the practice.

We want to make sure that practicing *asanas* never leads to fatigue and that participants are refreshed and peaceful after the class. We are always aware of their physical limitations and offer appropriate modification when required, always stressing that "It is not about how far you go, but how you go" (Mark Stephens[2]) (see Chapter 9 for precautions, contraindications, and things to watch for).

We may also have a variety of levels of ability in one class—cancer does not have a preference in picking yoga practitioners. It often happens that a yoga instructor sits next to someone with a very inflexible body who has never done yoga before. We usually explain that we use *asanas* not so much for the purpose of training, flexibility, and muscles, but for integrating awareness, breath, and energy with the body. Therefore, during the class, the emphasis is placed on the participant's awareness of their physical limits in the *asana*, breath, and awareness of the body. We watch in particular for limitations to movement resulting from scars, for example those caused by a lumpectomy or mastectomy. We strongly encourage a gentle approach, never forcing beyond the limits. We ask participants to feel their limit and to then back off a little into their comfort zone, and we offer modifications accordingly.

We usually sequence *asanas* as a posture and counter-posture, increasing the level of difficulty, remembering to always use relaxation between each *asana*. It is practical to choose two to three *asanas* for each category (supine, prone, sitting, standing) from the list below, slowly increasing the holding time, and always reminding participants to breathe deeply and to be aware of their body sensations and emotions at all times.

SUPINE POSITIONS

Jathara Parivartanasana (Revolved Abdomen Pose 1)

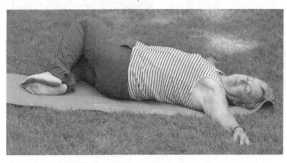

Jathara Parivartanasana (Revolved Abdomen Pose 1a)

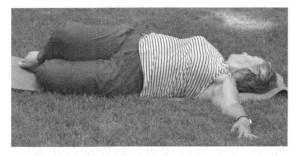

Jathara Parivartanasana (Revolved Abdomen Pose 2)

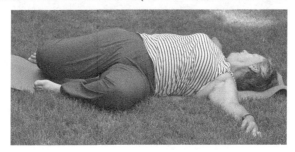

Jathara Parivartanasana (Revolved Abdomen Pose 2a)

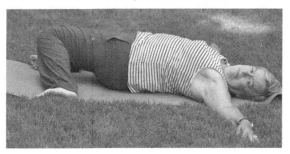

Ardha Halasana (Half Plough Pose)

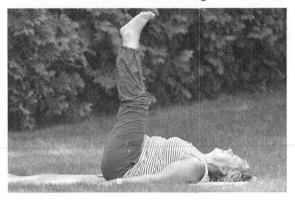

Ardha Pavanmultasana (Half Wind Relieving Pose)

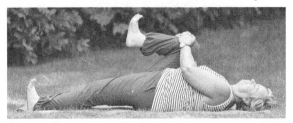

Pavanmultasana 1 (Wind Relieving Pose, easy)

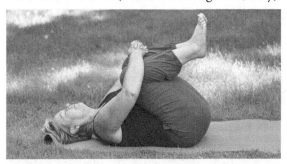

Pavanmultasana 2 (Wind Relieving Pose)

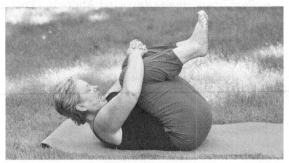

Matsyasana (Fish Pose)

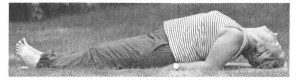

Naukasana 1 (Boat Pose, easy)

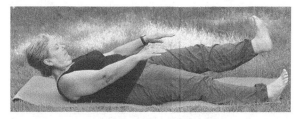

Naukasana 2 (Boat Pose)

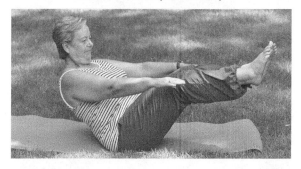

Setubandhasana (Bridge Pose)

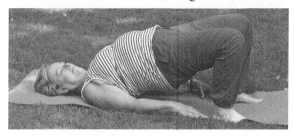

Shavasana (Corpse Pose, relax)

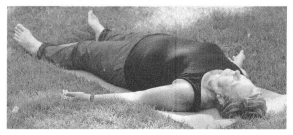

PRONE POSITIONS

Bhujangasana 1 (Cobra Pose, easy)

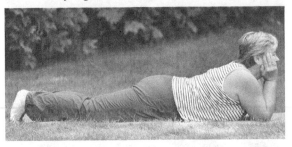

Bhujangasana 2 (Cobra Pose)

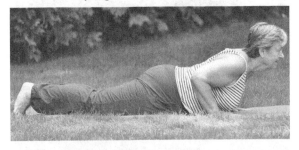

Naukasana coordination (Boat Pose, coordination)

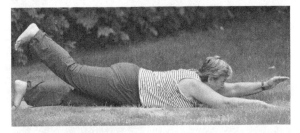

Ardha Salabasana (Half Locust Pose, easy)

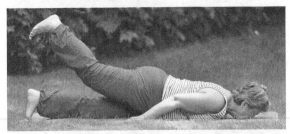

Marjyasana (Cat Pose)

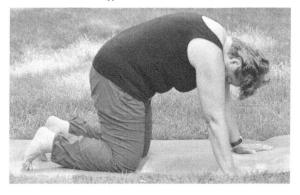

Bitilasana (Cow Pose)

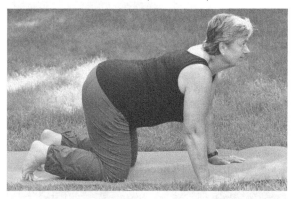

Dandayamana Bharmanasana (Balancing Table Pose)

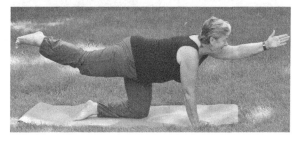

Makarasana (Crocodile Pose, relax)

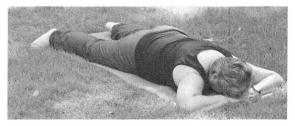

SITTING POSITIONS

Janu Shirsasana (Head Toward Knee Pose)

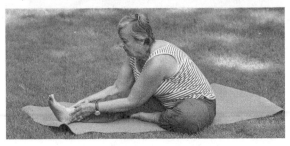

Paschimutasana (Seated Forward Bend Pose)

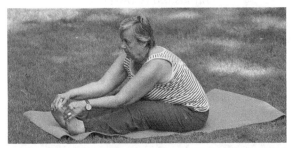

Vajrasana (Kneeling Thunderbolt)

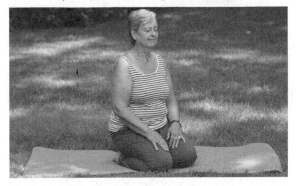

Ushtrasana (Camel Pose, easy)

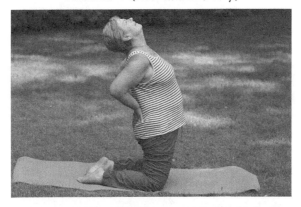

Yoga Mudraasana (Yoga Seal, kneeling)

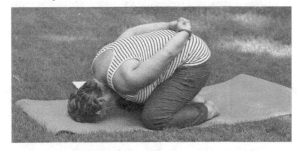

Gomukhasana (Cow Face Pose, legs)

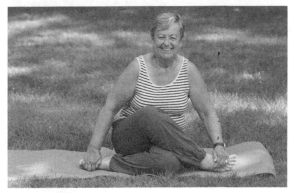

Vakrasana (Sitting Twist)

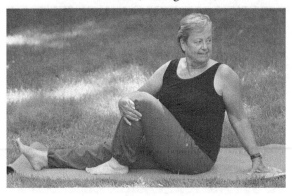

Baddha Konasana (Butterfly Pose)

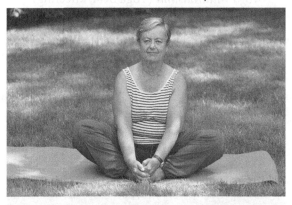

Dandasana (Staff Pose, easy, relax)

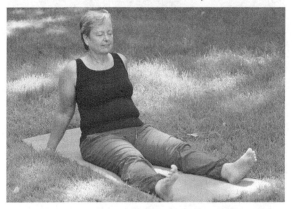

STANDING POSITIONS

Chakrasana (Side Bending)

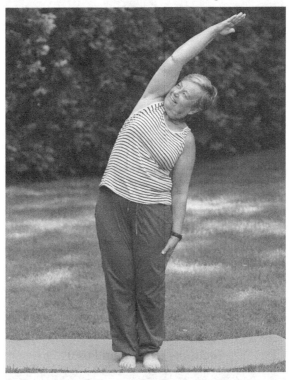

Trikonaṣana (Triangle Pose)

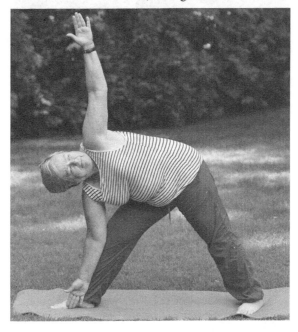

Virabhadrasana (Warrior 1 Pose)

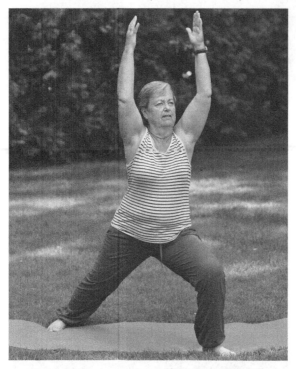

Tadasana (Mountain Pose)

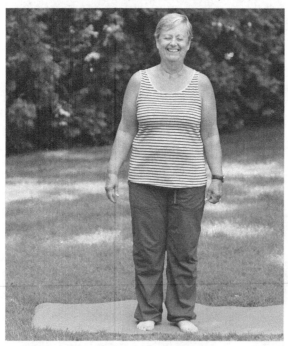

Utkasana (Chair Pose)

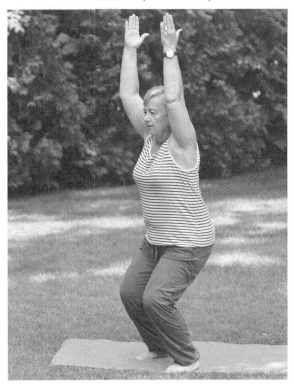

Vrkrasana 1 (Tree Pose, easy)

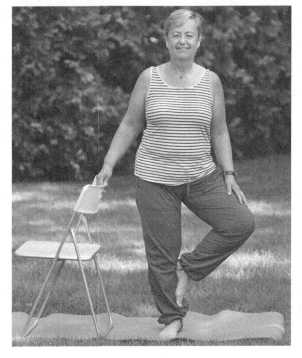

Vrkrasana (Tree Pose)

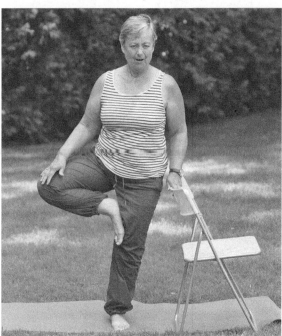

At the end we follow up with general relaxation and awareness in *shavasana* (Corpse Pose) for a few minutes. Then, in sitting position, with closed eyes, the participants bring their awareness to the state of their body, breath, mind, and emotions, noticing the difference before and after the *asana* class.

Pranayama

In the last 40 years researchers have confirmed the importance and the effects of slow breathing techniques, which are beneficial for the cardiovascular and autonomic nervous systems[3, 4] and cancer-related fatigue.[5] Another review[6] postulates that slowing down the breath to six breaths per minute causes rhythms of autonomous physiological functions (heart rate, blood pressure, blood flow to the brain) to act in coherence, reinforcing each other and resulting in better functioning of the immune system, reduction of inflammation, regulation of blood sugar levels, induced calmness, clarity of the mind, and a feeling of inner peace. On the other hand, specific *pranayamas* like *bhramari* practice produce a relaxed state, in which parasympathetic activity overrides the sympathetic activity.[7] Other research[8] has measured the effect of unilateral forced nostril breathing, showing the unique unilateral effects on the sympathetic stimulation of the heart.

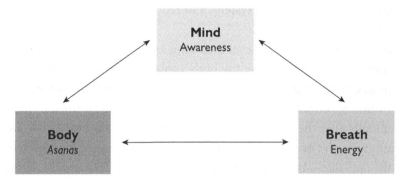

Interdependence of mind–body–breath rate

The function of breathing is, of course, involuntary, and as discussed before and as shown in the drawing above, the mind and body mutually influence it. Our ancient masters knew thousand of years ago that through the control of breath, every vital function, state of mind, and even longevity could be impacted. As evidenced by the ancient Vedic texts and more contemporary yogic texts such as the *Hatha Yoga Pradipika*, the power of *pranayama* is made explicit: "By proper practice of *prāṇāyāma*, etc., all diseases are eradicated. Through improper practice all diseases can arise."[9]

To appreciate the function of our breathing mechanism we need to consider that the goal of breathing is to deliver oxygen to our cells. Our breathing reflex is controlled and regulated by the levels of CO_2 in our blood. Our entire physiologic system is founded on the balance of O_2 and CO_2, which determines the basis for homeostasis and health. If our respiratory chemistry is balanced, our immune system, digestive system, cardiovascular system, and neurological system will function well.

"Breathing regularly in a way that maintains CO_2 at its healthy levels provides our ANS with a nice resilient buffer. However, if we develop a consistent pattern of over-breathing or hyperventilating, the medulla oblongata will reset, and over time this new pattern will become the norm. In other words, our brain 'gets used to' too much volume/rate of O_2 and too little CO_2," writes Robin Rothenberg in her pioneering book, *Restoring Prāṇa: A Guide to Prāṇāyāma and Healing Through the Breath for Yoga Therapists, Yoga Teachers, and Health-Care Practitioners*.

CO_2 acts as a natural antioxidant, reducing oxidative stress on our system. It also appears that reduction of CO_2 increases lactic acid, which promotes inflammation and fibrosis. Carbon dioxide has many other stabilizing actions, including protection against hypoxia (lower than normal levels of oxygen), calming of the central nervous system, and reducing inflammation. So how we breathe is crucial to our health!

Consistent practice of low-level breathing and breath retention to increase CO_2 is the only way to increase the body's tolerance of CO_2 and affect long-term, metabolic change. Practicing *pranayama* multiple times during the day in 10–15-minute chunks, in a reduced way, as suggested by the ancient yogis, will eventually alter the autonomic nervous system and the blood chemistry.

Breathing harder or faster does not increase oxygenation of the blood. In fact, it does the opposite—because of an imbalance between CO_2 and O_2, our ability to absorb oxygen is decreased and we feel the lack of air...so we breathe more quickly. And thus the vicious circle of hyperventilation starts. Hyperventilation is defined as breathing in excess of our metabolic capacity to produce CO_2. With heavy breathing, we don't gain O_2 but we lose CO_2 on every exhale, and thus the homeostasis is disturbed. Hyperventilation syndrome (HVS) is just one of several types of breathing pattern disorders, one of the most common and most commonly missed.

The list of symptoms associated with hyperventilation includes:[10]

Shortness of breath	Postural issues
Chest breathing	Heartburn (GERD)
Anxiety or panic	Migraines
Asthma, COPD	Muscle cramps
Insomnia	Multiple chemical sensitivities
Snoring or sleep apnea	Muscle pain
Restless leg syndrome	Myofascial pain
Anaphylactic reactions	Mood swings
TMJ (temporomandibular joint syndrome, also called TMD, temporomandibular joint disorder)	Poor exercise tolerance
	Poor immunity
	Poor memory
Chronic cough	Swollen lymph glands
Stuffy nose, sinusitis, hay fever	Dry skin, mouth, eyes
Anterior head carriage	High blood pressure

Food allergies

Constipation

Bloating

Excessive flatulence

Brain fatigue

Abdominal spasms

Anal irritation

Hemorrhoids

Food cravings

Sluggishness

Depression

Chronic fatigue

Osteoporosis

Seizure disorder

Dizziness

Cold hands or feet (Raynaud's syndrome)

High or low blood pressure

Recurrent bladder infections

Recurrent vaginal infections

Recurrent skin rashes.

Hyperventilation and breathing pattern disorders need to be considered as a causative factor, not simply a symptom. In other words, *breathe less, lighter, and through the nose.* The less breath is moving through the airways, the less inflammation and loss of CO_2 occurs. Just like my teacher, Shri O.P. Tiwariji of the Kaivalyadhama Yoga Institute, one of the last living *pranayama* masters, says, the less you can feel the breath moving in your nostrils, the better quality of *pranayama*.

There are indications that intermittent hypoxia (IH) stimulates neurogenesis, the formation of nervous tissue, and may be applicable as both a treatment and prevention of mental disorders.[11] To date, IH has been used specifically in the treatment of depression, anxiety, and stress, and there are some implications that it may be useful in treating schizophrenia and bipolar disorder.[12]

Over the last 30 years, IH has been used with approximately 2 million patients. It appears to curb free-radical production, acting as protection to the mitochondria and supporting ATP (adenosine triphosphate) production.[13] This translates into a stronger immune system, a decrease in systemic inflammation, and greater vitality. It seems that IH is being put forward as a means to improve the general resistance and resilience of an organism, with the potential to positively impact every level of the *panchamaya* (the five dimensions of human existence). Of course, this lies at the heart of *pranayama* practice.[14] Yoga incorporates many different breathing techniques that produce different results. Some are stimulating, some are relaxing, some balance the subtle energies, and some are warming or cooling.

The breathing itself regulates our autonomic nervous system, whether we know it or not. As we inhale, we stimulate the sympathetic nervous system, increasing the acidity of the body, which is connected to inflammatory, allergic, and malignant diseases. As we exhale, we stimulate the parasympathetic nervous system, enhancing digestion, increasing alkalinity of the body environment, and influencing the functioning of the gall bladder and glands; therefore, the management of the breathing ratio between inhale and exhale becomes very intentional for the effect we want to create.

In addition, breathing through one nostril activates the opposite hemisphere of the brain and activates the corresponding part of the autonomic nervous system. When we breathe through the left nostril we activate the left peripheral subtle energy channel (*ida nadi*) and right brain hemisphere, cooling the body and stimulating the parasympathetic nervous system. As a result, our brain wave frequency slows down, the pupils become small, there is an increase in salivation, the heart rate slows down and blood vessels are dilated, stomach secretion and pancreatic secretion are stimulated, and peristaltic movement increases. This is the healing and restorative state of the body.

When we breathe through the right nostril we activate the right peripheral subtle energy channel (*pingala nadi*) and left brain hemisphere, warming the body and stimulating the sympathetic nervous system. In such cases our brain increases in beta activity, the pupils widen, salivation is decreased, the heart rate increases and blood vessels constrict, the stomach and pancreatic secretion are reduced, and peristaltic movement and the whole immune system are suppressed. This is a catabolic non-healing state of the body, in which all energies are directed towards quick and effective action.

Therefore, if *pranayama* is used correctly, it can become a very potent tool to produce the desired healing effects. Yogic science seems to understand this very well, and gives us many *pranayama* techniques to manage the balance of physical, emotional, and mental states.

Most of our participants have never done *pranayama*. For most of them the notion of managed breath is also very foreign, and we spend the first couple of *pranayama* classes teaching slow, light breathing, with proper engagement of the diaphragm muscle. For many, this is a very revealing experience as the majority of our participants come with very quick and short (usually clavical) breath, indicating hyperventilation.

Consequently, we spend a lot of time on individual assessment and correction of breathing patterns. We make participants aware of the number of breaths per minute they take, the length of inhale and exhale, if the exhale or inhale is smooth or interrupted, and how deeply or shallowly they breathe.

When they are ready, and have learned to breathe with full engagement of just the diaphragm, we proceed to the next step. We teach them to breathe to a metronome, first with equal inhale to exhale. When they find the right count of beats and breathe comfortably, we ask them to double the exhale to the inhale ratio. This process may take several classes as for most of the participants the idea of consciously managing the breath is foreign, and we always need to go slowly with minimal effort.

When teaching *pranayama* we make sure that participants are seated with a straight back, either in a meditative *asana* on the floor or on a chair. In our retreats we may use the following *pranayama* techniques:

Kapalbhati

Chandra bhedan

Surya bhedan

Seetali (shitkari)

Nadi shuddhi (anuloma or viloma or alternate nostril breathing)

Ujjayi

Bhramari.

The vagus nerve (the main regulator of the parasympathetic nervous system) passes through the thorax with nerve endings that exert control over the constrictor muscle of the pharynx, creating greater vocal prosody for a more pleasing sound. This is part of the social engagement neural platform of polyvagal theory, which enhances the potential for positive social connection.

Additionally, during breath techniques such as *ujjai* or chanting, the longer exhalation and altered breathing rhythm activates the vagus nerve and parasympathetic system for body-wide systemic restoration, including effects for digestive health.

The classic text of yoga, *Hatha Yoga Pradipika*,[15] mentions in its second chapter, among others, the following *pranayamas* and their healing qualities:

- *Chandra bhedan*—cooling breath, activates the parasympathetic nervous system, relaxes the body, mind, and emotions.

- *Surya bhedan*—warming and energizing technique, activates the sympathetic nervous system, balances *vata*, improves circulation, rejuvenates cells, purifies blood, and removes parasites.

- *Sitali*—known as cooling breath balancing *pitta*, heals spleen disorder and is very effective for inflammation and any kind of tumor.

- *Nadi shuddhi*—known to balance subtle energy between *ida* and *pingala*.

- *Kapalbhati*—known as cleansing *kriya*, balancing *kapha* and an energizing *pranayama*, helps poor blood circulation, slows peristaltic movement, improves poor digestion, and energizes the body. In our case, we make sure that the strokes of breath are gentle and a maximum of 120/minute.

We start each *pranayama* session with the following *mudras* as preparation:

- *Agnisar*—three times.

- *Simhasana* with *jiva bandha*—five times.

- *Brahma mudra*—three times.

We slowly introduce different *pranayamas* over the following two weeks, closely monitoring clients for the proper use of the techniques. By the third week most of the clients can do the desired sequence of the *pranayama* session:

1. *Kapalbhati* (gentle, not quicker than 120 strokes/minute, and only if there are no contraindications)

2. *Nadi shuddhi*

3. *Chandra* or *surya bedhana*

4. *Sitali* (or *sitkari*)

5. *Ujjayi*

6. Ending with *brahmari*.

The duration of each breath as well as variations of techniques are, of course, tailored to every person. Saying that, however, we find that most of the clients, especially in cancer groups, are *pitta/vata*, and therefore the *pranayama* is often similar for the whole group. We put a special emphasis on *sitali*, as this "anti-inflammatory" breath is excellent for cancers and all NCDs.

Meditation

Our meditations are always preceded by either *pranayama* or chanting. This prepares participants by creating in them favorable states for meditation and/or contemplation. Although the groups will vary, in my experience I find that at noon, guided meditation is very effective, while in the evening after chanting, silent meditation is more appropriate.

In both meditation and *pranayama* class it is important that all are sitting in a circle and nobody sits outside of the circle. This helps to build energy and creates a strong and positive group resonance. It also helps to create cohesiveness in the group, and encourages relationship building.

Most of the participants who come to our retreats have never meditated. This means that either they do not know what meditation is or they have some preconceived ideas about what meditation "should be." Some fear that meditation is not for them. So before we start the class we gauge our participants' understanding to find out how much they know and what ideas they have about meditation. This allows us to manage their expectations effectively.

We start meditation by creating proper postures while sitting: if on a chair or the floor, the spine should be straight, maintaining natural curvature. (Some participants need to lie down and we make sure to offer them a bolster or blanket under their knees for comfort.) The posture needs to be adjusted so that they can sit comfortably for at least 15 minutes without any movement.

We then introduce participants to meditation as the process of inner exploration or inner journey, where you become physically still and go within, observing the breath, body, mind (passing thoughts), and/or emotions. Research reveals that mindful meditation practices of this type produce structural and functional changes in the brain and are involved with enhancing memory, learning, gaining perspective, and regulating thoughts and emotions.[16, 17]

Many novices have preconceived ideas that you only meditate when there is cessation of the thought process—so they struggle to "not have" thoughts in their mind. And this resistance creates all kind of problems. We encourage the posture of witness to the thoughts, as if you are standing in a room looking out of the window and watching a passer-by walking in and out of view. So we ask them to simply observe the thoughts coming in and out of awareness, not allowing themselves to be hijacked by any one particular thought. Simply observing impartially what is appearing and disappearing on the canvas of awareness.

In the beginning this may be challenging, and novices find themselves hijacked by emotions or simply bored.

We usually start the first week with guided mindfulness meditation and adding the "so hum" mantra in rhythm with the breath. The guidance is for a full 20 minutes at the beginning of the week, slowly increasing silence over the week. We find this to be an effective introduction to the process of meditation. By the end of the first week everyone usually feels comfortable with silence and is able to practice focusing on the breath and mantra on their own.

At the end of meditations we encourage people to share their experiences. It is important that we, as facilitators, stress that every meditation may be different and not to expect the same experiences the next time. Additionally, each person will have their own experiences, which should not be compared or expected by others.

Depending on the level of the group and participants' challenges at hand, we can also offer any particular guided meditation, choosing from samples provided in Appendix 1: mindfulness meditation, breath meditation, forgiveness or heart opening meditation, mantra meditation, or simply silent meditation.

In my experience, while dealing with participants of these programs I find that many are holding strong resentments, have anger directed inwardly or outwardly, and/or have difficulties forgiving others. We help them deal with these issues and emotions in the second week. We start to work on the emotions in *yoga nidra* and through forgiveness meditation. We use the "Feelings Wheel" (see Appendix 7) at the beginning of the second week of the program, to open conversations about feelings and emotions, the emotions that lurk in the subconscious, those we consciously suppress, that we do not want to feel and use distractions to avoid. What do they do to the body? What do they do to our mind? What do they do to our energy field?

It is important for participants to explore their feelings before (hopefully) they put themselves in the chair of forgiveness. Again, we fully guide the first two sessions and then increase moments of silence—patients find this very effective. There are other guided meditations provided in Appendix 1. We usually start with the simple ones and as we recognize the issues people are working with, we choose according to the need within the group.

Kirtan kriya

The first thing we do after commencing our daily activity in the afternoon is *kirtan kriya*. This 12-minute practice dispels afternoon sleepiness, provides a good energizer after a lunch break, and brings back alertness for the rest of the day.

Kirtan kriya comes from *Kundalini Yoga* as taught by *yogi Bhajan*. One of his disciples and a medical doctor, Dr Dharma Sing Khalsa, former president of Alzheimer's Research, conducted a series of studies[18] on *kirtan kriya* meditation. Daily 12-minute practice for eight weeks revealed many positive health benefits.

The outcomes of the research were divided into three categories, *mind*, *body*, and *spirit*, all of which optimize brain and body aging and fit very effectively in correcting the side effects of chemotherapy (brain) and expanding telomeres (connected to cancer and other diseases).

Staring with the mind, *kirtan kriya* improved memory, reduced stress, and lowered cortisol levels. It enhanced brain blood flow, which influences attention, concentration, focus, memory, depression, trauma, and resilience. It also improved communication between brain cells by increasing neurotransmitters.

At the body level, *kirtan kriya* increased telomerase by 44 percent (the biggest increase noted to date), down-regulated inflammatory genes, and improved the genes that boost the immune system. The experimental group also showed improvements in sleep.

At the spirit and wellbeing level, meditators reported discovery of clarity of purpose and psychological wellbeing such as acceptance, personal growth, and improvement in relationships.

(For a description of *kirtan kriya*, please see Appendix 6.)

Mudras and restorative yoga

The Sanskrit word *mudra* is usually defined as "energy seal or shortcut" or "circuit by-pass." *Mudras* signify a gesture with the eyes, body, and most commonly, with hands and fingers.

The use of *mudras* evolved during the time of Tantra (up to the 15th century CE). Shiva Tantric texts, such as *Hathapradipika, Nisha Satva Samhita Uttara Sutra, Dattatreya Yogashas, Goraksha Shataka, Shiva Samhita, Gheranda Samhita*, and many others, elaborate on different *mudras*, their application, and effects on subtle energy.[19] *Mudras* establish a subtle, non-intellectual connection with these areas. Each sets up a different link and has a correspondingly different effect on the body, mind, and *prana*.[20]

The finger *mudras* are said to guide the energy flow and reflexes of the brain. The yogis mapped out the hand areas, with each one connecting to a different part of the body and brain, representing different emotions and behaviors.[21] In Tantra it is believed that each finger relates to planetary energy and the quality that that planet represents. The thumb relates to the individual's persona.

For some, the importance of *mudras* was so great that they treated them as a separate limb[22] of yoga science. *Mudras* are regarded as higher practices, which lead to balancing of the subtle energy levels (*prana vayus* and *chakras*), awakening *kundalini*, and that can result in developing psychic powers in an advanced practitioner.

Until recently research on *mudras* was scarce due to lack of a sensitive enough apparatus. Although the Russians have been studying human consciousness and bio-energy with special interest for more than 80 years, the results were not published internationally in English-language journals because Russian research did not follow internationally recognized standards in study design, selection of endpoint, timelines, and therapy regimens, data analysis, and presentation of results.[23] Since 2000, however, we have started seeing the publication of such research in Western periodicals and conferences, which has introduced the use of new technology—electrophonic imaging (EPI).

EPI is a process that measures the energy fields of humans as well as plants, crystals, essential oils, and water. These images are captured by a highly specialized camera, referred to as a GDV (gas discharge visualization), EPC (electrophonic camera), or EPI. EPI is growing as a novel technique of health assessment and is being utilized in the fields of alternative medicine, conventional practices, psychophysiology, psychology, and consciousness studies.

In 2005 at the IEEE conference, a paper was presented which evaluated GDV as a possible medical diagnostic application.[24] The authors demonstrated the possibilities of providing holistic medical screening through measurement of bio-energy fields, which have both bio-physical and bio-physic bearings.

This led to a systematic review of research on EPI/GDV published in 2010.[25] The search yielded 136 articles addressing four different fields of medical and psychophysiologic applications of EPC (GDV). The reviewer concluded that this technology was easy to use and could be implemented as a quick and accurate method of assessment of treatment effectiveness and evaluating people's emotional and physical conditions.

This sparked the interest of researchers of yoga, and in 2018, the *International Journal of Yoga* published two papers back to back. The first, very interesting for us, paper[26] looked at EPI technology as a successful application for various conditions. It examined this approach relative to yoga theory, traditional medicine systems, and scientific developments in the field of gene expression and neuroplasticity. It also pointed to EPI as a translational technology between traditional medicine systems and modern medicine.

The second paper[27] looked at EPI-captured coronal discharge around the fingers as a result of electron capture from the 10 fingers during holding a finger *mudra*. The coronal discharge around each fingertip was then studied to understand the effect of the *mudra* on EPI parameters. The result of the *mudra* intervention showed statistically significant changes versus a control group. There are still many studies to be conducted before we will be able to fully understand and document the impact of *mudras* on human health, according to old yogic texts.

Perhaps the most popular use today of hand and finger *mudras* is for health or healing. According to yogic texts, their effects span from physical, energetic, psychological, and mental to spiritual levels. The mental focus of bringing the breath to the specific part of the body while holding a *mudra* enhances our awareness of the body and increases circulation in a chosen part of the body. As we channel the breath and attention, we learn to recognize and cultivate our sensitivity to subtle energy—*prana*—being energized or calmed. And as each *mudra* has its core qualities, we learn to evoke and feel these qualities within all levels of our existence.

We need to keep in mind that the effects of *mudras* are not immediate. In our retreats we practice the same set of four *mudras* for a week, holding each for approximately 10–15 minutes. We practice them sitting, lying down, or during restorative yogic position. The breath is natural and will be controlled by the *mudra* itself. Many of the *mudras* open the clients to experiencing the subtle energy system for the first time, which may be unfamiliar or even uncomfortable. Therefore we start with four superficial *mudras* in the first week as an introduction to deeper practices in the following weeks.

All *mudras* listed in Appendix 3 have been taken from the beautiful edition of *Mudras for Healing and Transformation* by Joseph Le Page and Lilia Le Page (2014). We slightly modified their corresponding meditations to fit the healing profile of the populations we work with during our retreats.[28]

We use a different set of four *mudras* for each week in the sequence outlined in Appendix 3. The sequence is designed to lead participants from superficial to deeper states as they progress. Each *mudra* has its own position—chosen from restorative yoga—and is held for the duration of the guided meditation (approximately 10–15 minutes). The positions, however, can be adjusted to meet the group's abilities.

The first and fourth *mudras* are usually performed in a sitting position since right after this session we start *yoga nidra* in *shavasana* (Corpse Pose). For the second and third *mudras* each week we typically use *jathara parivartanasana* (Revolved Abdomen Pose), *supta konasana* (legs in Butterfly), or *viparita karani* (Legs up the Wall Pose) (or on the chair). We may change the position based on our clients' abilities, comfort, and amount of support props we have at our disposal. Most important is that the clients are comfortable and not distracted during the guided meditations.

After each *mudra* and meditation we encourage clients to write their experiences in their diaries and to share with the group if they feel like it.

Yoga nidra

In the Tantric tradition *yoga nidra* entailed the systemic rotation of consciousness in the body called *nyasa* (which means "take the mind to that point"). *Nyasa* was practiced in a sitting posture and involved the use of specific mantras, which were placed, felt, or experienced at a different part of the body.

Swami Satyananda of the Bihar School of Yoga developed the practice based on *nyasa* in traditional texts into a seven-part process allowing the student to stay in deep relaxation between awakened and sleep states, and called this *yoga nidra*.

Richard Miller, PhD, founder of Integrative Restoration (iRest) Yoga Nidra Meditation, took *yoga nidra* a step further by developing the process into highly individualized meditation practices that support an individual's psychological, physical, and spiritual healing. He writes in his "iRest Program for Healing PTSD":

> [iRest] *Yoga Nidra* is made up of a sequence of meditation practices that help you feel connected to yourself, connected with others, and to the world around you… It is integrative, as it addresses both psychological and physical issues such as trauma, insomnia and pain in your body and mind. It helps you feel yourself as a fully functioning integrated and healthy human being. It is restorative because it helps you recover your inner resources of joy, peace and well-being… Research participants report a broad range of improvements including psychosomatic disorders like depression and anxiety, PTSD, MNS, Hypertension, Colitis, Asthma, Eczema, Arthritis and coronary diseases.[29]

We started by using *yoga nidra* based on Satyananda's model. Then we changed to iRest *Yoga nidra* and we found it to be much more individualized, allowing for much deeper experiences. We also found it more suited to the specific needs of cancer patients. Therefore, most of the following text, including the practices, was either taken directly from Richard Miller (2005) *Yoga Nidra: The Meditative Heart of Yoga* with the author's permission, or is based directly on iRest principles.

During 18 days the group goes through a very powerful process of learning to witness themselves. This enables participants to be deeply aware and able to reconnect with the deepest sense of being. We have prepared five texts that are changed every three days (see Appendix 2). Each text introduces a new element, taking participants into deeper layers of their being.

During the first week we help the clients to reconnect with their body by having them sense the breath and sensations manifesting within the body. This, in itself, can be a profound experience for some. We often find that in the process of chemotherapy many people disconnect from their body, as they don't want to deal with the severe side effects of treatment.

We teach the group to use healing visualizations while in states of deep relaxation. The two visualizations we included, the second one in particular, call on the individual creativity of each participant, who tend to really enjoy this freedom of the process.

In the second week participants start working with their feelings and emotions. This is a good time to introduce the "Feelings Wheel" (see Appendix 7) in order to help them identify their emotions. It is also a good time to introduce the concept of welcoming whatever "shows up," especially if these are the negative emotions.

Transformation only happens if the participant is willing to move into the unknown, into sometimes uncomfortable territory, where they can feel that they are "out on a limb," so to speak. The first step is to bring into awareness "what is," especially the strong negative emotion they may not want to feel. Following a deep state of relaxation, we help them to accept it without resistance, witnessing it in the mind, while locating it in the body as a sensation.

Witnessing with acceptance creates the opportunity to transcend or go beyond the emotion, and offers a constructive insight that enables participants to progress in ways they might not otherwise have imagined. In this process of dispassionate observing, the emotion seems to lose the power it had over the mind. It seems to lessen its grip, and becomes more externalized, and as such, much easier to handle.

Dr Miller writes:

> By welcoming each sensation, emotion, thought, person and situation—just as it is—you grow confident in the ability to respond in a way that "hits the mark". The more you welcome and respond to everything just as it is, in ways that feel right to you, the more confident and empowered you will feel. The more confident and empowered you feel, the more you are able to welcome and respond to all of life's challenges and release long standing negative patterns of emotions and thoughts.[30]

The second week of the retreat process teaches participants how to connect and feel the emotions as sensations in the body. It then teaches them to hold opposites—the negative emotion or sensation and its opposite (positive)—at the same time in their awareness and in the body. This is a very powerful process of bringing the negative emotions and beliefs from subconsciousness into awareness in a safe and relaxed manner. Moreover, it is a powerful way of teaching participants how to be aware of, while learning how to respond to, negative emotions and thought patterns.

The shifting between opposites "unlearns" conditioned patterns of reactive behavior and rewires new coping strategies into the brain.[31] Consequently, participants learn how to reinforce a stance of witnessing rather than being hijacked by any one strong emotion. This then allows them to choose suitable responsive actions in the moment instead of instinctive reactions.

Negative thoughts and emotions are expressions of mental conditionings that exist in the deeper layers of consciousness, seeking a channel to release. By allowing these negativities to emerge into consciousness we cleanse our mind from unconscious negative thoughts. With time and practice, negativity subsides and loosens the grip on habitual behaviors.

In the third week we continue to work with negative thought and belief patterns. We take the practice a step further, helping participants reconnect with feelings of deep joy, bliss, wellbeing, inner peace, and gratitude. The participants are given the opportunity to realize that these beautiful positive emotions are already within them, always there waiting to be discovered, so that at any time they can access them at their will.

The third week practices help participants to discover their undivided wholeness through experiencing the simple feeling of being, which is the universal felt-sense, or non-verbal inner knowing that we all experience.[32] It is always here in us, as the background waiting to be rediscovered.

Whether or not students hear the teacher's instructions does not matter. According to Swami Satyananda, when one is asleep, there remains a state of potentiality, a form of awareness, that is awake and fully alert to outside situations. It is natural for participants to miss some of the instructions because very often the conscious mind withdraws itself, allowing the subconscious mind to come to the forefront.

GUIDELINES FOR INSTRUCTIONS

Yoga nidra is usually practiced in a supine position—*shavasana*—as a position most conducive to deep relaxation. However, it can also be practiced in a sitting pose or any other comfortable position.

If a student feels any kind of tension, fear, negative emotion, or mental disturbance, we strongly encourage them to simply observe it without resistance, while focusing on a slow, deep breath and remembering that this is a temporary experience, and the next session will be better. In such a case, if needed, the posture can be adjusted, eyes can be opened, or they can doze off to sleep.

"Welcome" is the word we always keep displayed in a prominent place—on a white board or a poster on the wall. At the end of each session we encourage participants to write in their diaries and then share, voluntarily, their experiences. All experiences—positive and negative—should be validated, as they are simply manifestation of the participant's mind content.

Before we start the first session we help our participants to formulate a resolve (or affirmation). The resolve is very important and very potent when repeated in the state of total relaxation during *yoga nidra*. It has to be a positive, definite, and short statement made in the present tense. We discourage "weak" words such as try, want, or think, or negative statements such as "I don't want to have cancer," instead replacing them with positive ones—"I am healthy." The resolve may be changed or modified with time as the participant's awareness expands; however, it should always be the same at the beginning and end of the same practice.

PROCESS OF *YOGA NIDRA*

Below is a general outline of the session. In Appendix 2 we provide the texts to the sessions we use.

1. Relaxation and affirmation: After short relaxation the resolve or affirmation is repeated three times silently.

2. Rotation of awareness/body sensing: Relaxing the brain by relaxing the body. The brain is the physical mediator of the consciousness, linking mind, body, and emotions into one unit. In *yoga nidra* we start stimulation or clearing of the neuron paths in the brain by progressively rotating awareness through the individual parts of the body. We start with the most sensitive parts—the mouth, the ears, and the nostrils.

3. Breath sensing: After body sensing we further practice our ability to concentrate by watching the breath and counting it down.

4. Welcoming sensory experiences or opposite feelings and emotion or beliefs and thought patterns: The practice now shifts to arousal of feelings, then emotions, and finally thought patterns. The ability to experience the opposites (negative/positive) brings into simultaneous operation nerve circuits in the opposite hemispheres, which never usually operate at the same time.

5. Visualization or imagery—*Yoga nidra* uses symbols or visualization to bring out suppressed unconscious impressions, *samskaras*. The images can be universal symbols (as described by Jung)—such as mandalas, archetypes, or mantras. This part may also include relaxing or healing visualizations.

   There can also be symbols conditioned by society, culture, country, etc. Therefore, the selection of symbols for the audience is very important. We have provided a generic list but if you wish, you may simply ask the group for what is meaningful imagery for them. The process of visualization may bring about repressed associations from the subconscious mind, allowing purging of painful memories and fears, inhibitions, complexes, and neuroses to come forth into consciousness.

The law of awareness states that whatever we are willing to be with, we go beyond. Whatever we simply allow to be in our awareness without resistance dissolves and disappears. This way the negative experiences disappear or are simply integrated into consciousness. The energy that has been used for repressing unconscious feelings can now be released and channeled to other activities.

Some people whose minds are scattered may have difficulty with visualization. Remembering or recalling instead of visualizing might be easier in such cases. With time and practice, activity in the mind subsides and the mind becomes clear and steady enough to hold the image.

6. Meeting, greeting, welcoming, engaging: Noting whatever sensation, emotion, or feeling is arising without conceptual labels. Simply being with the sensation and noticing where it is located in the body:

   – Welcome the opposite sensation, emotion, or feeling, noticing where it is located in the body

   – Alternate between opposites

   – Experience both opposites at the same time

   – Become a witness to what is arising.

7. Accessing and welcoming joy, wellbeing, and inner peace: This step teaches participants that they are always able to access these positive emotions in any situation in life.

8. Resolve or affirmation: After visualization we ask participants to repeat the same resolve they had at the beginning.

9. Coming out: Finally, we bring the participants out in a very gentle and slow manner as some of them may go very deep and need some time to come out.

The following are the five consecutive *yoga nidra* samples that we use in our retreats. We start with number 1 and change the text every three days. Every new text introduces the more difficult aspect of inner work:

1. We start with simple healing visualization.

2. We introduce the list of items to be visualized and to invoke corresponding emotion, which is then correlated with sensation in a particular place in the body.

3. During visualizations, participants create in their mind a perfect place where they feel safe and happy. This place becomes their inner resource where they can go to at any time during *yoga nidra*.

    For the first time also they learn to find the felt-sensations in the body (such as tiredness or warmth) and then evoke its opposite and find its place in the body as well (tiredness—vitality, warmth—coolness, etc.). Finally, in the third step, they feel both sensations in the body at the same time. This is an introductory exercise to more advanced work with emotions and negative self-belief in the following classes.

4. In this class we change the breathing—instead of simply watching the breath, clients now do mental alternate nostril breathing *pranayama*, without using the hand, focusing only awareness of the working nostril.

    This is also the first class where clients start their work with emotions. Prior to beginning the class each participant will choose a negative emotion with which they will want to work—it may be anger, fear, anxiety, etc. They will now go through the same three steps with emotion as they did in number 3 with feeling sensations. First they feel and find the original emotion manifesting in the body. Then they feel and find the opposing emotion in the body, and finally they learn to hold and feel both emotions simultaneously in the body.

    Visualization includes healing the body with any creative method, using all imaginary tools the client is able to come up with.

5. In this class participants start working with a chosen negative self-belief, such as, "I am not good enough," "I am stupid," or "I can never do anything right." They now go through the same three steps with emotions, as they did in previous classes, feeling and finding the original emotion connected with negative belief manifesting in the body, then feeling and finding the emotion connected with an opposite belief, in the body, and finally holding and feeling both emotions simultaneously in the body.

    During the visualization clients learn to invoke the inner feeling of joy and wellbeing.

After each *yoga nidra* session we encourage clients to write about their experiences in their journals. All sessions can be found in Appendix 2.

Chanting

Chanting, singing, and dancing have been central to religious and cultural activities since time immemorial. They taught people to act collaboratively and cohesively within society and were central to community survival. The research suggests that creating music together evolved as a tool of social living—groups and tribes sang and danced together to build loyalty, transmit vital information, and ward off enemies.

Researchers became interested in the neural underpinning of these behaviors and their role in establishing group cohesion. They found that synchronized activities increase group cohesion and cause participants to like each other and behave more pro-socially toward each other.[33] Another pilot study of middle school students (aged 11–14) showed that the experimental group that chanted and sang for 12 weeks significantly increased their scores compared with the control group.[34]

Chanting in itself has its merits, but does it matter what we chant? J. Hertzell,[35] a researcher in the Basque Center on Cognition, Brain and Language, studied the effects of chanting Sanskrit mantras by 21 people using an MRI scan. He discovered that memorizing Vedic mantras increases the size of brain regions associated with cognitive function, including short- and long-term memory.

This finding corroborates the beliefs of the Indian tradition, which holds that reciting mantras enhances memory and thinking. But so do other mind–body techniques such as meditation, so the question now is, does chanting produce any different effects than other mind–body practices?

A recent review[36] suggests that meditation influences brain systems involved in attention, awareness, memory, sensory integration, and the cognitive regulation of emotion. However, some effects are specific to active-based meditation (meditations that include activity, such as moving part of the body or chanting) in brain areas involved in self-control, social cognition, language, speech, tactile stimulation, sensorimotor integration, and self-control. If such meditations are done in a group, the effects are multiplied by the synchronicity and entrainment of the participants.

GROUP RESONANCE

From a scientific point of view, the true power of coming together as a group stems from a collective resonance effect. Just as brain wave entrainment can occur between two individuals, it can also be established between group members chanting together. The electrical activity of each individual in the group begins to resonate on a common synchronized wavelength and in phase, a choir perfectly in tune. Like a coherent group of electrons that begins to vibrate as one giant electron, the group creates a resonance that magnifies the individual effect.

Collectively, such results suggest that chanting (active) meditation may be especially useful for brain fitness in aging adults. It provides enhancements in higher cognitive functions and social cognition, attention, memory, movement, and emotional regulation that can help in preventing mood, physical, and cognitive disorders of aging. Of course, we are also interested in such results from the point of view of chemotherapy and impaired neurogenesis in our clients.

The healing property of mantra chanting was confirmed by another study.[37] The results showed that when we repeat a mantra or prayer, we automatically adjust our breath to six or fewer breaths per minute. This frequency happens to be the natural rhythm of fluctuations of other biological functions (heart rate, blood pressure, blood flow to the brain). The result of this synchronization is that the rhythm of each function resonates in coherence with the other autonomous physiological functions, mutually reinforcing each other. This coherence produces health benefits:

- Better functioning of the immune system
- Reduction of inflammation
- Better regulation of blood sugar levels.

However, lack of coherence increases with age and is linked to high blood pressure, cardiac insufficiency, and complications from diabetes and cancer.

A recent study[38] looked specifically at the ability of chanting to create different effects to meditation or prayer. Researchers used neuroimaging and electrophysiological methods to measure brain activity during the chanting of a Buddhist mantra. The results suggested that the neurophysiological correlates of mantra chanting are different from those of meditation and prayer, and would possibly induce distinct psychotherapeutic effects in participants.

In this study, chanting the Gayatri mantra, one of the oldest and most popular Vedic mantras, was compared with chanting a poem. Sixty students (aged 12–14 years old) chanted the mantra for 10 minutes for five days (the experimental group) and the control group recited a poem. The experimental group showed significantly higher results than the control group.

Perhaps the most important yogic chant, mentioned even by Patanjali in his *Sutras*, is *pranava*, chanting "om." Studies have shown that chanting "om" modulates the brain regions involved in emotional processing and implicated in major depressive disorders,[39] deactivated limbic regions,[40] improved pulmonary function,[41] and induced a deep state of relaxation throughout the brain region.[42]

It may even protect the brain from harmful mobile phone radiation.[43] In short, it may prove effective in clinical setting for treating major depressive disorders and other stress-related problems.

This is, of course, of major interest for our clients as depression, anxiety, and tension are some of the most commonly occurring side effects of cancer treatment, aging, and chronic diseases. Hence we included in our retreats 30 minutes of chanting, followed by silent meditation by candlelight. This is a perfect ending to the day—after the silent meditation everyone leaves the room in silence and goes to rest.

In the yoga tradition there are three stages of chanting a mantra. You begin with chanting aloud (*vaikhari japa*) to learn proper pronunciation. After getting used to the mantra for sufficient time, you should then chant the mantra in a low, whispering voice (*upanshu japa*). The third stage, chanting the mantra silently in the mind (*manasa japa*), is regarded as a great achievement, as it requires constant inner awareness. If our participants are yoga teachers and know the mantra well, we may encourage them to either whisper or chant silently in their mind.

It is advantageous to chant mantras on one breath. It is also good to chant mantras in unison, together, when in a group. Therefore, when we lead the chant we adjust the rhythm and tempo of chanting to the average ability of people within the group. Some may have a very short breath and to help them extend their breath we usually explain the technique used by professional singers.

Being able to control airflow while singing is a very important skill for all classical Western singers. If you take a deep breath, then apply a gentle neck lock, you may have a feeling of air being "captured" in the body between the neck lock and the diaphragm. As you gently push on the diaphragm, this will create a little pressure. Then all you have to do is to control the outflow of the breath as you make a sound, making sure that flow is even throughout. Maintaining constant pressure between the neck lock and diaphragm does this.

Usually we blow out a lot of air at the very beginning of making the sound, and the flow becomes weaker and weaker. Singers make sure that they do not waste the air at the beginning and blow air out only as much as needed to make the desired volume of sound. This way they control the volume of their voice to express the musical phrase.

We take the breath through the mouth to be quick, yet fill the lungs completely. We make sure that we fully engage the diaphragm on inhales and that the belly bulges. This way we take a very deep, but quick, inhale and with control of exhale described above we can make a very long outflow during chanting.

WEEK 1

Most of our clients have never done yoga and are shy of singing or chanting. Hence we start very slowly by introducing the healing chant from *Kundalini Yoga*—"Raa Maa Daa Saa"—sung by Snatam Kaur. It is very melodic, easy to remember, and has very beautiful instrumentation. We find that even the most timid clients cannot resist and start chanting within the first 10 minutes of introducing it.[44]

- Raa invokes the energy of the Sun.

- Maa invokes the energy of the Moon.

- Daa invokes the energy of the Earth.

- Saa invokes the energy of Infinity.

- Say invokes the experience of totality.

- So-hung (hum)…"I am That"…is beyond any description.

Before we start chanting, we center within in a minute of silence. We then make participants aware of how they feel in their body, their emotions, and their thoughts.

At the end of the chant we again make people aware of any difference in the way they feel their body, emotions, and the mind compared with the beginning of the chant.

The mantra is truly beautiful and quickly becomes everyone's favorite.

WEEK 2

In the second week we introduce another healing mantra, this time from Veda and highly regarded by Hindus—Maha Mrityunjaya, also called the Trayambakam mantra. It is said to be beneficial for mental, emotional, and physical health, and to bestow longevity and immortality.[45] This mantra is addressed to Lord Shiva for warding off untimely death.[46] Whereas the Gayatri mantra is meant for purification and spiritual guidance, the Maha Mrityunjaya mantra is meant for healing, rejuvenation, and nurturance.[47]

Learning this mantra takes a little longer, and the first chant is spent on introducing and learning the pronunciation of the Sanskrit words. Typically after a couple of days everyone knows the words and the meaning, and can chant it by heart by candlelight:

Om tryambakam yajamahe sugandhim pushtivardhanam

urvaarukamiva bandhanaan mrityormukshiya maamritaat

Meaning (free translation): "We concentrate on our third eye which lies behind the two eyes and this gives us the power to feel you and by this we feel happy, satisfied, and peace in life. We know immortality is not possible but some extension can be given to our death by your powers, Lord Shiva."

The word for word translation:

- *Om*—the primeval ancient sound from which everything originated. This sacred syllable represents the entire manifested world and the unmanifest, and also that which lies beyond both the unmanifest and the manifest.

- *Tryambakam*—represents the three-eyed Lord Shiva, who sees what we can see but who also sees what we cannot see.

- *Yajamahe*—we honor, worship, adore.

- *Sugandhim*—sweet smelling, fragrant.

- *Pushthi*—a well-nourished condition, prosperous, thriving, the fullness of life. Reality nourishes (sustains) everything.

- *Vardhanam*—one who strengthens, nourishes, causes to increase (in wealth, health, wellbeing, wisdom, knowledge). On the spiritual path, our understanding increases day by day.

- *Urvaarukamiva*—like the cucumber. Here, it symbolizes each of us and our relationship to existence.

- *Bandhanaan*—from captivity.

- *Mrityormukshiya*—free, liberate from death, attain *moksha* (a blissful state of existence of a soul, completely free from karmic bondage).

- *Maamritaat*—may I never again be parted from the immortality.

As we chant these Sanskrit words we create vibrations within the body which balance our energy centers (the *chakras*). *Chakras* contain all of the Sanskrit alphabet in them, and when we chant these sounds, we automatically induce balance into the corresponding *chakra*. So even if we do not understand the mantra, it will still produce desirable effects on our subtle body, mind and emotions.

WEEK 3

By the third week everyone is used to chanting and most of the participants really enjoy it—it feels like a perfect ending to a busy day. At the beginning of the third week we introduce chanting —"om," perhaps the least liked, but the chant during which most of the participants have strong inner experiences. "Om" is the primeval ancient sound from which everything originated. This syllable, regarded as sacred by Hindus, represents the entire manifested world and that which lies beyond both the manifest and the non-manifest. We chant it in the group in a synchronized way, all together, for 30 minutes.

Group activities and lectures

According to adult learning theory, adults learn best when they are motivated by personal goals and when they understand that the training relates to their situation in the real world. Since the retreats are only the beginning of transformation and change in a client's life, we recognize the importance of providing information on what yogic practices we teach and why. We want clients to buy in to the yogic practices so that they practice at home after finishing a retreat. For that purpose we dedicate an hour and a half every day to lectures, films, and group work.

WEEK 1

In the first week we use the lecture time to explain in detail the anatomy and physiology of yoga. We cover most aspects of yoga—*asanas, pranayama* meditation, *kriyas*, and *mudras*—elaborating on their impact on all our body systems, and particularly our brain and nervous system. Most clients do not realize how encompassing the effects of yogic techniques are, and that the most important part is not the *asana*, but the brain and the development and reconditioning of our nervous system. We use videos prepared by Kaivalyadhama Yoga Institute, alongside discussions whenever clients have questions and want to go deeper. The goal is to interest them, explain the benefits of doing practices, and make them aware of their own transformational experiences they may have during the retreat.

WEEK 2

In the second week we discuss the main factors causing cancer and chronic lifestyle diseases. We connect the *prana* energy centers to nerve plexuses and major glands. We connect the effects of stress, diet, EMF (electromagnetic field), toxicity (internal and external), and other factors, to our endocrinal system and body regulation. We then look in particular at lifestyle, diet, environmental toxicity, and negative emotions and thought patterns, and recommend a list of changes. We discuss *yamas* and *niyamas* as lifestyle recommendations. During these discussions each client creates their own list of changes they will implement in their lifestyle, diet, and environment after returning home from the retreat. By the end of the second week each client has their own individual "Fridge List," as we call it. On the Fridge List they list three changes to be implemented every week over eight weeks, a total of 24 changes.

WEEK 3

Also during the second week we start to work in other classes with our emotions and negative self-beliefs. During this week a lot of "stuff" comes up and is processed. Especially powerful are the *yoga nidra* and forgiveness meditation we do that week. As one client said:

> *Yoga nidra* had perhaps the biggest impact on me from all the yogic tools we practiced. I felt most resistance to it at the beginning. But at the end I gained the most from the experiences I had during *nidra* sessions.
>
> Another practice that had profound impact on me was forgiveness meditation. It allowed to resolve a lot of my own internal issues and bring a closure within myself, with people I had issues with in the past. It was a process and I have to continue this process within myself. (J.)

Such work prepares them for the third week, when we start creating a roadmap for the future—planning how to implement all the information and tools in their life after the retreat. The clients are now going through a deeply meditative process of creating a life mandala, during which they examine their own core beliefs. The process is slow and as deep as the client is able and willing to be.

Mandalas

Mandalas have been used by many cultures as meaningful meditation tools and as an expression of personal healing and integration. They usually consist of a central point with a symmetric geometric shape around it. Many forms in nature are an expression of mandalas, for example, flowers (daisies, roses, etc.) and rings of a tree.

The exercise described in detail in Appendix 8 has the form of meditating inquiry. Participants will seek answers within to 16 questions. This process will take them deep within, in introspection and examining their core values and the meaning of their life. By asking these basic questions and meditating on them, one by one, they have the opportunity to get in touch with their soul's purpose and to understand what changes they will need to make in order to manifest it in their lives. The process usually takes two or three 1.5-hour sessions, and tends to stir patients deeply; people may have significant dreams or "aha" moments, or strong emotions may surface suddenly. (We encourage a daily diary, to follow their development.)

In this process the participant refocuses their energies and brings stability as they find their own compass or anchor in their life. The life mandala also becomes a roadmap in living the soul's purpose and finding meaning in the participant's life. I encourage them to frequently review their mandala after they return home, especially their inner circle. This roadmap is a living document, and with time and the participant's inner development, the roadmap may change, with new shortcuts and paths created.

We encounter participants with different levels of awareness. Our role is to encourage each to go as deep within as they are capable in the meditation process, and to come up with answers that are meaningful to them. We do this by listening carefully, and through questioning, encourage them to go even deeper. The whole process requires great sensitivity to ensure that we are meeting our client where they are, and know how to encourage them to go deeper. It also is a very intimate process and participants have to have a sense of their own space within the room to work individually on their mandala. We often encourage them to work in their own language if it is other than English. At the end of the process, if the group is cohesive, we encourage a voluntary sharing within the group of the most important "aha" moments or decisions made.

The end result of this work is a list of actionable items they will implement over the next 12 months in order to live healthier and be happier. In the words of one client:

> I still think back to the life mandala exercise that we did during the three-week retreat, remembering my action goals for how to bring my life into more balance and harmony. Thanks for that experience! (M.)

APPENDIX 1

Guided Meditations

In this section you will find samples of meditation scripts that we use. The scripts should be read slowly, with some longer pauses, indicated in the text by "…" or [long pause]. If you have patients who have never meditated before, start the first week with guided meditation, using the mantra "so hum" for mindfulness. This works very well. As the days pass and patients get used to sitting in meditation, increase the time of silent pauses until the last two days, and then ask them to meditate on their own, without your guidance.

The following week is the week of working with emotions. This is also a good time to start forgiveness meditation. Let patients bring people with whom they have difficult relationships, so they can work on unresolved issues and negative emotions.

Meditation on the breath with "so hum"[1]

Assume a comfortable posture, lying on your back or sitting. If you are sitting, keep the spine straight and let your shoulders drop.

Close your eyes if it feels comfortable. Begin watching your breath. At first… start by breathing normally, gradually letting your breath slow down until it is quiet, even, and the lengths of the breaths fairly long.

From the moment you sit down to the moment your breathing has become deep and silent, be conscious of everything that is happening in yourself…

Bring your attention to your belly, feeling it rise or expand gently on the in-breath and fall or recede on the out-breath.

Keep the focus on your breathing, "being with" each in-breath for its full duration and with each out-breath for its full duration, as if you were riding the waves of your own breathing.

Every time you notice that your mind has wandered off the breath, notice what it was that took you away, and then gently bring your attention back to your belly and the feeling of the breath coming in and out.

Your breath should be light, even, and flowing, like a thin stream of water running through the sand. Your breath should be very quiet, so quiet that a person sitting next to you cannot hear it; and your breath should flow gracefully, like a river, like a water snake crossing the water, and not like a chain of rugged mountains or the gallop of a horse. To master our breath is to be in control of our bodies and minds.

[Breath is a bridge between the body and the mind. When trying to meditate it is extremely common to have tension in the muscles and noisy thoughts in the mind. The nervous system is the arbiter between the tense body and the noisy mind. One of the best ways to regulate that nervous system, and in turn the body and mind, is through the breath.]

Now we will introduce a mantra to help us manage the mind, "so hum." This means "I am That"…"I am an indescribable Divine Principle within me." So, breathe in, breathe out, completely.

So—hum…

Slowly become aware of the sensations in your body… Of the room you are sitting in…and when you are ready, you can open your eyes.

Forgiveness 1

Relax… Close your eyes…

Focus your attention on your feet, on your ankles and your calves…and relax your muscles and ligaments… Take a deep breath…

Focus on your knees and thighs…and *relax* them now.

Move your attention to the belly…and all the organs within the belly…and relax.

Focus on your chest and all the organs within the chest…and relax them completely… Take a deep breath…

Now move the focus to your fingers, palms, and wrists… And relax all the muscles and ligaments…

Now focus on your elbows, arms, and shoulders… And relax all the ligaments and muscles of your elbows, arms, and shoulders…

Focus on your neck, face, and eyes… And relax all the ligaments and muscles of your neck, face, and eyes…

Now begin to observe your breathing…breathe in slowly and breathe out slowly…being completely conscious of the breath…follow every movement of the breath with your attention… And just enjoy the motion of breathing…

Now imagine that with every breath you breathe in the healing light from Universal Source. See the light filling your body, inhaling light, and as you exhale you distribute the light to every cell in your body… Inhaling light… Exhaling it into the body.

As you continue, see this healing light extending beyond the body and building a cocoon of light around your body.

As you breathe…intensify this light surrounding you…

See the light extending further to the front so that it encompasses an empty chair in front of you… Now the chair is included in the healing light.

Now imagine a person with whom you have a difficult relationship or you have to forgive; invite them into your circle of light, and ask them to sit in the chair in front of you.

The person feels the light around you—notice their reaction…

Now focus on intensifying the light surrounding you with every breath so that it also reaches the person sitting in front of you. They look at you and you look back at them.

Notice the facial expression of the person as they sit within your light. Allow for any exchange that may happen between you and the person…

If you can, and feel moved to…say to them, "I forgive you" and "I love you"…

Notice if the person says anything to you…

[Silence.]

Now thank the person for coming and being with you. Gently say goodbye to them and watch them go out of your sight.

[If there is time, you may repeat the process inviting another person.]

Slowly withdraw the light, now feeling it all inside of your own body.

Slowly close the image and become aware of sitting in the room with others.

Focus on your breath. Become aware of the body being supported by the floor or the chair.

Take a deep breath, and while exhaling, gently move your toes and fingers, and when you are ready, slowly open your eyes.

Forgiveness 2

Relax… Close your eyes… Sit in a comfortable position… Or you may be in a lying position…

Focus your attention on your feet, ankles, and calves…and relax all your muscles and ligaments… Take a deep breath…

Focus on your knees and thighs…and *relax* them now.

Move your attention to the belly…and all the organs within the belly…and relax.

Focus on your chest and all the organs within the chest…and relax them completely… Take a deep breath…

Now move the focus to your fingers, palms, and wrists… And relax all the muscles and ligaments…

Now your elbows, arms, and shoulders… And relax all the ligaments and muscles of your elbows, arms, and shoulders…

Focus on your neck, face, and eyes… And relax all the ligaments and muscles of your neck, face, and eyes…

Now begin to observe your breathing…breathe in slowly and breathe out slowly…being completely conscious of the breath…follow every movement of the breath with your attention… And just enjoy the motion of breathing…

Now imagine in your mind's eye a chair standing in front of you. On this chair you can see sitting a person whom you love very, very much. They are sitting and looking at you with a loving smile. You can feel your love growing in your heart as you watch the person smiling at you.

You are now filled to the brim with your own love for that person. Feel it vibrating in every cell of your body… See your love now extending out of your body and it now surrounds you. Pay full attention to yourself, as you slowly grow in intensity this feeling of love extending and surrounding you.

Notice that your feeling of love now encompasses the chair, but the chair is empty…the person has left. Nevertheless, you still are able to feel and grow even more the intensity of your love. Feel it vibrating in every cell now…

And now…bring into the picture the person you have a difficult relationship with. Watch that person now sitting on the chair in front of you. Visibly the person enjoys the energy of your love, which covers them and the chair.

Notice if the person is saying anything to you…

Now say to this person—"I am filled with love and I forgive you." Notice any response…

[Silence…]

Slowly let go of the image…still feeling the intensity of your own love…with no object in front of you…

Now slowly repeat this three times: "I am happy, I am strong, I am loving, and I am peaceful."

Take a deep breath, and as you exhale, slowly move your toes and fingers, and when you are ready, gently open your eyes.

Healing heart

Find a comfortable position and close your eyes. I am going to count slowly down from 10 to 1. Imagine the numbers as I count.

10, 9, 8, 7, 6, 5, 4, 3, 2, 1.

Now imagine moving into your own heart...

Imagine holding your own heart with the deepest compassion...

Ask your heart... What is it that you need to be healthy and whole? How can I help? What can I do?... Pause and listen.

Now imagine holding your heart between your hands. Imagine a stream of golden light going from one hand to the other and holding your heart in a cocoon of this golden healing light. Notice how your heart rejuvenates and revitalizes as it sits in this golden cocoon...

Now thank the heart and imagine it coming back to your chest. Relax and take a deep breath.

We have come together as a group for positive and constructive purposes.

In a moment I am going to count from 1 to 5. At the count of 5 you will open your eyes feeling wide awake, refreshed, and alert.

1...2...coming out slowly, 3...at the count of 5 you will be wide awake, alert, and refreshed, 4...5 eyes open, alert, and refreshed.

Open heart, compassion

Find a comfortable position and close your eyes. I will help you to enter your deeper levels by counting slowly from 10 to 1. Imagine the numbers as I count.

10, 9, 8, 7, 6, 5, 4, 3, 2, 1.

You are now at a deeper level of mind.

In order to help you relax and enhance your faculty of imagination, I am going to count from 1 to 3, and at the count of 3, project yourself mentally to a pleasant place of your choice for relaxation.

1...2...3...you are now in your place of relaxation. Think about the sights... the sounds...the smells...and the feeling there... Until you hear my voice again in a little while.

[45-second pause.]

Relax…take a deep breath…and we will continue. Remember that in case of interruption or an emergency you will open your eyes immediately and be wide awake and alert.

You are always in control at all levels of your mind.

If, for some reason, you need to end the exercise on your own, before the rest of us, all you need to do is take a deep breath and open your eyes and you will be wide awake, alert, and refreshed.

I may bring you out of this level of mind or a deeper level than this by counting to you, from 1 to 5, or by gently touching you on the shoulder.

Now start by focusing your breath on the heart…breathing in and out of your heart area.

Now imagine that you are breathing in love from Universal Source into your heart and as you exhale you distribute self-compassion and love into each and every cell in your body.

Now radiate compassion out from your heart to people and the world around you.

Send out compassion as radiance and care, with understanding for what people are going through.

Imagine the light of compassion lifting the hearts of others…your friends, your family, your enemies.

Relax and take a deep breath.

We have come together as a group for positive and constructive purposes.

We use these levels of the mind to help ourselves, help one another, to help any human being who needs help.

In a moment I am going to count from 1 to 5. At the count of 5 you will open your eyes feeling wide awake, refreshed, and alert.

1…2…coming out slowly, 3…at the count of 5 you will be wide awake, alert, and refreshed, 4…5 eyes open, alert, and refreshed.

Pain control

Take a deep breath and mentally repeat and visualize the number "3" three times.

Take another deep breath and mentally repeat and visualize the number "2" three times.

Take a deep breath and mentally repeat and visualize the number "1" three times.

Relax.

Slowly count from 10 to 1, every time feeling yourself going deeper and feeling more relaxed.

Concentrate your sense of awareness on your scalp. Sense the blood vessels—the feeling of warmth or tingling sensation caused by circulation.

Now release and relax all tensions from this part of your body completely, and place it in a deep state of relaxation.

Repeat focusing and relaxing with your:

- forehead
- eyelids
- face
- throat
- inside the throat and area around
- shoulders
- chest
- inside the chest and area around
- abdomen
- inside the abdomen and area around
- thighs
- knees
- calves
- heels
- soles of your feet and toes.

Now cause your feet to feel as if they do not belong to your body.

Cause your feet, ankles, calves, knees, and thighs to feel as if they do not belong to your body.

Cause your feet, ankles, calves, knees, thighs, waist, shoulders, arms, and hands to feel as if they do not belong to your body.

You are completely relaxed now your body feels as if it does not belong to you.

1. Point mentally to the exact location of your pain.

2. If the pain could fit in a container, what container size would be perfect for it (can, bottle, box, etc.)?

3. If the pain had a color, what color would it be? Feel the pain. What color is it?

4. If the pain had a taste, what would it taste like? Feel the pain. How does it taste?

5. If the pain had a smell, what would it smell like? Feel the pain. How does it smell?

Go through steps 1–5 again, noticing changes in the location, size, color, taste, and smell.

If there is still some pain left, repeat the cycle (steps 1–5) a few more times if necessary, until you can no longer locate or feel the pain.

You are very relaxed now.

[Coming out.]

Repeat mentally to yourself the following: "In a moment I will count from 1 to 5. At 5 I will open my eyes, be wide awake, feeling fine and in perfect health. Feeling much better than before."

Count slowly from 1 to 5 and at 5, repeat… "I am wide awake, feeling fine, and in perfect health. Feeling much better than before."

Headache and pain control

Find a nice, comfortable position…and allow your eyes to close…

And now, as you take a nice deep breath in…and let it out…and another slow, deep breath in…and let it out…just feel the discomfort in your body… Great…

And on a scale of 1 to 100, where 1 is the minimum and 100 is the maximum, just rate the intensity of the discomfort… At what level would you say it is right now?… Okay…

Now, in your mind's eye, see a part of you getting up…and going over and sitting in a chair across the room…and see the area of discomfort in the body of that part of you across the room… Great…

Now, give a color to the area of discomfort in the part of you across the room…or imagine what color it might be…and now see that color…

Next give a texture to that area of discomfort…or imagine what texture it might have…and now see the texture…

Next give a shape to that area of discomfort…or imagine what shape it might be…and now see the shape…

Next give the area a sound…or imagine what sound it might make…and now hear the sound…

Now see the size of that area of discomfort...

And so, seeing the color...and the texture...and the shape...hearing the sound...and noticing the size...

Now change the color to your favorite color, or a healing or soothing color... You can change the tone and the brightness until it is ideal... Good...

Now change the texture until it's smooth, or change it into a healing, soothing texture... Okay...

Now change the shape to your favorite shape, or into a healing, soothing shape... Great...

Now change the sound into a healing, soothing sound... Great...

And now reduce the size until the area disappears completely... Good...

And now see another part of you, a healing part of you, getting up...and going to the chair across the room...

See that healing part of you putting its hands on the area where there was discomfort in the first part of you across the room... And see that healing part of you giving your body across the room healing energy and healing light and love... Great...

Now see the healing part of you merge into the first part across the room...

And see that merged part get up from its chair, come back to you...

And feel it putting its healing, loving hands on the area of your body where the original discomfort was located...

Feel healing energy and light and love coming from its hands...permeating your body and your being...soothing, relaxing, and deeply healing you... Great...

And now feel the healing part merge with you...and when you are ready, knowing that this healing and integration will continue to take place perfectly and naturally on its own, gracefully and automatically within your body... effortlessly and easily...

Feeling rested and much more comfortable now...you may open your eyes, when you are ready... Great...

And on a scale of 1 to 100, go ahead and rate how you are feeling in your body... (Let the answer come)... Excellent... Great work!

Yoga Nidra

Nidra 1

Preparation

Take a deep breath and relax. Observe the natural breath and with every exhale, feel your body letting go and sinking deeper into the floor...[1]

As you watch your body breathing, notice that there is a little pause between exhale and inhale. Connect to this pause and make it comfortably longer... Notice what happens during that pause... How does your body feel then...?

Become now aware of the fact that you will practice *yoga nidra*. Mentally repeat to yourself, "I am aware... I am going to practice *yoga nidra*..."

Affirmation

Remember your resolve and repeat it to yourself mentally three times—fill it with conviction and awareness that this is already so.

Rotation of awareness: sensing the body

We now begin rotation of awareness around the body. Rotate your attention through your body while experiencing and welcoming sensations...

You may feel something, or little at all... Whatever your experience, it is perfect just as it is...

Sense your jaw...mouth...teeth...lips and gums...tongue...the entire inside of your mouth...the entire jaw and mouth...as a sensation...

Give up thinking and simply welcome the sensation in your jaw and mouth...

Sense your left ear...right ear...welcoming both ears at the same time...as a sensation...

Sense your left nostril…right nostril…the flow of air and the sensation inside both nostrils…

Feel the sensation of the left eye…eyebrow…temple…cheekbone…the entire left side of your face…

Right eye…eyebrow…temple…cheekbone…the entire right side of your face…

Welcome both eyes at the same time…as a sensation…

Without thinking, just feeling…the sensation of the forehead…scalp…back of the head…neck…the entire face…head…and neck as a sensation…

Sense your left shoulder…left upper arm…forearm…wrist…palm and fingers…the sensation of your entire left arm and hand…

Right shoulder…right upper arm…forearm…wrist…palm and fingers…the sensation of your entire right arm and hand…

Welcoming both arms and hands at the same time as a radiant sensation…

Sense the upper chest…mid chest…belly…the sensation of the upper back…mid back…lower back…the entire back of the torso…entire front of the torso…the entire torso, front and back…inside and outside…as a shimmering sensation…

Bring attention into the pelvis…left hip…left thigh…knee…calf muscle… ankle…foot…the sensation of the entire left foot…leg and hip…

Be awake…attentive…yet relaxed and at ease…

Sensing the right hip…right thigh…knee…calf muscle…ankle…and foot… the sensation of the entire right foot, leg, and hip…

Welcome both hips…legs…and feet…all together as a radiant sensation…

Welcome the entire front of the body…as a radiant sensation…back of the body…left side of the body…right side…inside the body…outside the body… the entire body as a shimmering sensation…

Note how you are the observer…watching all of these sensations coming and going, everything just as it is…

Feel yourself being non-judging awareness, in which all of these sensations are coming and going…

Silently affirm to yourself, "I am practicing *yoga nidra*…my body is deeply at rest…but I am aware…at ease…attentive and awake…"

[Long pause]

Breathing

Now become aware of your body breathing…

Feel the flow of the breath in and out of your lungs…

Do not try to breathe; just watch your body breathing...

Now focus your awareness on your navel moving up and down with the breath...

Now start counting your breath from 10 down to 1—10 navel rising, 10 navel falling, 9 navel raising, 9 navel falling, etc.... Say the words mentally to yourself as you count the breaths.

If you make a mistake, start counting from 10 again... [Long pause]

Awareness of the breath and counting... [Long pause]

Now stop your counting and move your attention from your navel to your chest...

Watch your chest rising and falling as your body breathes...

Continue watching the movement of the chest and start counting your breath from 10 down to 1—10 navel rising, 10 navel falling...just like before... [Long pause]

Keep on with the practice, counting and awareness, awareness and counting... [Long pause]

Now cease your counting and move your attention from your chest to your throat...

Focus on the sensation of air coming in and going out as your body breathes...

Continue watching the movement of breath and start counting your breath from 10 down to 1—10 navel rising, 10 navel falling... [Long pause]

Keep on with the practice and continue to count your breaths in the throat... [Long pause]

Now stop your counting and move your attention from your throat to your nostrils...

Focus on the sensation of air coming in and going out through the nostrils as your body breathes...

Continue watching the movement of breath and start counting your breath from 10 down to 1—10 navel rising, 10 navel falling... [Long pause]

Keep on with the practice and continue to count your breaths in the nostrils... [Long pause]

Image visualization

Stop your counting and now we come to visualization...

See yourself walking on the beach by the ocean. The beach is small and empty, the temperature is just right, and you feel a light breeze on your skin. The ocean is calm, of a beautiful turquoise color, and the waves are moving slowly through the deep water. Above is a beautiful, clear blue sky. Observe the ocean and the waves and be aware what, if anything, is showing up in your emotions... Welcome whatever emotion comes...

Now stop by the edge of the ocean and let the waves come to your feet. The water is warm and you feel an urge to go deeper into the water... Walk slowly, feeling the warmth of the water...stop when the water reaches your chest...and lie down on the water... The ocean is very salty and you effortlessly float on the surface... You feel safe and calm...your breath is slow and deep...and you watch yourself from above, floating freely in the water...

Look closer and you see that with every exhale the body expels dark cells that flow down and are absorbed by the bottom of the ocean... Notice that these are cancer (diseased) cells, which your body is getting rid of... Now see them floating continuously from the whole surface of the body, forming a funnel, whirling down to the point at the bottom of the ocean and disappearing... Watch this process as the ocean absorbs all the diseased cells and you know that with every minute you are getting healthier...lighter...more energized...and you feel better and better... Stay there for some time...enjoying witnessing your body getting rid of the cancer (disease)... [Long pause]

Look down at your body and notice that the flow of diseased cells to the bottom of the ocean has stopped as your body has now completely cleansed itself. Slowly come out of the ocean and sit on the warm sand. Experience the feeling of wellbeing and joy in your body... It expands throughout your entire body...every cell in your body is welcoming its natural sense of joy and wellbeing... Perhaps the experience of an inner smile is coming from your heart...throughout your entire body...your lips gently smiling...joy, wellbeing, and an inner smile flowing throughout your body...face...torso...arms...legs... your entire body alive with the feeling of wellbeing and joy... [Long pause]

Affirmation

Now is the time for you to repeat the affirmation. Repeat it silently three times with full conviction and awareness...

Finish

Relax all efforts and simply be, observing your body as it breathes. Become aware of the whole body lying on the floor...

Become aware of the sounds in the room...

And sounds coming into the room from outside...

Visualize the room you're in...

Take a deep breath and as you exhale, gently move your fingers and toes....

Turn to the side and lift yourself to a sitting position, opening your eyes when you are ready.

Nidra 2

Preparation

Lie down in *shavasana* (Corpse Pose) and adjust your position to be as comfortable as possible. Take a deep breath and relax. Observe the natural breath and with every exhale, feel your body letting go and sinking deeper into the floor.

Nothing to do... Nowhere to go...

As you watch your body breathing, notice that there is a little pause between exhale and inhale. Connect to this pause and make it comfortably longer... Notice what happens during that pause... How does your body feel then...?

Affirmation

Remember your affirmation and repeat it to yourself mentally three times—filled with conviction and awareness that this is already so.

Rotation of awareness: sensing the body

We now begin rotation of awareness around the body. Rotate your attention through your body while experiencing and welcoming sensations...

You may feel something, or little at all... Whatever your experience, it is perfect just as it is...

Sense your jaw...mouth...teeth...lips and gums...tongue...the entire inside of your mouth...the entire jaw and mouth...as a sensation...

Give up thinking and simply welcome the sensation in your jaw and mouth...

Sense your left ear...right ear...welcoming both ears at the same time...as a sensation...

Sense your left nostril...right nostril...the flow of air and the sensation inside both nostrils...

Feel the sensation of the left eye...eyebrow...temple...cheekbone...the entire left side...

Right eye...eyebrow...temple...cheekbone...the entire right side... Welcome both eyes at the same time...as a sensation...

Without thinking, just feeling...the sensation of the forehead...scalp...back of the head...neck...the entire face...head...and neck as a sensation...

Sense your left shoulder…left upper arm…forearm…wrist…palm and fingers…the sensation of your entire left arm and hand…

Right shoulder…right upper arm…forearm…wrist…palm and fingers…the sensation of your entire right arm and hand… Welcoming both arms and hands at the same time as a radiant sensation…

Sense the upper chest…mid chest…belly…the sensation of the upper back…mid back…lower back…the entire back of the torso…entire front of the torso…the entire torso, front and back…inside and outside…as a shimmering sensation…

Bring attention into the pelvis…left hip…left thigh…knee…calf muscle…ankle…foot…the sensation of your entire left foot…leg and hip…

Be awake…attentive…yet relaxed and at ease…

Sensing the right hip…right thigh…knee…calf muscle…ankle…and foot…the sensation of the entire right foot, leg, and hip…

Welcome both hips…legs…and feet…all together as a radiant sensation…

Welcome the entire front of the body…as a radiant sensation…back of the body…left side of the body…right side…inside the body…outside the body…the entire body as a shimmering sensation…

Note how you are the observer…watching all of these sensations coming and going, everything just as it is…

Feel yourself being non-judging awareness, in which all of these sensations are coming and going…

Silently affirm to yourself, "I am practicing *yoga nidra*…my body is deeply at rest…but I am aware…at ease…attentive and awake." [Long pause]

Breathing

Now become aware of your body breathing…

Feel the flow of your breath in and out of your lungs… Do not try to breathe; just watch your body breathing…

During each exhalation feel a deep release of tension throughout your body and with each inhalation simply stay with the feeling of release, welcoming a deep sense of relaxation…

Sense the breath moving along the passage between the navel and the throat…on inhalation it rises from the navel to the throat…on exhalation it descends from the throat to the navel…throat to navel and navel to throat; follow the breath, sensing its movement…

Maintain awareness of this movement and count the breaths, starting from 10 down to 1. Inhale 10, exhale 10, inhale 9, exhale 9, and so on… Count to yourself mentally as you watch the movement of breath between the throat and navel... [Long pause]

Total awareness of breathing and counting...

Image visualization

Stop your counting and now we come to visualization...

I will be bringing in images and feelings to your awareness. I want you to visualize each one, feel each one, and be aware of any sensations in your body and welcome the emotions that each image may bring.

[Read very slowly, repeating two or three times] House you grew up in
Grandmother; The dog; Childhood friend; Grandfather
Beautiful meadow
Shop with all the goodies you used to frequent; Your favorite teacher
Peaceful ocean with clear water; Cousins playing together; Beautiful sunrise
Mother; Blue sky
Monsoon with torrential rains
Storm with lightning and thunder; White clouds in the sky
Loss of a close one
Beautiful sunset across the sky; Emotional abuse
Addiction of a close one; Overbearing parent; Distant parent
Slow waves across a peaceful sea; Father
[Long pause]

Awareness of sensations

- *Heaviness:* Awaken the feeling of heaviness in your body, perhaps remember a situation when your body felt very heavy...become aware of every single part of your body being so heavy that you are unable to move it...your body is so heavy that you are sinking into the floor...the hands... legs...torso and head...awareness of heaviness...

- *Lightness:* Now awaken the feeling of lightness in your body...or perhaps remember a moment in which your body felt weightless... A sensation of weightlessness in the body...see if you can locate a place of lightness in your body...your body feels so light that it starts floating above the floor... awareness of lightness... Now as you hold lightness, bring in the heaviness and hold both in your body simultaneously...

- *Heat:* Invoke an experience of warmth in the body…recall any kind of heat you experienced in the past…recollect the feeling of warmth and notice where and how it feels in the body…

- *Coolness:* Recollect the feeling of coolness, any kind of coolness, physical or psychological… Make it real, make it vivid… Notice where and how in the body it feels…stay with it for a while, just witnessing the sensations in the body… Now as you hold coolness, bring in the heat and hold both together in your body simultaneously…

Affirmation

Now come back to the breath and just observe your body breathing… It is time for you to repeat the affirmation. Repeat it silently three times with full conviction and awareness…

Finish

Relax all efforts and simply rest in your being, observing your body breathing, become aware of the whole body lying on the floor… [Long pause]

Become aware of the sounds in the room…

And sounds coming into the room from outside… Visualize the room you're in…

Take a deep breath and as you exhale, gently move your fingers and toes…

Turn to the side and lift yourself to a sitting position, opening your eyes when you are ready.

Nidra 3

Before you start this session, please check with participants if they need to change their affirmation—either modify the old one or create a new one…

Preparation

Lie down in *shavasana* (Corpse Pose) or you may choose to sit… Adjust your position to be as comfortable as possible. Take a deep breath and relax. Observe the natural breath and with every exhale, feel your body letting go and sinking deeper into the floor.

As you watch your body breathing, notice that there is a little pause between exhale and inhale. Connect to this pause and make it comfortably longer... Notice what happens during that pause... How does your body feel then...?

Mentally repeat to yourself, "I am aware... I am going to practice *yoga nidra...*"

Affirmation

Remember your affirmation and repeat it to yourself mentally three times, filled with conviction and awareness that this is already so.

Rotation of awareness: sensing the body

You will follow my voice moving your awareness from one part of the body to another. Rotate your attention through your body while experiencing and welcoming sensations...

You may feel something, or little at all... Whatever your experience, it is perfect just as it is...

Sense your jaw...mouth...teeth...lips and gums...tongue...the entire inside of your mouth...the entire jaw and mouth...as a sensation...

Give up thinking and simply welcome the sensation in your jaw and mouth...

Sense your left ear...right ear...welcoming both ears at the same time...as a sensation...

Sense your left nostril...right nostril...the flow of air and the sensation inside both nostrils...

Feel the sensation of the left eye...eyebrow...temple...cheekbone...the entire left side...

Right eye...eyebrow...temple...cheekbone...the entire right side... Welcome both eyes at the same time...as a sensation...

Without thinking, just feeling...the sensation of the forehead...scalp...back of the head...neck...the entire face...head...and neck as a sensation...

Sense your left shoulder...left upper arm...forearm...wrist...palm and fingers...the sensation of your entire left arm and hand...

Right shoulder...right upper arm...forearm...wrist...palm and fingers...the sensation of your entire right arm and hand... Welcoming both arms and hands at the same time as a radiant sensation...

Sense the upper chest...mid chest...belly...the sensation of the upper back...mid back...lower back...the entire back of the torso...entire front of the torso...the entire torso, front and back...inside and outside...as a shimmering sensation...

Bring attention into the pelvis...left hip...left thigh...knee...calf muscle...ankle...foot...the sensation of the entire left foot...leg and hip...

Be awake...attentive...yet relaxed and at ease...

Sensing the right hip...right thigh...knee...calf muscle...ankle...and foot...the sensation of the entire right foot, leg, and hip...

Welcome both hips...legs...and feet...all together as a radiant sensation...

Welcome the entire front of the body...as a radiant sensation...back of the body...left side of the body...right side...inside the body...outside the body...the entire body as a shimmering sensation...

Note how you are the observer...watching all of these sensations coming and going, everything just as it is...

Feel yourself being non-judging awareness, in which all of these sensations are coming and going...

Silently affirm to yourself, "I am practicing *yoga nidra*...my body is deeply at rest...but I am aware, attentive, and awake."

[Long pause]

Breathing

Now become aware of your body breathing...

Feel the flow of your breath in and out of your lungs...

During each exhalation feel a deep release of tension throughout your body and with each inhalation simply stay with the feeling of release, welcoming a deep sense of relaxation...

Sense the breath moving along the passage between the navel and the throat...on inhalation it rises from the navel to the throat...on exhalation it descends from the throat to the navel...throat to navel and navel to throat...follow the breath, sensing its movement...

Maintain awareness of this movement and count the breaths starting from 10 down to 1. Inhale 10, exhale 10, inhale 9, exhale 9, and so on... Count to yourself mentally as you watch the movement of breath between throat and navel... [Long pause]

Total awareness of breathing and counting...

Image visualization: perfect place and inner resource

Stop your counting and now we come to visualization…

I want you to go back in your memory and search for a time when you were completely happy. Perhaps a brief moment that still lingers deep in your memory of complete safety, love, and inner peace…

Bring that moment from your memory when you were perhaps accepted by everyone…surrounded by love… And felt totally safe… It might have been in nature…or a moment with your friends or loved ones…perhaps a fleeting moment or a longer period of time… But it felt like a time of inner peace and complete fulfillment…

If you found it…hold on to it, make it vivid in your imagination, see the colors…smell the smells…hear the sounds…and notice every detail in this picture…

[Only read the following the first time:

Or if you have difficulty finding such a moment in your memory, you may want to create anew a place in your imagination, a place where you are completely safe and filled with inner peace…

You may imagine that you are sitting by the bank of a river with a beautiful shore and vista to the other side…

Or in a stunning meadow full of blooming flowers and a shimmering stream…

Or on top of a mountain watching the breathtaking view…

Or you may be sitting on a beach by the turquoise sea, watching the rays of sun dancing on the water…

Or you may create any other place that invokes in you a feeling of inner peace, complete safety, and fulfillment…

Make it vivid in your imagination… See the colors…smell the smells…hear the sounds…notice every detail in this picture…]

Now I want you to place yourself in the middle of this scenery or place, and as you are there, notice how it feels in your body… Do you feel any sensations arising in your body?

How does it feel to be there in the middle of your favorite place? Take a moment to focus on the sensations arising in your body as you bask in this perfect place of your memory or imagination…

These sensations and emotions of inner peace, acceptance, safety, and joy are your inner resource…they are always there…waiting for you…beckoning you to come back and feel them again…your inner resource…

And the place in your memory or imagination is a perfect healing place, the place where you can go to any time you need to access your inner resource... The feelings of peace and fulfillment...

Take a moment now just to be in this place...being aware of any sensations in your body...feeling completely safe, filled with inner peace and joy...

[Long pause]

Opposite feelings

Now stop the visualization. Feelings are any physical sensations you feel in the body. I want you now to scan your body and become aware if you feel anything, any sensations...

Welcome whatever you notice...whatever is present...perhaps a feeling of warmth or the feeling of being at ease...tiredness...heaviness...or deep relaxation... Whatever is present, welcome it just as it is without any desire to change anything...

Now locate the opposite feeling, if you felt warmth...find coldness; if heaviness...find lightness, if you felt relaxed, then find tension...if tiredness, then vigor...without going into thinking...just sensing your body...and feeling the opposite to your first feeling...where do you sense it in your body?...

Now I want you to bring in the inner resource, the feeling you felt when you were in your perfect place, completely safe, fulfilled, and in peace...

Then come back to the original feeling...then go back to the opposite feeling again...

And when you are ready, move back and forth between the opposites at your own pace... Finally welcome both opposites at the same time...

Feeling them simultaneously...

Become aware how this impacts your entire body and mind...not with thinking...just sensing and experiencing...

Become an observer who is witnessing all these feelings that are coming and going in your awareness... Not engaging in judging or choosing one over the other...just simply being non-judgmental awareness in which all these movements are coming and going...

Affirmation

Now come back to the breath and just observe your body breathing... It is time for you to repeat your affirmation. Repeat it silently three times with full conviction and awareness...

Finish

Relax all efforts and simply rest in your being, observing your body breathing...
Become aware of the whole body lying on the floor... [Long pause]

Become aware of the sounds in the room...

And sounds coming into the room from outside...

Take a deep breath and as you exhale, gently move your fingers and toes...

Turn to the side and lift yourself to a sitting position, opening your eyes when you are ready.

Nidra 4

At the beginning of this session we ask each participant to choose a negative emotion that they may be struggling with or that they may simply want to work with—such as jealousy, fear, hatred, or anger. Once this choice is made, we then ask each client to decide what is the opposite emotion to the chosen one. Each person may have a different idea as to what the opposite emotion to fear or anger or jealousy may be.

Preparation

Lie down in *shavasana* (Corpse Pose) and adjust your position to be as comfortable as possible. Take a deep breath and relax. Observe the natural breath and with every exhale, feel your body.

As you watch your body breathing, notice that there is a little pause between exhale and inhale. Connect to this pause and make it comfortably longer... Notice what happens during that pause... How does your body feel then...? Letting go and sinking deeper into the floor....

Affirmation

And now it is time for the affirmation. Remember your resolve and repeat it to yourself mentally three times—feel and affirm it with your entire body and mind as true in this moment...

Rotation of awareness: sensing the body

And we begin rotation of our awareness around the body sensing each part of the body separately. Rotate your attention through your body while experiencing and welcoming sensations...

You may feel something, or little at all... Whatever your experience, it is perfect just as it is...

Sense your jaw...mouth...teeth...lips and gums...tongue...the entire inside of your mouth...the entire jaw and mouth...as a sensation...

Give up thinking and simply welcome the sensation in your jaw and mouth...

Sense your left ear...right ear...welcoming both ears at the same time...as a sensation...

Sense your left nostril...right nostril...the flow of air and sensation inside both nostrils...

Feel the sensation of the left eye...eyebrow...temple...cheekbone...the entire left side...

Right eye...eyebrow...temple...cheekbone...the entire right side...

Welcome both eyes at the same time...as a sensation...

Without thinking, just feeling...the sensation of the forehead...scalp...back of the head...neck...the entire face...head...and neck as a sensation...

Sense your left shoulder...left upper arm...forearm...wrist...palm and fingers...the sensation of your entire left arm and hand...

Right shoulder...right upper arm...forearm...wrist...palm and fingers...the sensation of your entire right arm and hand... Welcoming both arms and hands at the same time as a radiant sensation...

Sense the upper chest...mid chest...belly...the sensation of the upper back...mid back...lower back...the entire back of the torso...entire front of the torso...the entire torso, front and back...inside and outside...as a shimmering sensation...

Bring attention into the pelvis...left hip...left thigh...knee...calf muscle... ankle...foot...the sensation of the entire left foot...leg and hip...

Be awake...attentive...yet relaxed and at ease...

Sensing the right hip...right thigh...knee...calf muscle...ankle...and foot... the sensation of the entire right foot, leg, and hip...

Welcome both hips...legs...and feet...all together as a radiant sensation...

Welcome the entire front of the body...as a radiant sensation...back of the body...left side of the body...right side...inside the body...outside the body... the entire body as a shimmering sensation...

Note how you are the observer...watching all of these sensations coming and going, everything just as it is...

Feel yourself being non-judging awareness, in which all of these sensations are coming and going...

Silently affirm to yourself, "I am practicing *yoga nidra*...my body is deeply at rest...but I am aware...at ease...attentive and awake."

[Long pause]

Breathing

Now become aware of your body breathing…simply observe. Feel the flow of your breath in and out of your lungs…

No effort…just witnessing what is…nothing to do, nowhere to go…no one to be…

During each exhalation feel a deep release of tension throughout your body and with each inhalation simply stay with the feeling of release, welcoming a deep sense of relaxation…

We will start now with *anuloma viloma* (alternate nostril breathing), directing the breath with our awareness, without using the hand. In the next exhalation focus your awareness on your left nostril and then inhale, keeping your awareness on your left nostril… In the next exhale change your focus to your right nostril… Inhale, keeping your awareness on your right nostril…

Exhale and inhale through one nostril, change, and exhale and inhale through the other one… Watch for any sensations in the body as you do this…

Maintain awareness of this movement and count the breaths starting from 10 down to 1. Inhale 10, exhale 10, inhale 9, exhale 9, and so on… Count to yourself mentally as you watch the movement of breath between the nostrils…

Total awareness of breathing and counting… [Long pause]

Opposite emotions

We will work now with emotions. Emotions such as fearful or courageous, calm or anxious, peaceful or angry are states that arise in response to circumstances and relationships. So now I want you to become aware of and welcome any emotion that is present in your body…or recall an emotion you are working with in your life…

Remember that you are in safe space to feel whatever you need to feel…

And if you are sensing an emotion…where and how does it feel in your body?

Are there thoughts and any other emotions accompanying this emotion? And remember, welcome this experience just as it is, without judging or trying to change it…

Now I want you to bring in the inner resource, the emotions you feel when you are in your perfect place, completely safe, happy, and in peace…

Now locate an opposite emotion to the original one and become aware where and how you experience this opposite in the body… If it is helpful, recall a memory that will help you to invite this opposite emotion more fully into your body…

And go back to the original emotion again…

When it feels right…move back and forth between the opposite emotions, experiencing first one and then its opposite in your own time…and as you do this, sense how each emotion affects your body and mind…

And now hold and sense both emotions at the same time…being aware how this affects your entire body and mind…

Become an observer who is witnessing all these emotions that are coming and going in your awareness… Not engaging in judging or choosing one over the other…just simply being non-judgmental awareness in which all these movements are coming and going…

Be aware of yourself witnessing all that is present in your consciousness… awake and aware… Sensations…thoughts…images…

Affirm to yourself, "I am awake and aware… I am practicing *yoga nidra*… and resting at ease."

Slowly withdraw your attention from the sensations and become aware of the breath coming in and out…

Image visualization

We come to visualization now… I want you to see your body lying on the floor. In your mind's eye come closer and closer and finally penetrate the skin and find yourself inside your body. Look around and see your cells…some are healthy and some are not. Move through the body to the location of the diseased cells…

Start working now on the elimination of the diseased cells from your body. Imagine an unlimited supply of tools and white blood cells at your disposal, and watch them destroying all the diseased cells around your body…

Take some time to make sure you have eliminated all the sick cells in your body…

I will be sounding the gong gently just in case your mind wanders off—to remind you to go back to working with your image.

[Long pause, 10 minutes]

Now check if the body is clean… So many cells were eliminated, so now fill the vacant space with healthy, vibrant cells…

And now fill your whole body with bright white or yellow healing light. Let this light fill in your whole body and invigorate every cell…do it for some time to make sure that you work around the whole body.

Affirmation

Now cease the visualization and come back to your breath…this is the time for you to repeat the affirmation. Repeat it silently three times with full conviction and awareness…

Finish

Relax all efforts and simply rest in your being, observing your body as it breathes. Become aware of the whole body lying on the floor… [Long pause]

Visualize the room you're in…

Become aware of the sounds in the room…

And sounds coming into the room from outside…

Take a deep breath and as you exhale, gently move your fingers and toes…

Turn to the side and lift yourself to a sitting position, opening your eyes when you are ready.

Nidra 5

Before you begin this *nidra*, introduce the subject of working with limiting beliefs about ourselves. Ask participants to take a minute to think what limiting beliefs they have about themselves: "Not good enough," "Not smart enough," "Unlovable," "Have no right to exist," "Guilty," etc. Ask each one to choose one statement with which they will be working during *yoga nidra*.

Preparation

Lie down in *shavasana* (Corpse Pose) and adjust your position to be as comfortable as possible. Take a deep breath and relax. Observe the natural breath and with every exhale, feel your body letting go and sinking deeper into the floor.

As you watch your body breathing, notice that there is a little pause between the exhale and inhale. Connect to this pause and make it comfortably longer… Notice what happens during that pause… How does your body feel then?…

Now become aware of the fact that you will practice *yoga nidra*. Mentally repeat to yourself, "I am aware… I am going to practice *yoga nidra*…"

Affirmation

Remember your affirmation and repeat it to yourself mentally three times… filled with conviction and awareness that this is already so.

Rotation of awareness: sensing the body

We now begin rotation of awareness around the body.

Rotate your attention through your body while experiencing and welcoming sensations…

You may feel something, or little at all… Whatever your experience, it is perfect just as it is…

Sense your jaw…mouth…teeth…lips and gums…tongue…the entire inside of your mouth…the entire jaw and mouth…as a sensation…

Give up thinking and simply welcome the sensation in the jaw and mouth…

Sense your left ear…right ear…welcoming both ears at the same time…as a sensation…

Sense your left nostril…right nostril…the flow of air and sensation inside both nostrils…

Feel the sensation of the left eye…eyebrow…temple…cheekbone…the entire left side…

Right eye…eyebrow…temple…cheekbone…the entire right side… Welcome both eyes at the same time…as a sensation…

Without thinking, just feeling…the sensation of the forehead…scalp…back of the head…neck…the entire face…head…and neck as a sensation…

Sense your left shoulder…left upper arm…forearm…wrist…palm and fingers…the sensation of your entire left arm and hand…

Right shoulder…right upper arm…forearm…wrist…palm and fingers…the sensation of your entire right arm and hand… Welcoming both arms and hands at the same time as a radiant sensation…

Sense the upper chest…mid chest…belly…the sensation of the upper back…mid back…lower back…the entire back of the torso…entire front of the torso…the entire torso, front and back…inside and outside…as a shimmering sensation…

Bring attention into the pelvis…left hip…left thigh…knee…calf muscle…ankle…foot…the sensation of the entire left foot…leg and hip…

Be awake…attentive…yet relaxed and at ease…

Sensing the right hip…right thigh…knee…calf muscle…ankle…and foot…the sensation of the entire right foot, leg, and hip…

Welcome both hips…legs…and feet…all together as a radiant sensation…

Welcome the entire front of the body…as a radiant sensation…back of the body…left side of the body…right side…inside the body…outside the body…the entire body as a shimmering sensation…

Note how you are the observer…watching all of these sensations coming and going, everything just as it is…

Feel yourself being non-judging awareness, in which all of these sensations are coming and going…

Silently affirm to yourself, :I am practicing *yoga nidra*…my body is deeply at rest…but I am aware…at ease…attentive and awake…"

[Long pause]

Breathing

Now become aware of your body breathing…

Feel the flow of your breath in and out of your lungs…

No effort…just witnessing what is…nothing to do, nowhere to go…

We will start now with alternate nostril breathing (*nadi shuddhi*), directing the breath with our awareness. In the next exhalation focus your awareness on the left nostril and slowly inhale, exhale, and change your focus to the right nostril… Stay with the right nostril as you inhale…exhaling, change your focus to the opposite nostril and hold it there during inhale as well.

Exhale and inhale through one nostril, change, and exhale and inhale through the other one… Watch for any sensations in the body as you do this…

Maintain awareness of this movement and count the breaths starting from 10 down to 1. Just like before…

Total awareness of breathing and counting… [Long pause] Stop the counting…

Welcoming opposite beliefs

If it feels right, welcome a particular thought or belief or self-judgment you take to be true about yourself and believe at times… A judgment that you would like to work today with—it may be "I am worthless"…"I am never good enough …"I am unlovable"…

Notice where and how you feel it in your body when you take it to be true…

Welcome memories, emotions, and sensations that naturally arise, without resisting them or engaging in judgment or trying to change them… Remember that at any moment you can go to your inner resource and bring the feeling of safety, inner peace, and joy.

And if this belief had an opposite…what might its opposite be? Bring to mind the opposite to your belief or self-judgment… Where and how do you feel it in your body when you take this opposite belief to be true?

Now return to the original belief or judgment…welcoming this experience with curiosity and openness…

Now at your own pace go back and forth several times between these opposites, experiencing first one, then the other, with your entire body, emotions, and mind...

When it feels right, welcome both beliefs at the same time, experiencing them simultaneously in your body and mind...

And be aware of all that's in your awareness right now...sensing how you are a witness to all that is arising in your awareness...awake...and aware...of sensations...emotions...thoughts...

Affirm to yourself, "I am aware...and awake... Practicing *yoga nidra*...and resting at ease..."

Joy and wellbeing

Bring your attention to the sensation in your body of wellbeing or of joy... or recall a memory of a particular situation that invites the feeling of joy and wellbeing... Locate it in your body...

Now experience that feeling of wellbeing and joy expanding throughout your body...experience how every cell in your body is welcoming a natural sense of joy and wellbeing...

Perhaps experience an inner smile that is coming from your heart and extending throughout the body...your lips gently smiling...joy, wellbeing, and inner smile are flowing throughout your entire body...face...torso...arms...and legs... Your entire body feels alive with wellbeing and joy...

And you are aware of all that is right now in your awareness, while you are dissolving into spacious openness in which all these changing activities are coming and going...

And be aware of all that is now in your awareness...being an observer of all that is arising in you...awake...aware of the sensations...aware of emotions... thoughts...aware of the joy and wellbeing...

Affirm to yourself, "I am awake...and aware... I am practicing *yoga nidra*... and resting at ease..." [Long pause]

Affirmation

Now return your focus to your breath. Simply watch your body breathing rhythmically... Now is the time for you to repeat the resolve. Repeat it silently three times with full conviction and awareness...

Finish

Relax all efforts and simply rest in your being…

Become aware of the whole body lying on the floor… [Long pause] Become aware of the sounds in the room…

And sounds coming into the room from outside… Visualize the room you're in…

Take a deep breath and as you exhale, gently move your fingers and toes… Lift your hands up and stretch, making yourself as long as you can…

Turn to the side and lift yourself to a sitting position, opening your eyes when you are ready.

APPENDIX 3

Mudra Practices

Week 1

Purna swara mudra–Complete breath

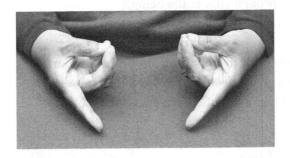

Position: Heart opening.

Core quality: Complete breathing.

Helpful for:

- Facilitating full yogic breath

- Releasing tension from the entire torso

- Supporting healing of all systems of the body

- Integrating body, mind, and spirit.

Drop down to the center of your being and become aware of any feelings or sensations coming up in you.

Notice how your breath flows freely from the base of the body up to your neck and then smoothly back again.

Sense your inhalation awakening each area of the body.

As you exhale, sense the breath flowing downward, instilling a deep release.

Notice a wave-like motion of your breath flowing throughout your being, evoking a sense of integration and harmony.

As your breathing flows more freely, you naturally become more sensitive to the expansion of each part of your lungs.

As you inhale, sense the base of your lungs expanding, followed by the middle lungs, and finally filling the very top of your lungs (or the opposite way).

Sense your exhalation releasing the air gradually, beginning at one part of the body, emptying the middle lungs, and finally releasing from the rest of the lungs.

Connect to the pause between the exhale and inhale, and make it comfortably longer.

Now notice how your breath is nourishing the back, front, and sides of your lungs evenly, instilling the feeling of fullness and vitality.

As your breath flows more easily, any blockages in your breathing are released, allowing the vital energy to flow through your entire being.

Now sense your complete breathing instilling integration and harmony within your being.

Affirm your free breathing, repeating the following three times to yourself: "I experience complete relaxation with my deep and slow breathing now."

Gently release the *mudra* and take a minute to integrate the experience.

Bhramara mudra–Gesture of bee

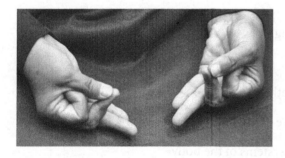

Position: Legs up the wall.

Core quality: Healthy immunity.

Helpful for:

- Balancing the immune system
- Establishing personal boundaries
- Cultivating a positive attitude.

Drop down to the center of your being and become aware of any feelings or sensations coming up in you.

Notice how your breath is gently directed to your upper chest, neck, and head, instilling a sense of clearing throughout your breathing passages.

As you breathe more easily you are able to sense the breath expanding beyond your physical body, allowing for greater sensitivity to your energetic being.

You may notice that the contours of your body naturally expand with each inhalation and soften with each exhalation.

Explore these boundaries as you experience the subtle field surrounding your being.

Your experience of energetic boundaries is a reflection of how you relate to the world. If your sense of boundaries is too rigid, you may overreact to life's challenges.

If your boundaries are too porous, you lose the ability to distinguish "me" from "not me," allowing invaders to challenge your integrity.

When your boundaries are balanced comfortably you welcome all that is healthy while maintaining an energetic shield that protects you adequately.

Now take a minute to sense if your energetic boundaries are perhaps too porous, too rigid, or balanced.

Envision the changes you could make to your relationships and all your activities that would support greater balance in your energetic boundaries.

With healthy boundaries you are safe against the threats that compromise your body's integrity, allowing your immune system to function optimally.

With optimal immunity you find a natural balance between giving and receiving.

Affirm your healthy immunity and balance, repeating the following three times: "With healthy boundaries my immune system functions optimally." [The leader repeats the affirmation twice.]

Gently release the *mudra* and take a minute to integrate the experience.

Svadistana mudra–Inner dwelling place

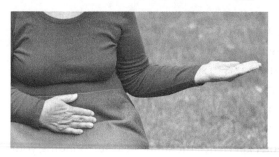

Position: *Shavasana* (Corpse Pose), legs in *baddha konasana* (Butterfly Pose), right hand below the belly button, left open with the elbow by the body.

Core quality: Self-nourishment.

Helpful for:

- Cultivating self-nourishment

- Supporting the health of the urinary and reproductive systems

- Releasing tension from the lower back

- Enhancing our sense of being at home with ourselves.

Drop down to the center of your being and become aware of any feelings or sensations coming up in you.

Notice how your right hand instills a sense of comfort and inner nourishment.

Sense how your left hand is naturally open to receive universal healing energy, channeling it to your inner dwelling place through your right hand.

With your next inhalation, attune to your inner dwelling place opening to receive the quality of fluidity. As you exhale, a sense of fluidity flows from your pelvis to your entire being.

With the quality of fluidity you naturally develop an ability to easily flow with life's cycles and seasons.

Now with your next inhalation return to your inner being and as you exhale, allow the quality of equanimity to naturally unfold within you.

Sense the equanimity deepening, naturally instilling calmness in you no matter what is happening in your surroundings.

And now with greater fluidity and equanimity, healthy relationships unfold naturally because when you are at home within your own being you are able to be with others in complete comfort and safety.

With your next inhalation allow a sense of deep self-nourishment to unfold naturally within you.

Let this feeling of self-nourishment permeate your entire being, supporting you lovingly in caring for yourself and for others.

Affirm your self-nourishment repeating the following three times and feeling it in the body: "At home in my being I experience deep self-nourishment and healing now." [The leader repeats the affirmation twice.]

Gently release the *mudra* and take a minute to integrate the experience.

Dvimukham mudra–Deep relaxation

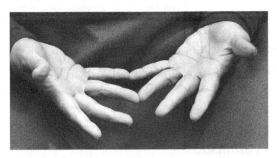

Position: Sitting with hands facing upward, supported below the navel.

Core quality: Deep relaxation.

Helpful for:

- Reducing stress and blood pressure

- Supporting the health of the urinary, reproductive, and eliminatory systems

- Supporting treatment of anxiety and insomnia.

Drop down to the center of your being and become aware of any feelings or sensations coming up in you.

Notice how your breath is directed into your pelvis and lower abdomen, becoming slow and deep, allowing you to relax completely.

To relax even more deeply, visualize yourself being by the tranquil sea with gentle waves flowing softly.

With the next inhalation, relax your feet and legs, and with exhalation, release any tension from these parts.

With the next inhalation, relax your pelvis, abdomen, lower, and mid back. As you exhale, release all tension from these areas.

With the next inhalation, relax your chest and upper back. As you exhale, release all tension down and out of your body.

Take a few moments to sense and enjoy complete relaxation from your chest down to your feet.

With the next inhalation, relax your hands all the way to your shoulders. As you exhale, sense all tension being released from your hands.

Take a moment to feel the area from your hands to the soles of your feet completely relaxed.

Now relax your head and neck, allowing your forehead, jaw, mouth, and eyes to become completely calm.

With your entire body relaxed and at ease, allow your mind to rest completely within your inner being.

Affirm your absolute relaxation by repeating the following three times: "My entire being relaxes completely now." [The leader repeats the affirmation twice.]

Gently release the *mudra* and take a minute to integrate the experience.

Week 2

Kapota mudra–Non-violence, ahimsa

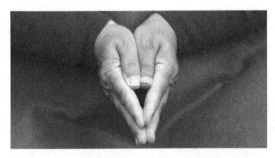

Position: Sitting with hands supported in front of the solar plexus.

Core quality: Non-violence.

Helpful for:

- Cultivating non-violence towards self and inner peace at all levels of being

- Supporting the health of the immune system

- Cultivating self-care and self-healing

- Facilitating introspection and inner listening.

Drop down to the center of your being and become aware of any feelings or sensations coming up in you.

Direct the breath to your heart, filling it with inner peace.

Create the intention to listen to your body's messages at all times and to exercise greater self-care and self-healing.

Make a vow of peace towards your body by silently chanting "om shanti" three times.

Create the intention to be aware of and to welcome your thoughts and emotions without any judgment.

Make a vow of peace towards your challenging thought patterns and emotions by silently chanting "om shanti" three times.

Resting in your heart, invoke loving kindness towards your body and mind, towards yourself.

Now include in your loving kindness your family, your friends, and community.

Visualize your loving kindness now enveloping the entire natural world and all living beings.

Holding this image in your mind, reconnect again with the center of your being.

From that place invoke a peaceful unity with everyone and everything.

Affirm this unity with all by repeating the following silently three times: "I live in complete inner and outer harmony now!" [The leader repeats the affirmation twice.]

Gently release the *mudra* and take a minute to integrate the experience.

Anamika mudra–Ring finger

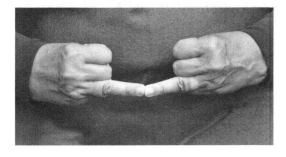

Position: *Shavasana* (Corpse Pose) with legs in *baddha konasana* (Butterfly Pose), hands supported in front of the solar plexus.

Core quality: Self healing.

Helpful for:

- Cultivating self-healing and self-nourishment

- Sense of coming home to yourself

- Supporting the health of the urinary and reproductive systems.

Drop down to the center of your being and become aware of any feelings or sensations coming up in your body.

Focus on the incoming and outgoing slow, deep breath, and notice the gap between exhalation and inhalation.

With every inhale, visualize a healing light or energy coming into your feet and your legs.

With the next inhalation, direct this healing light or energy to nourish your abdomen, solar plexus, lower, and mid back.

Now move the healing energy or light to your heart, lungs, chest, and upper back.

With the next inhalation, direct this healing light or energy to nourish the shoulders, hands, palms, and fingers.

Finally move this healing energy or light to your neck and head.

Feeling the healing light or energy encompassing all levels of your being, visualize all diseased (cancer) cells disappearing and the complete healing taking place now!

Now cease the visualization and rest in your being, filled with peace and harmony.

It's time to affirm your self-healing by repeating the following three times, feeling it in your body: "I experience complete healing on all levels of my being now." [The leader repeats the affirmation twice.]

Gently release the *mudra* and take a minute to integrate the experience.

Avahana mudra–Heartfelt acceptance

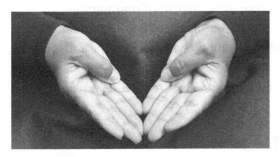

Position: Legs up the wall, hands in front of the solar plexus.

Core quality: Heartfelt acceptance.

Helpful for:

- Opening the heart to welcome all situations as a learning and a blessing

- Learning to welcome challenges as opportunities

- Supporting the healthy functioning of the immune system

- Exposing and releasing limiting beliefs.

Drop down to the center of your being and become aware of any feelings or sensations coming up in your body.

Notice how your breath flows gently upwards from your solar plexus to your chest, bringing a sense of ease and openness.

Take a few moments to welcome everything you notice in your natural surroundings.

Now embrace different facets of your personality, welcoming your habits and tendencies with empathy and full acceptance.

Welcome *all* aspects of your personality, especially the ones you do not like!

Now openly embrace others and their points of view, learning from different ways of seeing and being.

As you embrace others more openly, release any tendencies to be critical or demanding.

And now you are open to embrace your own life history, understanding that each chapter in your life has been an essential part in the process of your own transformation and healing.

Welcome every chapter of your life wholeheartedly by recognizing that even the greatest challenges actually turned out to be blessings.

Finally welcome life as a whole, including the cancer journey, recognizing that everything that occurs has its own meaning within your journey.

Affirm your heartfelt acceptance by repeating the following affirmation three times: "I accept wholeheartedly all situations in my life now!" [The leader repeats the affirmation twice.]

Gently release the *mudra* and take a minute to integrate the experience.

Ratna prabha mudra–Radiant jewel

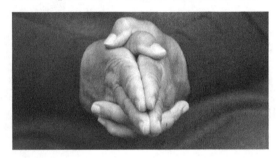

Position: Sitting with palms supported in front of the solar plexus.

Core quality: Vitality.

Helpful for:

- Enhancing enthusiasm and vitality

- Activating digestion

- Building self-esteem

- Creating a clear sense of life purpose.

Drop down to the center of your being and become aware of any feelings or sensations coming up in your body.

Notice how your breath flows naturally into your solar plexus and chest, enhancing the sense of vitality.

Visualize the source of vitality as a brilliant jewel at the center of your solar plexus and notice its color, shape, size, and clarity, allowing its luminosity to radiate throughout your body.

With each inhalation the light of your inner jewel shines more brightly, and with each exhalation you fill your body with its radiance.

Now allow this light to fill your digestive system with the vital energy.

Move the light to fill your respiratory system, clearing away any congestion.

Now let your inner jewel naturally illuminate your mind with self-acceptance and self-esteem.

As the light of your inner jewel infuses your body at all levels, sense your life as a field of infinite possibilities.

Allow this radiant light to illuminate all of your healing possibilities, while providing the energy to manifest them completely.

Affirm your healing vitality as you repeat the following three times, experiencing it in your body: "I am filled with healing vitality on all levels of my being now!" [The leader repeats the affirmation twice.]

Gently release the *mudra* and take a minute to integrate the experience.

Week 3

Pranidhana mudra–Learning to let go

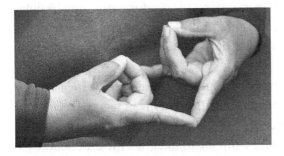

Position: Sitting, hands below the navel.

Core quality: Letting go.

Helpful for:

- Surrendering to life's flow

- Letting go of the need to control or possess

- Attuning to your essential being

- Reducing stress and blood pressure.

Drop down to the center of your being and become aware of any feelings or sensations coming up in your body.

Notice how your breath is gently directed down to the base of the body, cultivating a sense of release.

With the next inhale, gently tense all of your body parts—from your head to your feet.

Now slowly begin to release the tension starting from your feet and legs and continuing up the body, part by part, ending at the scalp, so that at the end of the process you feel a complete release.

With greater relaxation and ease, notice how your breath naturally flows more smoothly and easily.

Now envision having this level of relaxation and release in all of your daily activities.

Begin by visualizing yourself letting go of the need to be constantly doing and achieving.

In the space created by this release, sense yourself appreciating the simple things, allowing you to live fully and joyfully.

Living with greater ease you naturally let go of self-judgments and self-criticism.

Embracing yourself with ease allows you to let go of the need to control and judge others, and to focus on your own process of transformation and healing.

With greater acceptance of yourself and others you naturally surrender deeply to your own inner being, allowing it to guide your healing journey with equanimity.

Affirm your ability to surrender to your inner guidance, repeating the following three times: "As I surrender, I am attuned to my inner guidance." [The leader repeats the affirmation twice.]

Gently release the *mudra* and take a minute to integrate the experience.

Jayashala mudra–The lake

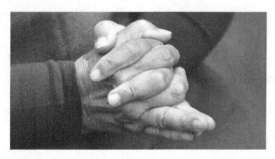

Position: Lying, legs in *baddha konasana* (Butterfly Pose), base of the hands joined below the navel.

Core quality: Serenity.

Helpful for:

- Releasing a tendency towards judgment

- Instilling a cooling effect to relieve inflammation

- Releasing tension in the body

- Calming the mind.

Drop down to the center of your being and become aware of any feelings or sensations coming up in your body.

Notice how your breath is directed into your pelvis and the base of your body, evoking a feeling of ease and serenity.

To deepen the sense of serenity, visualize yourself near a calm lake surrounded by green trees and wild flowers swaying in the soft breeze.

Sense yourself within that scene. The water is warm, the sandy, clean bottom is inviting you to enter in complete comfort and safety.

As you bathe effortlessly in this lake of serenity, you receive all its essential nourishing qualities.

Begin by absorbing the quality of release, sensing yourself letting go and simply be, without need to control or change anything.

As you allow things to simply be, your breathing becomes even more calm and serene.

With a greater sense of calmness and serenity, contentment unfolds naturally. You know you already possess everything you need for your healing.

Resting in contentment, you naturally enjoy all of life's simple things.

And now attuned to the present moment, evoke a feeling of oneness with the natural world.

Holding the experience of oneness, take a moment to let loving compassion unfold naturally.

With a greater sense of loving compassion and unity, you envision the harmonious cooperation of all your body systems resulting in complete healing.

Affirm your complete healing by repeating the following three times, feeling it in your body: "With all my systems in harmony I am completely healed now." [The leader repeats the affirmation twice.]

Gently release the *mudra* and take a minute to integrate the experience.

Brahma mudra–Creative energy

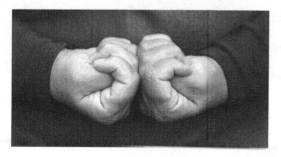

Position: Legs up the wall, folded fists in front of the solar plexus.

Core quality: Awakening of energy and vitality.

Helpful for:

- Expanding the free flow of creative energy throughout the body

- Supporting optimal health and healing

- Cultivating vitality

- Building self-esteem and self-mastery.

Drop down to the center of your being and become aware of any feelings or sensations coming up in your body.

Notice how your breath flows smoothly to your chest, ribs, and upper back, naturally deepening your sensitivity to the breathing process.

As you attune to your breathing, your awareness of its four phases expands naturally.

With each inhalation your chest expands fully to receive vital energy followed by a pause in which your lungs absorb the life force.

With each exhalation you experience a sense of release followed by a pause, allowing you to rest deeply.

As you sense this wave-like movement, comfortably lengthen each phase of breathing now.

As your vital energy expands, you are able to channel it to each part of your body.

Begin by inhaling deeply and with exhalation, direct the creative energy down to your pelvis, legs, and feet.

Take a moment to notice these areas expanding and releasing energetically, in synch with your inhale and exhale.

As your lower body breathes completely, sense this area nourished and vitalized by creative energy.

Take another slow and deep breath, and while exhaling, direct the creative energy to your abdomen, solar plexus, lower, and mid back.

And notice these areas expanding and releasing energetically in synch with your breath.

As your middle region breathes completely, sense this area nourished and vitalized by the energy.

Take another slow and deep breath and while exhaling, direct creative energy to your chest, upper back, shoulders, and hands.

And notice these areas expanding and releasing energetically, in synch with your breath.

As these parts of your body breathe completely, sense this area vitalized by the energy.

With another slow and deep breath and while exhaling, direct creative energy to your neck, head, and brain. Feel your mind infused with clarity and vitality.

Finally sense your entire body expanding with every inhale and releasing with every exhale, allowing creative energy to revitalize your entire being.

Affirm the power of the life force by repeating the following three times: "As the energy fills my entire being I am healed now." [The leader repeats the affirmation twice.]

Gently release the *mudra* and take a moment to integrate the experience.

Hakini mudra–Integration

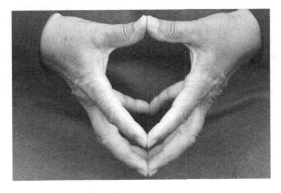

Position: Sitting with hands facing each other, at the solar plexus.

Core quality: Integration.

Helpful for:

- Optimizing integration and healing at all dimensions of being

- Connecting to inner wisdom

- Overall integration at physical and subtle levels

- Supporting overall health and healing.

Drop down to the center of your being and become aware of any feelings or sensations coming up in your body.

Notice how each inhalation flows upward from the base of the body to your collarbones, and how each exhalation smoothly descends, releasing all tension in the body.

And sense how this deep breath naturally cultivates integration and harmony in your being.

In a moment you will enhance this integration by directing your breath into various parts of your body individually, culminating in an experience of unity and healing.

Begin by directing your breath to the left side of your body, sensing how it awakens the receptive and intuitive aspects of your being.

Now direct the breath into the right side of the body, sensing how it naturally awakens your active, dynamic polarity.

Now let the breath flow to both—left and right—sides of the body evenly, integrating them as harmonious unity.

With left and right sides integrated completely, now direct the breath into the back of your entire body.

Sense how this breathing attunes you to subconscious dimensions of your being which hold deep beliefs.

Now direct your breath to the front of your entire body, attuning to the conscious aspects of your being, the qualities that make your personality.

Now let the breath flow into both—back and front—planes of the entire body evenly, integrating the subconscious and conscious as a seamless unity.

With back and front, left and right planes integrated completely, start directing your breath towards the lower part of the body, creating the sense of being grounded in your physical being.

Now direct the breath towards the upper part of your body, allowing you to attune to the subtle dimensions of your being.

Now breathe into your lower and upper body evenly, harmonizing the material and subtle dimensions of your being.

Finally breathe fully and freely throughout your entire body, sensing left and right, back and front, bottom and top, integrated as a harmonious unity.

Affirm your complete integration by repeating the following three times: "With my being fully integrated I feel completely healed now." [The leader repeats the affirmation twice.]

Gently release the *mudra* and take a minute to integrate the experience.

Home Plan, Template

Morning practice

1. Kriyas–before asanas

Jala neti (nasal cleansing with water): Daily.

Sutra neti (nasal cleaning with thread): Twice a week.

2. Asanas

Daily in the morning, before breakfast.

Before starting *asanas* you may do simple joint movements—wrists, elbows, shoulders, ankles, and knees. While doing *asanas* please move in and out of the posture in a very slow and controlled manner. Always take at least a 30-second break between each *asana* (in *shavasana* (Corpse Pose), *jathara parivartanasana* (Revolved Abdomen Pose), sitting, or standing positions). Always engage *slow, deep yogic breathing*. Keep your focus and awareness on your body, emotions, and mind. If you find your mind racing, mentally connect the mantra "so hum" to your breath.

You may choose three to four *asanas* for your daily practice, alternating them every day. The whole *asana* practice should take no more than an hour. After practice always relax in *shavasana* for at least 8 minutes.

SUPINE

Jathara parivartanasana (Revolved Abdomen Pose)

Ardahalasana (Half Plough)

Satubandhasana (Bridge Pose)

Pavanmuktasana (Wind Relieving Pose)

Viparita karani (Legs up the Wall Pose) with *ashwini mudra*

Halansa (Plough Pose)

Matsyasana (Fish Pose)

Naukasana (Boat Pose)

Relax in *shavasana* (Corpse Pose)

PRONE

Makarasana (Crocodile Pose)

Niralambasana (Pillar Pose)

Naukasana coordination (Coordinated Boat Pose)

Bhujangasana (Cobra Pose)

Shalabasana (and *ardha halasana*) (Locust Pose)

Marjarasana (Cat–Cow Pose)

Relax in *makarasana* (Crocodile Pose)

SITTING

Janushirasana (Head to Knee Pose)

Paschimottanasana (Seated Forward Bend)

Supta vajrasana (Reclining Hero Pose)

Ushtrasana (Camel Pose)

Yoga mudra

Gomukhasana (Cow Face Pose)

Vakrasana (Simple Spinal Twist)

Bhadrasana (Butterfly Pose)

Relax in *dandasana* (Staff Pose)

STANDING

Surya namaskar (Sun Salutations)

Chakrasana (Side Bending)

Tadasana (Mountain Pose)

Trikonasana (Triangle Pose)

Virabhadrasana (Warrior Pose)

Konasana (Bound Angle Pose)

Utkasana (Chair Pose)

Vriksasana (Tree Pose)

Garudasana (Eagle Pose)

3. Mudras (preparation for pranayama)

Agnisar kriya

Simhasana (Lion Pose) with *jiva bandha* x 5

Brahma mudra x 3

4. Pranayama

At the beginning, the inhale to exhale ratio is 1:2 with no suspension of the breath. Precision is important, so use a metronome. Always seek the guidance of an experienced teacher before advancing your routine.

Kapalbhati 20 x 3, or to capacity, increasing weekly by a maximum of 5 to 100 breath strokes

Anuloma viloma (alternate nostril) x 10

Surya bhedana (right nostril) x 10

Sitali (cooling breath) x 15

Ujjayi (victorious breath) x 15

Chandra bhedana (left nostril) x 10

Bhramari (humming bee breath) x 15

5. Meditation

Sit for at least half an hour daily in meditation, at the same time of day (with an empty stomach), before meals, in the same place. Choose a comfortable position and do not move for the duration of the meditation.

Recommended: 10-day *Vipassana* course.

6. Mantra chanting–Trayambakam

Evening practice

Yoga nidra 2 x week

Bhramari x 20 (daily, before bed)

Sitali x 20

During the day

While sitting at your desk or computer, make sure that you take a break every two hours, and do the following:

Parvatasana (Seated Mountain Pose): hold for 2 minutes

Uttana mandukasana (Extended Frog Pose): hold for 15 seconds each side

Vertical arms swing x 15

Sample for an Individual *Asana* Sequence

Begin in a comfortable seated position or in *shavasana* (Corpse Pose). Allow for some time to connect with your breath. Follow the natural flow of inhales and exhales, and begin to relax into your exhalations. Slowly begin to connect to the pause between exhale and inhale, and make it comfortably longer, gently softening and deepening your breath with each exhalation. In-between *asanas* use resting poses, such as *shavasana, jathara parivartanasana, balasana* (Corpse Pose, Revolved Abdomen Pose, Child Pose).

Supine

Ardha pavanmuktasana/pavanmuktasana (Half Wind Relieving Pose/Wind Relieving Pose): Begin with the right knee held into the chest and then move to the left knee being guided into the chest and hold in position, focusing on exhalations. Then hug and bring both knees into the chest for three breaths each leg and three breaths with both legs.

Setubandhasana (Shoulder Bridge Pose): Three to five times, rolling down with control, keeping feet and heels hip-distance apart and firmly grounded into the mat, shoulders rolled under to support the neck. To activate the thyroid gland, gently direct your chin to the heart.

Jathara parivartanasana (Revolved Abdomen Pose) variation

Supine Twist: Bring your arms to shoulder height, palms facing down (fingers in line with shoulders). Bring your knees and feet onto the floor, and keeping your knees stacked on your exhale, twist to the left side and look to the right hand, if your neck allows. Stay here for three to five breaths. Relaxing into your exhalations, focus on releasing your spine with each breath. Inhale to the center, look to the center, and repeat on the right side.

(When completing crocodile variation, turn your body to the left side and lie in *jathara parivartanasana*.)

Prone

Makarasana (Crocodile Pose): Rest with your forehead on the back of your hands and your legs apart, heels facing each other and toes out, for three breaths.

Transition pose, *Supta Tadasana* (Reclined Mountain Pose): Lengthen your arms out straight and legs together, with your forehead on the floor.

Niralambasana (Pillar Pose): This has three variations; choose one each day:

1. Slide your arms back and bend your elbows and rest your chin in your palms; elbows should be in line with your shoulders. Allow for space in your neck (as if you were holding an apple). Shoulders rest away from your ears, shoulder blades back. Hold for three to five breaths, relaxing into your exhalations.

2. Alternate leg raises: Bend your right knee and bring your foot to your buttock, and then lower to the floor. Bend your left knee and repeat on your left side. Remember to inhale, leg up, and exhale, leg down. Repeat two times each side.

3. Raise both feet to the buttocks, knees bent. Repeat two times with the breath, inhale up and exhale down.

Makarasana (resting pose): Awareness on the breath for three breaths.

Bhujangasana (Baby Cobra Pose): Bring the shoulder blades back and open up through the chest. No more than three times.

Marjarasana (Cat–Cow Pose): Come onto all fours, wrists in line with shoulders and knees in line with hips. Inhale, eyes, hips, and neck up to the ceiling, exhale, bring your eyes into your belly and arch your spine, relaxing your shoulders away from your ears. Repeat three to five full repetitions, with full breath awareness.

Balasana (Child Pose): You may either bring your knees together and lower your hips to your heels and forehead to the mat or separate your knees, mat distance apart (big toes touching), and then lower your forehead to the mat. Wrap your arms around your body to rest your shoulders, or extend your arms out straight to stretch your shoulders, arms, and side body. Rest here, breathing into your back body. Feel your back open and expand on the inhale and relax and fall on the exhale.

Sitting

Vakrasana (Seated Twist): Take a long sitting position, hands by the side of the body, palms on the ground. Fold your right leg at the knee and place the sole on the ground by the side of the left knee; the folded knee should point upwards. Take the right hand backwards and place the palm on the ground at a distance of around 10 inches, in line with the spine. Take the left hand towards the right side of the right knee and place the palm on the ground. Pushing the right knee towards the left side, twist your head back. Come back in reverse order. Repeat on the other side.

Ushtrasana (Camel Pose): Kneel on the floor with your knees and thighs hip-width apart and firm, but don't harden your buttocks, and keep your outer hips as soft as possible. Press your shins and the tops of your feet firmly into the floor. Rest your hands on the back of your pelvis, bases of the palms on the tops of the buttocks, fingers pointing down. Use your hands to spread the back pelvis and lengthen it down through your tailbone. Make sure that your hips are stable and are not pressing forward. Inhale and lift your heart by pressing the shoulder blades back. For the duration of the pose, keep your head up, chin down in the direction of your heart, and your hands on the pelvis. Beginners: come into a gentle back bend, lifting up through the chest. If you're not able to touch your feet without compressing your lower back, turn your toes under and elevate your heels.

Paschimottanasana (Seated Forward Bend): Sit on the mat with the sitting bones connected to the floor. Move any flesh away from the sitting bones. With straight legs, press your heels out and flex your toes back towards you. Inhale, lift up through the chest, directing the heart to the ceiling, lean forward, nice and long, and begin bending from the hip crease (not the waist). Exhale, begin to lower the ribs down in the direction of the thighs, chest lifted. If you are able, take hold of the sides of your feet with your hands, elbows extended. Relax and hold for three to five breaths. Then, if you wish, you may let go and round the back and relax to your thighs. Inhale, lift up through the chest, keeping a long spine, and as you are lifting, shoulders are back, beginning to raise the torso up.

Standing ——————————————————————————————

Tadasana (Mountain Pose, Palm Tree variation): Root your feet into the mat. Engage the thighs and draw the belly into the spine. Lift up through the chest and roll the shoulders back, shoulder blades together. The neck is long, with the crown of the head towards the ceiling. As you inhale, raise your arms up to shoulder height, fingertips in line with your shoulders. Turn your palms facing up, and with the next inhale, raise your arms up until your biceps are parallel with your ears. Relax the shoulders away from the ears. Keep your feet grounded on the floor as you lift up through the body on your inhalations, grounding on the exhalations. Come back in the same form with the exhale.

Utthita trikonasana (Extended Triangle Pose, variation): Part your legs in a standing position. Then turn the right foot sideways, 90 degrees to the right, and turn the left foot slightly to the right. Keep both knees tight and bend to the right side from the waist. Place your right palm on the ground behind your right foot. Stretch the spine, opening the chest, twist up, spreading your arms. Look at your left arm. Maintain the position for 30 seconds to a minute. Then do the same posture the other way round.

Utkatasana (Chair Pose): Stand in *tadasana* (Mountain Pose). Inhale and raise your arms perpendicular to the floor. For shoulder problems lower your arms to shoulder height, parallel to the floor. Exhale and bend your knees, trying to take the thighs as parallel to the floor as possible. Align your knees to the ankles and the torso will lean slightly forward over the thighs, until the front torso forms a right angle with the tops of the thighs. Keep the inner thighs parallel to each other and press the heads of the thigh bones down toward the heels. Bring your shoulder blades back. Take your tailbone down toward the floor and in toward your pubis, to keep the lower back long. Stay for 30 seconds to a minute. To come out of this pose, straighten your knees with an inhalation, lifting strongly through the arms. Exhale and release your arms to your sides into *tadasana*.

End the practice in *shavasana* (Corpse Pose) for 5–8 minutes.

Kirtan Kriya

Kirtan kriya is performed in a sitting position, either on the floor or on a chair. It uses a four-syllable mantra—chanting, whispering, and silent repetition—in synchrony and simultaneously with four *mudras*. Each repetition of the entire mantra takes 3–4 seconds.

Mantra

The mantra means:

- *Saa:* infinity, cosmos, beginning

- *Taa:* life existence

- *Naa:* death, change, transformation

- *Maa:* rebirth.

Repeat the mantra in the following manner:

- 2 minutes chanting

- 2 minutes audible whisper

- 4 minutes repeating mentally in silence

- 2 minutes whisper

- 2 minutes chanting.

(This can be modified if time permits for longer segments, but the ratio should always be kept as 1:1:2:1:1.)

Mudras

The most used *mudras* for this practice are *gyan*, *shuni*, *surya*, and *buddhi*, done simultaneously with two hands and changing each syllable in synchrony with the mantra.

- *Saa: gyan mudra*, representing knowledge (thumb and first finger, Jupiter).

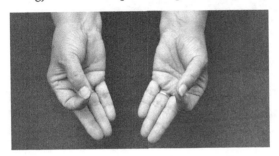

- *Taa: shuni mudra*, representing wisdom, intelligence and patience (thumb and middle finger, Saturn).

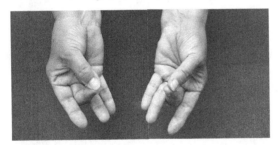

- *Naa: surya mudra*, representing vitality and energy of life (thumb and ring finger, Sun).

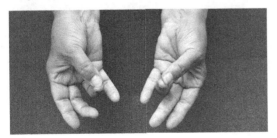

- *Maa: buddhi mudra*, representing ability to communicate (thumb and little finger, Mercury).

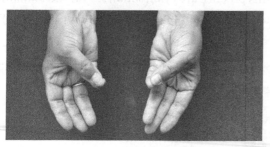

The elbows should be straight and the thumb touching the fingertip (not fingernail) with firm pressure.

When finished, follow with a minute of silence.

Feelings Wheel

English teacher Kaitlin Robbs created a vocabulary wheel that helps narrow down the exact word that best describes your feelings. We explain how we use this in Chapter 13.

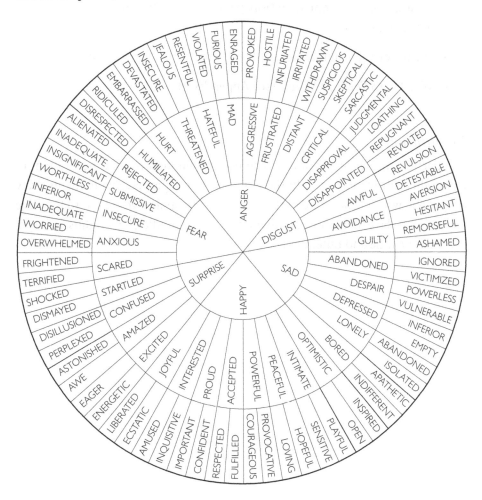

Life Mandala

Instructions

What is needed

- 1 large sheet of construction paper (24" x 36" or bigger) for each participant

- 1 pack of colorful markers to share (1 pack for 2 participants)

- Sheet with Feelings Wheel (see Appendix 7)

Preparation

The participants sit on the floor; each one has enough room around them to feel in their intimate space. On the large sheet of paper have your clients draw a big circle with a little circle in the center and 16 spokes going out to the edge (see below). Have them draw another circle in the middle of the radius, half way between the little and outer circles.

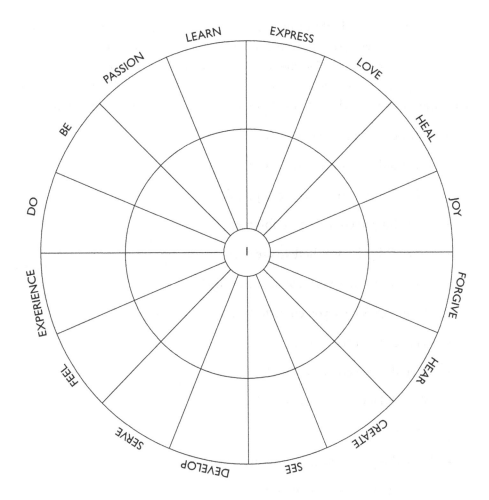

Outside of the big circle have them write the following words for each spoke: learn, heal, express, forgive, create, develop, serve, see, do, be, joy, hear, feel, passion, experience, love. In the little circle in the middle have them write: "I am here"—this is where they presently are in life.

Exercise

SESSION 1

The process in this exercise is based on meditative contemplation of the questions listed below. Start with a short meditation, to relax everyone. Then read the first question to them, and let them go back into a meditative state to listen or look for the answer. The questions mainly pertain to the discovery the client has made about him/herself during the course, much less to their expectations before coming here. The answers usually come as a first thought, and it is important not to allow for self-doubt or over-analyzing. It is also important to wait and listen to the answer arising from deep within rather than quickly "knowing" the answer in your head. The clients write the answer in the bigger circle under the appropriate word. Once a client is ready after writing down the answer, encourage them to go back to meditation to wait until the whole group is done.

- What did you come here to learn?

- What did you come here to heal?

- What did you come here to express?

- Who did you come here to forgive?

- What did you come here to create?

- What talents have you come to develop?

- What causes have you come to serve?

- What did you come here to see?

- What did you come here to do?

- What did you come here to be?

- What brings you joy?

- What did you come here to hear?

- What did you come here to feel?

- Where is your passion?

- What did you come here to experience?

- Who did you come here to love?

Repeat this process with the next question, taking your time—wait until everyone is ready before going on to the next question. It usually takes one session to answer the outer circle and one or two sessions to fill in the smaller circle.

Session 2 (and 3)

At the beginning the clients look through the questions *and* answers to the questions written the day before, and review them once again, one by one, to see if there are any changes or additions to be made to yesterday's notes. When ready, they start working on the inner circle. This process continues with meditative contemplation, but this time everyone works in silence or independently. Here the clients list the actions they need to take in order to achieve what they listed in the outer circle. It may be appointments to make, courses to enroll on, *sadhana* to be performed daily, money to be saved, people to be contacted, apologies to be made, and anything else that they need to do to "move" the "I" from the small circle in the middle to achieve the goal listed in the outer circle.

The final step is listing all the activities from the inner circle on one sheet. You could ask them to do this on their computer for ease of editing. There will be repetitions, and the more an activity is repeated, the higher on the list its position should be, as the more important it is to do it in order to achieve the goal.

To end the process, if the group is cohesive, I encourage a voluntary sharing within the group of the most important "aha" moments, decisions made, or simply the usefulness of the process.

Bibliography

Thomas Ashley-Farrand (2006) *Chakra Mantras: Liberate Your Spiritual Genius Through Chanting*. San Francisco, CA: Red Wheel/Weiser LLC.

Sri Aurobindo (1998) *Essays on Philosophy and Yoga* (Vol. 13). Pondicherry, India: Sri Aurobindo Ashram Publication Department.

Ananda B. Bavanani (2013) *Yoga Chikitsa: Application of Yoga as a Therapy*. Puducherry, India: Divyananda Creations.

Sharadchandra Bhalekar (2017) *Pranayama, Mudra and Meditation: Traditional Approach and Scientific View*. Lonavala, India: Kaivalyadhama.

Linda Carlson and Michael Speca (2010) *Mindfulness-Based Cancer Recovery*. Oakville, CA: New Harbinger Publications Inc.

Stephen Cope (2007) *The Wisdom of Yoga: A Seeker's Guide to Extraordinary Living*. New York: Bantam Dell.

Stephen Cope (2017) *Soul Friends: The Transforming Power of Deep Human Connection*. Carlsbad, CA: Hay House.

Richard J. Davidson and Sharon Begley (2012) *The Emotional Life of Your Brain: How Its Unique Patterns Affect the Way You Think, Feel, and Live—and How You Can Change Them*. London: Penguin.

Swami Degambaraji (ed.) (1990) *Hathapradipika of Swatmarama*. Lonavala, India: Kaivalyadhama.

Georg Feuerstein (2001) *The Yoga Tradition: Its History, Literature, Philosophy and Practice*. Prescott, AZ: Hohm Press.

Swami Gitananda Giri (1994) *Ashtanga Yoga of Patanjali*. Pondicherry, India: Satya Press.

Elliott Goldberg (2016) *The Path of Modern Yoga: The History of an Embodied Spiritual Practice*. Rochester, VT: Inner Traditions.

David R. Hawkins (2014) *Power vs. Force: The Hidden Determinations of Human Behavior*. Carlsbad, CA: Hay House.

David R. Hawkins (2015) *Healing and Recovery*. Carlsbad, CA: Hay House.

Patricia Joudry and Rafaele Joudry (1999) *Sound Therapy: Music to Recharge Your Brain*. A Success Stream Book. Albion Park Rail, NSW: Sound Therapy International.

Sat Dharam Kaur (2003) *The Complete Natural Medicine Guide to Breast Cancer: A Practical Manual for Understanding, Prevention and Care*. Toronto, ON: Robert Rose Inc.

Sat Bir Khalsa, Lorenzo Cohen, Timothy McCall and Shirley Telles (2016) *The Principles and Practice of Yoga in Health Care*. Fountainhall, UK: Handspring Publishing, Chapter 1.

Swami Kuvalayananda (2010) *Pranayama*. Lonavala, India: Kaivalyadhama.

Swami Kuvalayananda (2012) *Asanas*. Lonavala, India: Kaivalyadhama.

Swami Kuvalayananda and S.L. Vinekar (2011) *Yogic Therapy: Its Basic Principles and Methods*. Lonavala, India: Kaivalyadhama.

Vasant Lad (2006) *Secrets of the Pulse: The Ancient Art of Ayurvedic Pulse Diagnosis*, 2nd edn. Albuquerque, NM: The Ayurvedic Press.

Joseph Le Page and Lilia Le Page (2013) *Mudras for Healing and Transformation*. Sebastopol, CA: Integrative Yoga Therapy.

Yangping Li, Josje Schoufour, Klodian Wang, Dong D. Dhana *et al.* (2020) "Healthy lifestyle and life expectancy free of cancer, cardiovascular disease, and type 2 diabetes: prospective cohort study." British Medical Journal. doi: https://doi.org/10.1136/bmj.l6669

Sir James Mallinson (2017) *Roots of Yoga* (Penguin Classics). London: Penguin.

Richard C. Miller (2015) *The iRest Program for Healing PTSD: A Proven-Effective Approach to Using Yoga Nidra Meditation and Deep Relaxation Techniques to Overcome Trauma*. San Rafael, CA: iRest.

Ollie Minton, Alison Richardson, Michael Sharpe, Matthew Hotopf and Paddy Stone (2008) "A systematic review and meta-analysis of the pharmacological treatment of cancer-related fatigue." *Journal of the National Cancer Institute 11*, 16, 1155–1166.

Siddhartha Mukherjee (2011) *The Emperor of All Maladies: A Biography of Cancer*. London: Fourth Estate.

Swami Nirmalayananda (2010) *Yogic Management of Cancer*. Munger, India: Bihar School of Yoga.

Richard Nisbett (2004) *Geography of Thought: How Asians and Westerners Think Differently... and Why*. New York: Free Press.

Dean Ornish and Anne Ornish (2019) *UnDo It! How Simple Lifestyle Changes Can Reverse Most Chronic Diseases*. New York: Ballantine Books.

Frederica P. Perera, V. Rauh, R.M. Whyatt, D. Tang *et al.* (2005) "A summary of recent findings on birth outcomes and developmental effects of prenatal ETS, PAH, and pesticide exposures." *Neurotoxicology 26*, 4, 573–587.

Tari Prinster and Cyndi Lee (2014) *Yoga for Cancer: A Guide to Managing Side Effects, Boosting Immunity, and Improving Recovery for Cancer Survivors*. Rochester, VT: Healing Arts Press.

Richard Rohr (2019) "Daily Meditations." Center for Action and Contemplation (www.cac.org).

Robin Rothenberg (2019) *Restoring Prana: A Guide to Pranayama and Healing through the Breath for Yoga Therapists, Yoga Teachers, and Health-Care Practitioners*. London and Philadelphia, PA: Singing Dragon.

Dilip Sarkar (2017) *Yoga Therapy, Ayurveda, and Western Medicine: A Healthy Convergence*. Morrisville, NC: Lulu Publishing Services.

Sivananda Saraswati (2009) *Bliss Divine: A Book of Spiritual Essays on the Lofty Purpose of Human Life*. Rishikesh, India: Divine Life Society.

Swami Niranjananda Saraswati (2014) *Mudra Vigyan: Philosophy and Practice of Yogic Gestures*. Munger, India: Bihar School of Yoga.

Swami Satyananda Saraswati (2006) *Four Chapters On Freedom: Commentary on the Yoga Sutras of Patanjali*. Munger, India: Yoga Publications Trust.

Swami Satyananda Saraswati (2008) *Asana Pranayama Mudra Bandha*. Munger, India: Bihar School of Yoga.

Mark Singleton (2010) *Yoga Body: The Origins of Modern Posture Practice*. Oxford: Oxford University Press.

K.L. Spalding, O. Bergmann, K. Alkass, D.C. Mash *et al.* (2013) "Dynamics of Hippocampal Neurogenesis in Adult Humans." *Cell 153*, 6, 1219–1227.

Mark Stephens (2017) *Yoga Therapy: Foundations, Methods, and Practices for Common Ailments*. Berkeley, CA: North Atlantic Books.

Makunda Stiles (2008) *Ayurvedic Yoga Therapy*. Twin Lakes, WI: Lotus Press.

Marlysa Sullivan (2020) *Understanding Yoga Therapy: Applied Philosophy and Science for Health and Well-Being*. Oxfordshire: Routledge.

Matthew J. Taylor (2018) *Yoga Therapy as a Creative Response to Pain*. London and Philadelphia, PA: Singing Dragon.

Swami Yogapratap (2009) *Exploring Yoga and Cancer*. Munger, India: Yoga Publishing Trust.

Endnotes

PART 1

1   An expression coined by arguably one of the greatest Western yoga scholars to date, Georg Feuerstein, PhD. See Feuerstein, G. (2001) *The Yoga Tradition: Its History, Literature,* *Philosophy and Practice*. Prescott, AZ: Hohm Press.

2   Taylor, M.J. (2018) *Yoga Therapy as a Creative Response to Pain*. London and Philadelphia, PA: Singing Dragon, p.61.

CHAPTER 1

1   The dates mentioned here are approximate.

2   The oldest known collection of hymns and sacred teachings in Sanskrit, considered the fundamental scriptures of Hinduism.

3   "The Song of the Divine," often referred to as the *Gita*, is a 700-verse Sanskrit text, part of the *Mahabarata*.

4   The perspective from the compilation of these teachings is Vedanta, based on the essential abstracts and extracts of the *Vedas*.

5   A collection of 196 aphorisms on the theory and practice of yoga, compiled by Patanjali.

6   Feuerstein, G. (2008) *The Yoga Tradition: Its History, Literature, Philosophy and Practice,* 3rd edn. Prescott, AZ: Hohm Press.

7   A group of Shaivist monks who emerged around the 13th century. Their tradition is known as *Nath Sampradaya*.

8   An influential classic Sanskrit text on Hatha Yoga: Swami Svatmarama (1990) *The Yoga of Light: Hatha-Yoga-Pradipika*. London: Routledge.

9   Swami Niranjanananda Saraswati (2012) *Gheranda Samhita: Commentary on the Yoga Teachings of Maharshi Gheranda*. Munger, India: Bihar School of Yoga, a classic text from Northern India on *Hatha Yoga*.

10 www.kym.org

11 www.icyer.com

12 www.svyasa.edu.in

13 www.kdham.com

14 www.ym-kdham.in

15 Iyengar, B.K.S. (1966) *Light on Yoga: The Definitive Guide to Yoga Practice*. Crows Nest, NSW, Australia: George Allen & Unwin.

16 www.icyer.com

17 www.sbvu.ac.in/cyter

18 An overview of the studies can be read at Ramanathan, M. and Bhavanani, A.B. (2017) "Understanding how yoga works: A short review of findings from CYTER, Pondicherry, India." *European Journal of Pharmaceutical and Medical Research 4,* 1, 256–262.

19 Gitananda Giri Swami (1983) "Yoga Chikitsa – Yoga therapy." *Yoga Life 14,* 3–18.

20 Ibid.

21 Ibid.

22 This is a classic yoga text, named after the sage Vasistha, and has been estimated to be dated some where between the 6th century to as late as the 14th century, but it is likely that a version of the text existed in the first millennium.

23 *Shiva Swarodaya* is a Sanskrit tantric text that enables us to understand the nature of breath and its influence on the body as different modes of breathing lead to different types of actions—physical, mental, and spiritual.

24 *Swara Yoga* describes a special mode of analysis and practice of breathing.

25 The Ministry of Ayurveda, Yoga & Naturopathy, Unani, Siddha and Homoeopathy (AYUSH) was founded in 2014 as a governmental body in India, purposed with developing education and research in the field of alternative medicine.

26 Read more at Nataraj, P. (2018, November 20) "Ayush therapy for borderline lifestyle ailments." *Deccan Herald*. Available at www.deccanherald. com/state/ayush-therapy-govt-centres-703910. html

27 www.yogaiya.in/integrated-cancer-project-i-cap

Chapter 2

1 One of the major Indian concepts of disease causation is the imbalance of *tridosha*. This is found in numerous classic texts of yoga and Ayurveda, such as *Shiva Swarodaya*, *Sushruta Samhita*, *Charaka Samhita*, and *Tirumandiram*. According to the Dravidian poet saint Tiruvalluvar, disease results from *tridosha* imbalance (*miginum kuraiyinum noiseyyum noolor valimudhalaa enniya moondru*; *Thirukkural* 941). *Vata* is the energy of the body that moves like the wind and causes flow in the body. It may be related to the nervous system as well as to joints that enable us to move. *Pitta* is related to bilious secretion and is the cause of heat in the body. It is the energy of catabolism that is essential for digestion. *Kapha* is the glue that holds everything together and is the energy of anabolism, helping generative and regenerative processes. According to Mark Halpern, Founder-Director of the California College of Ayurveda in the US, the *tridosha* constantly fluctuate. As they move out of balance, they affect particular areas of our bodies in characteristic ways. When *vata* is out of balance—typically in excess—we are prone to diseases of the large intestines, such as constipation and gas, along with diseases of the nervous system, immune system, and joints. When *pitta* is in excess, we are prone to diseases of the small intestines, such as diarrhea, along with diseases of the liver, spleen, thyroid, blood, skin, and eyes. When *kapha* is in excess, we are prone to diseases of the stomach and lungs, most notably mucous conditions, along with diseases of water metabolism, such as swelling.

2 An ancient seminal textual source of yoga, which has teachings of yoga by Lord Krishna, who is also known as the Divine Source of Yoga (Yogeshwar).

3 The concept of the four phases of psychosomatic disorders is elaborated by Yogacharya Dr Ananda Balayogi Bhavanani: see Bhavanani, A.B. (2013) *Yoga Chikitsa: Application of Yoga as a Therapy*. Pondicherry, India: Dhivyananda Creations. Available at www.icyer.in

4 *Heyam dukkham anagatham*; Maharishi Patanjali's *Yoga-darshana*, Sadhana Pada, verse 16.

5 Mary Galantino, Robyn Galbavy, and Lauren Quinn published a systematic review of the literature on the therapeutic effects of yoga for children: see Galantino, M.L., Galbavy, R and Quinn, L.D. (2008) "Therapeutic effects of yoga on children: A systematic review of the literature." *Pediatric Physical Therapy 20*, 1, 66–80.

6 Ibid.

7 One of the oldest available collections of Dravidian (Tamil) poems from Sangam literature (200 bce–100 ce).

8 The *pancha prana vayus* (five major life forces) are described in *Shiva Samhita*, an ancient text, as, "*Hridi prano gude apanah samano nabhi mandaley udanah kantha desastho vyanah sarva shariragah.*" *Prana* is based in the heart region and governs cardiorespiratory function; *apana* is based in the pelvic region and governs the eliminatory function; *samana* is based in the navel region and governs digestion and assimilation; *udana* in the throat region governs communication and thought processes; while *vyana* pervades the entire body, enabling healthy circulation and neuronal activity.

9 Bhavanani, A.B. (2014) "Role of yoga in health and disease." *Journal of Symptoms and Signs 3*, 5, 399–406.

10 The *Gitananda Yoga* teachings in the *Rishiculture Ashtanga Yoga* tradition have a large number of practices that involve visualization of the bipolar flows of energy (*prana* and *apana*) in the human body. These dynamic mental practices are termed the *kriyas* and *prakriyas* of *Jnana* and *Raja Yoga*. Detailed explanations for them can be found in "Yoga: Step-by-Step," a correspondence course offered by ICYER (www.icyer.com). Dr Bhavanani has also discussed them in a video on YouTube: www.youtube.com/watch?v=OWhX7eZbdHk

11 Gitananda Swami (2008) *Pranayama: The Fourth Limb of Ashtanga Yoga*. Pondicherry, India: Satya Press.

12 Bhavanani, A.B. (2007) "Swarodaya vijnan: A scientific study of the nasal cycle." *Yoga-Mīmāṃsā 39*, 1 and 2, 32–38.

13 Venkatesananda, S. (2007) *The Supreme Yoga: Yoga Vashista*. Delhi, India: Motilal Banarsidass Pub. Pvt. Ltd.

14 Bhatt, G.P. (ed.) (2004) *The Forceful Yoga: Being the Translation of the Hathayoga-Pradipika, Gheranda-Samhita and Siva-Samhita*. Translated by P. Sinh and R.B.S.C. Vasu. Delhi, India: Motilal Banarsidass Pub. Pvt. Ltd.

15 Sovik, R. and Bhavanani, A.B. (2016) "History, Philosophy, and Practice of Yoga." In S.B. Khalsa, L. Cohen, T. McCall and S. Telles (eds) *The Principles and Practice of Yoga in Health Care* (pp.17–29). Fountainhall, UK: Handspring.

16 Samiti, K.S.M.Y.M. (1970) *The Hatha Yoga Pradipika*. Lonavala, India: Kaivalyadhama.

17 *Pranava pranayama* is an important technique of the Gitananda tradition that involves slow and deep inhalation with conscious use of complete yogic breathing followed by the audible vibratory resonance of a prolonged AUM chant with one-third of the time allotted for making the sounds AAAA, UUUU, and MMM. This technique is one of the regular practices taught in comprehensive yoga therapy at CYTER, Sri Balaji Vidyapeeth, Puducherry, India. See www.sbvu.ac.in/cyter

18 Iyengar, B.K.S. (1981) *Light on Pranayama*. London: George Allen & Unwin Ltd.

19 Gitananda Swami (2008) *Pranayama: The Fourth Limb of Ashtanga Yoga*. Pondicherry, India: Satya Press.

20 Dr Bhavanani gives a clear and scientifically valid explanation of this in a YouTube video: www.youtube.com/watch?v=Av7oPL7Vads

21 Dr Bhavanani has written about this concept extensively, including articles published in *Yoga Therapy Today* (2011; 7, 26–28) and the *International Journal of Yoga* (2012; 5, 157–158). As suggested during his recent keynote speech at the Symposium on Yoga Therapy and Research (SYTAR) in 2018, he is not against yogopathy, as it may no doubt be useful, but he suggests it be differentiated from real yoga therapy that takes a holistic approach to the whole person.

22 www.dictionary.com/browse/-pathy

23 Antonovsky, A. (1979) *Health, Stress and Coping*. San Francisco, CA: Jossey-Bass.

24 Acharya Sushrut, ca. 600 BCE, *Sushruta Samhita* (15:41).

25 Ornish, D. and Ornish, A. (2019) *UnDo It! How Simple Lifestyle Changes Can Reverse Most Chronic Diseases*. New York: Ballantine Books.

26 Bhavanani, A.B. (2016) "A brief qualitative survey on the utilization of yoga research resources by yoga teachers." *Journal of Intercultural Ethnopharmacology 5*, 2, 168–173.

27 Li, Y., Schoufour, J., Wang, D.D, Dhana, K. *et al.* (2020) "Healthy lifestyle and life expectancy free of cancer, cardiovascular disease, and type 2 diabetes: prospective cohort study." British Medical Journal. doi: https://doi.org/10.1136/bmj.l6669

CHAPTER 3

1 Turner, K. (2014) *Radical Remission: Surviving Cancer Against All Odds*. New York: HarperCollins.

2 Marmot, M.G. and Syme, S.L. (1976) "Acculturation and coronary heart disease in Japanese-Americans." *American Journal of Epidemiology 104*, 3, 225–247.

3 Holt-Lunstad, J., Smith, T.B. and Layton, J.B. (2010) "Social relationships and mortality risk: A meta-analytic review." *PLOS Medicine*. Available at https://doi.org/10.1371/journal.pmed.1000316

4 Hawton, A., Green, C., Dickens, A.P., Richards, S.H., *et al.* (2010) "The impact of social isolation on the health status of older people." *Quality of Life Research 20*, 1, 57–67.

5 Brofman, M. (2003) *Anything Can Be Healed*. Moray, UK: Findhorn Press Ltd.

6 www.who.int

7 www.ym-kdham.in

8 Jeter, P.E., Slutsky, J., Singh, N. and Khalsa, S.B.S. (2015) "Yoga as a therapeutic intervention: A bibliometric analysis of published research studies from 1967 to 2013." *Journal of Alternative and Complementary Medicine 21*, 10, 586–592.

9 Niventhita, L., Mooventhan, A. and Manjunath, N.K. (2016) "Effects of various *prāṇāyāma*

on cardiovascular and autonomic variables." *Ancient Science of Life 36*, 2, 72–77.

10 Kuppusamy, M., Kamaldeen, D., Pitani, R., Amaldas, J. and Shanmugam, P. (2017) "Effects of *Bhramari Pranayama* on health—A systematic review." *Journal of Traditional and Complementary Medicine 8*, 1, 11–16.

11 Chakrabarty, J., Vidyasagar, M., Fernandes, D., Joisa, G., Varghese, P. and Mayya, S. (2015) "Effectiveness of *pranayama* on cancer-related fatigue in breast cancer patients undergoing radiation therapy: A randomized controlled trial." *International Journal of Yoga 8*, 1, 47–53.

12 Punita, P., Trakroo, M., Palamlai, S.R., Subramanian, S.K., Bhavanani, A.B. and Madhavan, C. (2016) "Randomized controlled trial of 12-week yoga therapy as lifestyle intervention in patients of essential hypertension and cardiac autonomic function tests." *National Journal of Physiology, Pharmacy and Pharmacology 6*, 1, 19–26.

13 Bhavanani, A.B., Madanmohan, T. and Sanjay, Z. (2012) "Immediate effect of *chandra nadi pranayama* (left unilateral forced nostril breathing) on cardiovascular parameters in hypertensive patients." *International Journal of Yoga 5*, 2, 108–111.

14 Bernardi, L., Porta, C., Gabutti, A. Spicuzza, L. and Sleight, P. (2001) "Modulatory effects of respiration." *Autonomic Neuroscience: Basic & Clinical 90*, 1–2, 27–56.

15 Koenig, H.G., King, D.E. and Carson, V.B. (2001) *Handbook of Religion and Health.* Oxford: Oxford University Press.

16 Bonelli, R.M. and Koenig, H.G. (2013) "Mental disorders, religion and spirituality 1990 to 2010: A systematic evidence-based review." *Journal of Religion and Health 52*, 2, 657–673.

17 Koenig, H.G., King, D.E. and Carson, V.B. (2012) *Handbook of Religion and Health*, 2nd edn. Oxford: Oxford University Press.

18 Koenig, H.G. (2015) "Religion, spirituality and health: A review and update." *Advances in Mind-Body Medicine 29*, 3, 19–26.

19 Moreira-Almeida, A., Koenig, H.G. and Lucchetti, G. (2014) "Clinical implications of spirituality to mental health: Review of evidence and practical guidelines." *Revista brasileira de psiqiuatria 36*, 176–182.

20 Otis-Green, S., Sherman, R., Perez, M. and Baird, R.P. (2002) "An integrated psychosocial-spiritual model for cancer pain management." *Cancer Practice 10*, Suppl. 1, S58–S65.

21 Clark, C.C. and Hunter, J. (2018) "Spirituality, spiritual well-being and spiritual coping in advanced heart failure: Review of the literature." *Journal of Holistic Nursing 37*, 1, 56–73.

22 McCabe, R., Murray, R., Austin, P. and Sidall, P.J. (2018) "Spiritual and existential factors predict pain relief in a pain management program with a meaning-based component." *Journal of Pain Management 11*, 2.

23 Koenig (2015), op. cit.

24 Vyasa commentary on the 6th *Sutra* of the third chapter of Patanjali's *Yoga Sutras*, as translated by the authors. See Mallinson, J. and Singleton, M. (2017) *Roots of Yoga* (Penguin Classics). London, UK: Penguin.

25 Daaleman, T., Perera, S. and Studenski, S.A. (2004) "Religion, spirituality and health status in geriatric outpatients." *Annals of Family Medicine 2*, 1, 49–53.

26 Lee, M. (2019) "Missing the forest for the trees? Yoga therapy's promise as a transformational practice." *Yoga Therapy Today* Winter, 40–42. Available at https://cdn.ymaws.com/www.iayt. org/resource/resmgr/docs_pubs_ytt/2019_ytt_ pubs/ytt_winter_2019_feature_mich.pdf

27 Sarkar, D. (2017) *Yoga Therapy, Ayurveda and Western Medicine: A Healthy Convergence.* Morrisville, NC: Lulu Publishing Services.

28 Kuvalayananda, S. and Vinekar, S.L. (1963) *Yogic Therapy: Its Basic Principles and Methods.* Central Health Education Bureau, Government of India.

29 Lee, M. (2019) "Missing the forest for the trees? Yoga therapy's promise as a transformational practice." *Yoga Therapy Today* Winter, 40–42. Available at https://cdn.ymaws.com/www.iayt. org/resource/resmgr/docs_pubs_ytt/2019_ytt_ pubs/ytt_winter_2019_feature_mich.pdf

30 Desikachar, T.K.V. (1995) *The Heart of Yoga: Developing a Personal Practice.* Rochester, VT: Inner Traditions International.

31 Sivananda Saraswati (2009) *Bliss Divine: A Book of Spiritual Essays on the Lofty Purpose of Human Life.* Rishikesh, India: Divine Life Society.

32 Sri Aurobindo (1998) *Essays on Philosophy and Yoga* (Vol. 13). Pondicherry, India: Sri Aurobindo Ashram Publication Department.

33 Filliozat, J. (1991) "The Origins of an Indian Mystical Technique." In *Religion, Philosophy, Yoga: A Selection of Articles* (pp.293–306). Delhi, India: Motilal Banarsidass Pub. Pvt. Ltd.

34 Stephens, M. (2017) *Yoga Therapy: Foundations, Methods and Practices for Common Ailments.* London: Penguin.

35 Nizard, C. (2018) "Is Yoga a Spiritual Path?" Annual Conference of the European Association for the Study of Religions (EASR), June 17–21, Bern, Switzerland.

36 Smith, J.A., Greer, T., Sheets, T. and Watson, S. (2011) "Is there more to yoga than exercise?" *Alternative Therapies in Health and Medicine 17*, 3, 22–29.

37 Daaleman *et al.* (2004), op. cit.

38 Wu, Y., Johnson, B.T., Acabchuk, R.L., Chen, S. *et al.* (2019) "Yoga as antihypertensive lifestyle therapy: A systematic review and meta-analysis." *Mayo Clinic Proceedings 94*, 3, 432–446.

39 Turner, K.A. (2015) *Radical Remission: Surviving Cancer Against All Odds.* New York: HarperCollins.

40 Griera, M. (2016) "Yoga in penitentiary settings: Transcendence, spirituality and self-improvement." *Human Studies 40*, 1, 77–100.

41 Smith, B.R. (2007) "Body, mind and spirit? Towards an analysis of the practice of yoga." *Body & Society 13*, 2, 25–46, p.40.

42 Griera (2016), op. cit.

43 Wilson, S.R. and Spencer, R.C. (1990) "Intense personal experience: Subjective effects, interpretations and after-effects." *Journal of Clinical Psychology 46*, 5, 565–573.

44 Smith, K.B. and Pukall, C.F. (2009) "An evidence-based review of yoga as a complementary intervention for patients with cancer." *Psycho-oncology 18*, 5, 465–475.

45 Danhauer, S.C., Mihalko, S.L., Russell, G.B., Campbell, C.R., *et al.* (2009) "Restorative yoga for women with breast cancer: Findings from a randomized pilot study." *Psycho-oncology 18*, 4, 360–368.

46 Büssing, A., Hedstück, H., Khalsa, S.B.S., Ostermann, T. and Heusser, P. (2012) "Development of specific aspects of spirituality during a 6-month intensive yoga practice." *Evidence-Based Complementary and Alternative Medicine.* Available at www.hindawi.com/journals/ecam/2012/981523

47 Weaver, A.J. and Koenig, H. (2006) "Religion, Spirituality, and Their Relevance to Medicine: An Update." *American Family Physician 73*, 8, 1336–1337.

48 Saguil, A. and Phelps, K. (2012) "The Spiritual Assessment." *American Family Physician 86*, 6, 546–550.

49 Sarkar, D. (2017) *Yoga Therapy, Ayurveda and Western Medicine: A Healthy Convergence.* Morrisville, NC: Lulu Publishing Services, p.13.

50 Do not mistake Patanjali's "ashtanga Yoga" as outlined in his *Yoga Sutras* with Pattabhi Jois" *Ashtanga Yoga*, a student of Krishnamacharya who began the lineage called *Ashtanga Yoga* in India in the 20th century.

51 Sarbacker, S.R. and Kimple, K. (2015) *The Eight Limbs of Yoga: A Handbook for Living Yoga Philosophy.* New York: North Point Press.

52 Lee, M. (2019) "Missing the forest for the trees? Yoga therapy's promise as a transformational practice." *Yoga Therapy Today* Winter, 40–42. Available at https://cdn.ymaws.com/www.iayt.org/resource/resmgr/docs_pubs_ytt/2019_ytt_pubs/ytt_winter_2019_feature_mich.pdf

Chapter 4

1 "Sadhana Pada," the second chapter in Maharishi Patanjali's *Yoga Darshan* (*Yoga Sutras*), gives us the philosophical basis of the yoga therapy template through the concepts of *heya-hetu* and *hana-upaya*. These are derived from the following verses:

2.16: Prevent those miseries that are yet to occur (*heyam duhkham anagatam*).

2.17: Suffering is caused by mis-union between the observer and the observed (*drashtri drishyayoh samyogah heya hetuh*).

2.23: This union enables us to experience and attain mastery of our true self (*sva svami saktyoh svarupa upalabdhi hetuh samyogah*).

2.24: This union is caused by ignorance (*tasya hetuh avidya*).

2.25: Dissolution of ignorance breaks this union and enables emancipation (*tat abhavat samyogah abhavah hanam tat drishi kaivalyam*).

2.26: Constant and conscious discerning intellect dissolves ignorance (*viveka khyatih aviplava hana upayah*).

2 BMI is an estimate of body fat and a good gauge of risk for diseases that can occur with more body fat. The higher the BMI, the higher the risk for certain diseases such as heart disease, high blood pressure, type 2 diabetes, gallstones, breathing problems, and certain cancers. See

www.nhlbi.nih.gov/health/educational/lose_wt/risk.htm

3   An eminent physician, medical educator, and former Vice Chancellor of Sri Balaji Vidyapeeth in Pondicherry, India

4   Sethuraman, K.R. (2016) "Yoga for Holistic Wellness (Salutogenesis)." In International Symposium on Yoga and Wellbeing, CYTER, Sri Balaji Vidyapeeth, Pondicherry, India, 12 August 2016. Available at www.slideshare.net/anandabhavanani/yoga-for-holistic-wellness-salutogenesis-by-prof-kr-sethuraman

5   Yogamaharishi Swami Kanakananda Brighu was the yoga *guru* of Swami Gitananda Giri. He codified the teachings of mantra, yantra, and tantra that are today part and parcel of the *Rishiculture Ashtanga Yoga* tradition taught at ICYER at the Ananda Ashram in Pondicherry, India (www.icyer.com). He is mentioned in Swami Yogananda's book, *Autobiography of a Yogi*, as Ram Gopal Muzumdar, the sleepless saint.

6   "Yatho mana tatho prana" is a well-known yogic adage that reiterates the subtle interconnectivity between mind (*mana*) and energy (*prana*). You can watch a detailed video by Dr Bhavanani on this at: www.youtube.com/watch?v=8o2HD-YLr6Y

7   An excellent website with information on this aspect is: www.ayurvedichealth.com

8   Dr Bhavanani has written a detailed article on this. See Bhavanani, A.B. (2006) "Classification of actions according to the gunas." *Yoga-Mīmāṃsā XXXVII*, 3–4, 176–181.

9   Dr Bhavanani has given a detailed explanation of the 12 yogic diagnostic tools (*dwadasha rogalakshana anukrama*) as taught by his illustrious father-guru Dr Swami Gitananda Giri. See www.youtube.com/watch?v=bqF8tM3Psrk

10 The Optimal State assessment tools are detailed at https://amywheeler.com/online-yoga-courses

11 This method was created by the secretary of Kaivalyadhama Yoga Institute (www.kdhham.com), Shri O.P. Tiwariji, to be used as the evaluation tool for his *pranayama* courses.

12 Fernandez, A.M., Santi, A. and Torres Aleman, I. (2018) "Insulin peptides as mediators of the impact of lifestyle in Alzheimer's disease." *Brain Plasticity 4*, 1, 3–15.

13 Davidson, R.J. and Begley, S. (2013) *The Emotional Life of Your Brain: How Its Unique Patterns Affect the Way You Think, Feel, And Live—And How You Can Change Them*. London, UK: Plume.

CHAPTER 5

1   www.yogajournal.com/page/yogainamerica study

2   Montigny, D. "The unstoppable trend of yoga." Available at www.yogitimes.com/article/unstoppable-trend-yoga-infographic-business

3   See www.iayt.org

4   Greenlee, H., DuPont-Reyes, M., Balneaves, L.G., Carlson, L.E., et al. (2017) "Clinical practice guidelines on the evidence-based use of integrative therapies during and after breast cancer treatment." *CA: A Cancer Journal for Clinicians 67*, 3, 194–232. Available at https://onlinelibrary.wiley.com/doi/full/10.3322/caac.21397

5   Rohr, R. (2019) "Daily Meditations." Center for Action and Contemplation (www.cac.org).

6   Vyasa commentary on the 6th *Sutra* of the third chapter of Patanjali's *Yoga Sutras*, as translated by the authors. See Mallinson, J. and Singleton, M. (2017) *Roots of Yoga* (Penguin Classics). London: Penguin.

7   The following has been reprinted with permission of the publisher.

PART 2

1   Khalsa, S.B.S., Cohen, L., McCall, T. and Telles, S. (2016) *The Principles and Practice of Yoga in Health Care*. Fountainhall, UK: Handspring Publishing. (Emphasis added)

2   Taylor, M.J. (2018) *Yoga Therapy as a Creative Response to Pain*. London and Philadelphia, PA: Singing Dragon. (Emphasis added)

3   www.who.int/chp/about/integrated_cd/en

4   https://ourworldindata.org/burden-of-disease

5   https://en.wikipedia.org/wiki/Ikigai

6   https://moayush.wordpress.com/2017/05/09/the-yoga-of-responsibility

7   Vaandrager, L. and Kennedy, L. (2016) "The Application of Salutogenesis in Communities and Neighborhoods." In M.B. Mittelmark, S. Sagy, M. Eriksson, G.F. Bauer, *et al.* (eds)

The Handbook of Salutogenesis (Chapter 17). Springer. Available at www.ncbi.nlm.nih.gov/books/NBK435839

8 Ospina, M.B., Bond, K., Karkhaneh, M., Tjosvold, L., *et al.* (2007) "Meditation practices for health: State of the research." *Evidence Report/Technology Assessment 155*, 1–263.

9 Streeter, C.C., Gerbarg, P.L., Saper, R.B., Ciraulo, D.A. and Brown, R.P. (2012) "Effects of yoga on the autonomic nervous system, gamma-aminobutyric-acid, and allostasis in epilepsy, depression, and post-traumatic stress disorder." *Medical Hypotheses 78*, 5, 571–579.

10 www.slideshare.net/anandabhavanani/managing-stress-through-yoga-concepts-and-methods-137454901

CHAPTER 6

1 A statement by Swami Gitananda Giri in his classic book, *Yoga for Breathing Disorders*, revised and republished by Dr Bhavanani in 2008. Available at www.icyer.in

2 www.who.int/respiratory/about_topic/en

3 Singh, V. (1987) "Effect of respiratory exercises on asthma. The Pink City lung exerciser." *Journal of Asthma 24*, 355–359.

4 Tandon, M.K. (1978) "Adjunct treatment with yoga in chronic severe airways obstruction." *Thorax 33*, 514–517.

5 *Mukha bhastrika* is a specialized yogic practice, *pranayama*, described in *Yoga for Breathing Disorders*, revised and republished by Dr Bhavanani in 2008. It is available at www.icyer.in

6 All of these *pranayamas* have been explained in detail in Swami Gitananda's book on *pranayama* that is available from www.icyer.in

7 Nagarathna, R. and Nagendra, H.R. (1985) "Yoga for bronchial asthma: A controlled study." *BMJ 291*, 1077–1079.

8 Vempati, R., Bijlani, R.L. and Deepak, K.K. (2009) "The efficacy of a comprehensive lifestyle modification programme based on yoga in the management of bronchial asthma: A randomized controlled trial." *BMC Pulmonary Medicine 30*, 9, 37.

9 Satyaprabha, T.N., Murthy, H. and Murthy, B.T.C. (2001) "Efficacy of naturopathy and yoga in bronchial asthma: A self-controlled matched scientific study." *Indian Journal of Physiology and Pharmacology 45*, 80–86.

10 Two of these studies are: Bernardi, L., Passino, C., Wilmerding, V., Dallam, G.M., *et al.* (2001) "Breathing patterns and cardiovascular autonomic modulation during hypoxia induced by simulated altitude." *Journal of Hypertension 19*, 947–958; and Spicuzza, L., Gabutti, A., Porta, C., Montano, N. and Bernardi, L. (2000) "Yoga and chemoreflex response to hypoxia and hypercapnia." *The Lancet 356*, 1495–1496.

CHAPTER 7

1 Roth, G. (2019) "World Health Organization cardiovascular disease risk charts: Revised models to estimate risk in 21 global regions." *The Lancet Global Health*, September 2. Available at www.healthdata.org/research-article/world-health-organization-cardiovascular-disease-risk-charts-revised-models

2 Li, Y., Pan, A., Wang, D.D., Liu, X., *et al.* (2018) "Impact of healthy lifestyle factors on life expectancies in the US population." *Circulation 138*, 4, 345–355.

3 The two excellent reviews by Dr Innes include her work with H.K. Vincent (2007) "The influence of yoga-based programs on risk profiles in adults with type 2 diabetes mellitus: A systematic review." *Evidence-Based Complementary and Alternative Medicine 4*, 469–486; and her work with C. Bourguignon and A.G. Taylor (2005) "Risk indices associated with the insulin resistance syndrome, cardiovascular disease, and possible protection with yoga: A systematic review." *Journal of the American Board of Family Practice 18*, 491–519.

4 Ornish, D., Brown, S.E., Scherwitz, L.W., Billings, J.H., *et al.* (1990) "Can lifestyle changes reverse coronary heart disease? The Lifestyle Heart Trial." *The Lancet 336*, 8708, 129–133.

5 Ornish, D., Scherwitz, L.W., Billings, J.H., Brown, S.E., *et al.* (1998) "Intensive lifestyle changes for reversal of coronary heart disease." *JAMA 280*, 23, 2001–2007; Ornish, D. (1998) "Avoiding revascularization with lifestyle changes: The Multicenter Lifestyle Demonstration Project." *American Journal of Cardiology 82*, 10B, 72T–76T; Ornish, D., Lin, J., Daubenmier, J., Weidner, G., *et al.*

(2008) "Increased telomerase activity and comprehensive lifestyle changes: A pilot study." *Lancet Oncology 9*, 11, 1048–1057.

6   Ornish, D. and Ornish, A. (2019) *UnDo It! How Simple Lifestyle Changes Can Reverse Most Chronic Diseases.* New York: Ballantine Books.

7   Innes and Vincent (2007), op. cit.

8   Selvamurthy, W., Sridharan, K., Ray, U.S., Tiwary, R.S., *et al.* (1998) "A new physiological approach to control essential hypertension." *Indian Journal of Physiology and Pharmacology 42*, 205–213.

9   Bhavanani, A.B., Sanjay, Z. and Madanmohan, T. (2011) "Immediate effect of *sukha pranayama* on cardiovascular variables in patients of hypertension." *International Journal of Yoga Therapy 21*, 4–7.

10 Bhavanani, A.B., Sanjay, Z. and Madanmohan, T. (2012) "Immediate effect of *chandranadi pranayama* (left unilateral forced nostril breathing) on cardiovascular parameters in hypertensive patients." *International Journal of Yoga 5*, 108–111.

11 Bhavanani, A.B., Madanmohan, T., Sanjay, Z. and Basavaraddi, I.V. (2012) "Immediate cardiovascular effects of *pranava pranayama*

in hypertensive patients." *Indian Journal of Physiology and Pharmacology 56*, 3, 273–278.

12 Bhavanani, A.B., Madanmohan, T., Sanjay, Z. and Vithiyalakshmi, L. (2012) "Immediate cardiovascular effects of *pranava* relaxation in patients of hypertension and diabetes." *Biomedical Human Kinetics 4*, 66–69.

13 The sacred chant of the Shiva worshippers is the "om nama shivaya" known as the great chant (*maha mantra*). It is explained in more detail at http://allsaivism.com/articles/panchakshara.aspx

14 Bhavanani, A.B., Raj, J.B., Ramanathan, M. and Trakroo, M. (2016) "Effect of different *pranayamas* on respiratory sinus arrhythmia." *Journal of Clinical and Diagnostic Research 10*, CC04–CC06.

15 Bernardi, L., Sleight, P., Bandinelli, G., Cencetti, S., *et al.* (2001) "Effect of rosary prayer and yoga mantras on autonomic cardiovascular rhythms: Comparative study." *BMJ 323*, 7327, 1446–1449.

16 Critchley, H.D., Nicotra, A., Chiesa, P.A., Nagai, Y., *et al.* (2005) "Slow breathing and hypoxic challenge: Cardiorespiratory consequences and their central neural substrates." *PLOS One 10*, 5, e0127082.

Chapter 8

1   www.who.int/news-room/fact-sheets/detail/diabetes

2   Bijlani, R.L., Vempati, R.P., Yadav, R.K., Ray, R.B., *et al.* (2005) "A brief but comprehensive lifestyle education program based on yoga reduces risk factors for cardiovascular disease and diabetes mellitus." *Journal of Alternative and Complementary Medicine 11*, 267–274.

3   Yang, K. (2007) "A review of yoga programs for four leading risk factors of chronic diseases." *Evidence-Based Complementary and Alternative Medicine 4*, 4, 487–491.

4   Bernardi, L., Gordin, D., Bordino, M., Rosengård-Bärlund, M., *et al.* (2017) "Oxygen-induced impairment in arterial function is corrected by slow breathing in patients with type 1 diabetes." *Scientific Reports 7*, 1, 6001.

5   Rosengård-Bärlund, M., Bernardi, L., Holmqvist, J., Debarbieri, G., *et al.* (2011) "Deep breathing improves blunted baroreflex sensitivity even after 30 years of type 1 diabetes." *Diabetologia 54*, 7, 1862–1870.

6   Innes, K.E. and Vincent, H.K. (2007) "The influence of yoga-based programs on risk profiles in adults with type 2 diabetes mellitus: A systematic review." *Evidence-Based Complementary and Alternative Medicine 4*, 469–486.

7   Ibid.

8   Manjunatha, S., Vempati, R.P., Ghosh, D. and Bijlani, R.L. (2005) "An investigation into the acute and long-term effects of selected yogic postures on fasting and postprandial glycemia and insulinemia in healthy young subjects." *Indian Journal of Physiology and Pharmacology 49*, 319–324.

9   Chaya, M.S., Ramakrishnan, G., Shastry, S., Kishore, R.P., *et al.* (2008) "Insulin sensitivity and cardiac autonomic function in young male practitioners of yoga." *The National Medical Journal of India 21*, 5, 217–221.

CHAPTER 9

1   www.who.int/cancer/en
2   Ibid.
3   www.who.int/cancer/en
4   https://surveillance.cancer.gov/devcan
5   American Association for Cancer Research (AACR) (2018) *Cancer Progress Report, 2018*. Philadelphia, PA. Available at www.cancerprogressreport.org
6   *The Lancet Oncology* (2019) "Editorial: Prevention, treatment, and profit: An unsustainable alliance." *20*, 3, 311. Available at www.thelancet.com/journals/lanonc/article/PIIS1470-2045(19)30111-1/fulltext
7   www.who.int/cancer/en
8   Perera, F.P., Rauh, V., Whyatt, R.M., Tang, D. *et al.* (2005) "A summary of recent findings on birth outcomes and developmental effects of prenatal ETS, PAH, and pesticide exposures." *Neurotoxicology 26*, 4, 573–587.
9   See www.burzynskiclinic.com
10 Clavo, B., Pérez, J.L., López, L., Suárez, G., *et al.* (2004) "Ozone therapy for tumor oxygenation." *Evidence-Based Complementary and Alternative Medicine 1*, 1, 93–98.
11 Kienle, G.S., Mussler, M., Fuchs, D. and Kiene, H. (2016) "Intravenous mistletoe treatment in integrative cancer care." *Evidence-Based Complementary and Alternative Medicine.* Available at www.hindawi.com/journals/ecam/2016/4628287
12 Hurwitz, M. and Stauffer, P. (2014) "Hyperthermia, radiation and chemotherapy: The role of heat in multidisciplinary cancer care." *Seminars in Oncology 41*, 6, 714–729.
13 Abrams, D.I. (2016) "Integrating cannabis into clinical cancer care." *Current Oncology 23*, S8–S14. Available at https://current-oncology.com/index.php/oncology/article/view/3099/2084
14 Zitvogel, L., Galluzzi, L., Viaud, S., Vétizou, M., *et al.* (2015) "Cancer and the gut microbiota: An unexpected link." *Science Translational Medicine 7*, 271.
15 www.bcct.ngo
16 www.nobelprize.org/prizes/medicine/2018/summary
17 AACR (2018), op. cit.
18 Ibid.
19 Ornish, D. and Ornish, A. (2019) *UnDo It! How Simple Lifestyle Changes Can Reverse Most Chronic Diseases*. New York: Ballantine Books.
20 Harris Insights & Analytics (2017) *National Cancer Opinion Survey*. Prepared for the American Society of Clinical Oncology (ASCO). Available at www.asco.org/sites/new-www.asco.org/files/content-files/research-and-progress/documents/ASCO-National-Cancer-Opinion-Survey-Results.pdf
21 Steele, C.B., Thomas, C.C., Henley, S.J., Massetti, G.M., *et al.* (2017) "Vital signs: Trends in incidence of cancers associated with overweight and obesity—United States, 2005–2014." *Morbidity and Mortality Weekly Report 66*, 39, 1052–1058.
22 www.yogajournal.com/page/yogainamerica study
23 *Kirtan kriya* is described in Chapter 13 and Appendix 6.
24 The variety of meditations we use is detailed in Appendix 1.
25 Khalsa, D.S., Amen, D., Hanks, C., Money, N. and Newberg, A. (2009) "Cerebral blood flow changes during chanting meditation." *Nuclear Medicine Communications 30*, 12, 956–961.
26 Cramer, H., Lauche, R., Klose, P., Lange, S., Langhorst, J. and Dubos, G.J. (2017) "Yoga for improving health-related quality of life, mental health and cancer-related symptoms in women diagnosed with breast cancer." *The Cochrane Database of Systematic Reviews.* Available at www.ncbi.nlm.nih.gov/pubmed/28045199
27 Kleckner, I.R., Kamen, C., Gewandter, J.S., Mohile, N.A., *et al.* (2017) "Effects of exercise during chemotherapy on chemotherapy-induced peripheral neuropathy: A multicenter randomized controlled trial." *Supportive Care in Cancer 26*, 4, 1019–1028.
28 Remski, M. (2019) *Practice and All is Coming: Abuse, Cult Dynamics, and Healing in Yoga and Beyond*. Rangiora, New Zealand: Embodied Wisdom Publishing.
29 Bhavanani, A.B., Majewski, L. and Tiwari, S. (2016) "Effects of an intensive 3-week yoga retreat on sense of well being in cancer survivors." *Alternative Medical Journal*, December.
30 Spalding, K.L., Bergmann, O., Alkass, K., Mash, D.C. *et al.* (2013) "Dynamics of Hippocampal Neurogenesis in Adult Humans." *Cell 153*, 6, 1219–1227.
31 See https://yip.guru/
32 Fishman, L., Saltonstall, E. and Genis, S. (2009) "Understanding and preventing yoga injuries." *International Journal of Yoga Therapy 19*, 1, 47–53.

CHAPTER 10

1   You can contact me at info@yogaforhealth.
    institute

2   www.yogaforhealth.institute

3   *Psychology Today* (2019) "How yoga and
    breathing help the brain unwind." January
    16. Available at www.psychologytoday.com/
    us/blog/psychiatry-the-people/201901/
    how-yoga-and-breathing-help-the-
    brain-unwind?fbclid=IwAR0_jvjFTtMW
    qZc1KZ9wOidWoSQkRpSdti QCIIBx_1C
    Wu9QHCbIJ Y23bQp7o

4   Bernardi, N.F., Bordino, M., Bianchi, I., and
    Bernardi, L. (2017) "Acute fall and long-
    term rise in oxygen saturation in response to
    meditation." *Psychophysiology 54*, 12, 1951–
    1966. Available at www.ncbi.nlm.nih.gov/
    pubmed/28840941

5   Nivethita, L., Mooventhan, A. and Manjunath,
    N.K. (2016) "Effects of various *prāṇāyāma* on
    cardiovascular and autonomic variables."
    Ancient Science of Life 36, 2, 72–77.

6   Kuppusamy, M., Kamaldeen, D., Pitani,
    R., Amaldas, J. and Shanmugam, P. (2017)
    "Effects of *bhramari pranayama* on health: A
    systematic review." *Journal of Traditional and
    Complementary Medicine 8*, 1, 11–16.

7   Greenlee, H., Baineaves, L.G., Carlson, L.E.,
    Cohen, M., *et al.* (2014) "Clinical practice
    guidelines on the use of integrative therapies
    as supportive care in patients treated for breast
    cancer." *Journal of the National Cancer Institute
    50*, 346–358.

8   Desai, R., Tailor, A. and Bhatt, T. (2015)
    "Effects of yoga on brain waves and structural
    activation: A review." *Complementary Therapies
    in Clinical Practice 21*, 2, 112–118.

9   Kerr, C.E., Jones, S.R., Wan, Q., Pritchett, D.L.,
    et al. (2011) "Effects of mindfulness meditation
    training on anticipatory alpha modulation in
    primary somatosensory cortex." *Brain Research
    Bulletin 85*, 3–4, 96–103. Available at www.ncbi.
    nlm.nih.gov/pubmed/21501665

10 Nahum, M., Lee, H. and Merzenich, M.M.
    (2013) "Principles of neuroplasticity-based
    rehabilitation." *Progress in Brain Research 207*,
    141–171.

11 Wallington, M., Saxon, E.B., Bomb, M.,
    Smittenaar, R., *et al.* (2016) '30-day mortality
    after systemic anticancer treatment for breast
    and lung cancer in England: A population-
    based, observational study." *The Lancet 17*, 9,
    1203–1216.

12 Sprod, L.K., Fernandez, I.D., Janelsins, M.C.,
    Peppone, L.J., *et al.* (2015) "Effects of yoga on
    cancer-related fatigue and global side-effect
    burden in older cancer survivors." *Journal of
    Geriatric Oncology 6*, 1, 8–14.

13 Rani, K., Tiwari, S., Singh, U., Agrawal,
    G., Ghildyal, A. and Srivasteva, N. (2011)
    "Impact of Yoga Nidra on psychological
    general wellbeing in patients with menstrual
    irregularities: A randomized controlled trial."
    International Journal of Yoga 4, 1, 20–25.
    Available at www.ncbi.nlm.nih.gov/pmc/
    articles/PMC3099097

14 Rao, N.P., Deshpande, P., Gangadhar, K.B.,
    Arasappar, R., *et al.* (2018) "Directional brain
    networks underlying OM chanting." *Asian
    Journal of Psychiatry 37*, 20–25. Available at
    www.ncbi.nlm.nih.gov/pubmed/30099280

15 Solano, J.P., Gomes, B. and Higginson, I.J.
    (2006) "A comparison of symptom prevalence
    in far advanced cancer, AIDS, heart disease,
    chronic obstructive pulmonary disease and
    renal disease." *Journal of Pain and Symptom
    Management 31*, 1, 58–69.

16 Cramp, F. and Daniel, J. (2008) "Exercise for
    the management of cancer-related fatigue
    in adults." *Cochrane Database of Systematic
    Reviews*, April 23; Minton, O., Richardson, A.,
    Sharpe, M., Hotopf, M. and Stone, P. (2008)
    "A systematic review and meta-analysis of the
    pharmacological treatment of cancer-related
    fatigue." *Journal of the National Cancer Institute
    11*, 16, 1155–1166.

PART 3

1   Taylor, M.J. (2018) *Yoga Therapy as a Creative
    Response to Pain.* London and Philadelphia, PA:
    Singing Dragon.

CHAPTER 11

1 Yoga postulates that dis-ease begins in our mental space—first, through an unhealthy belief system, negative thoughts and/or emotions. If this is not resolved, the abnormality then moves to the subtle energy system (*prana*) creating blocks, and finally manifests as a disease in the physical body.

2 For more information on these retreats, see www.yogaforhealth.institute

3 Taylor, M. (2006) "Harvesting the full potential of group yoga therapy classes." *International Journal of Yoga Therapy 16*, 1, 33–37.

4 www.who.int/substance_abuse/research_tools/whoqolbref/en

5 Danhauer, S.C., Addington, E.L., Sohl, S.J. and Chaoul, A. (2017) "Review of yoga therapy during cancer treatment." *Support Care Cancer 25*, 4, 1357–1372.

6 Majewski, L. and Bhavanani, A.B. (2014) "A novel rejuvenation program for cancer patients at Kaivalyadhama, India." *Yoga-Mimamsa 46*, 1, 20–24.

7 Bhavanani, A.B., Majewski, L. and Tiwari, S. (2016) "Effects of an intensive 3-week yoga retreat on sense of well being in cancer survivors." *Journal of Alternative Medical Research 2*, 2, 116.

CHAPTER 12

1 Kleckner, I.R., Kamen, C., Gewandter, J.S. and Mohile, N.A. (2017) "Effects of exercise during chemotherapy on chemotherapy-induced peripheral neuropathy: A multicenter, randomized controlled trial." *Supportive Cancer Care 26*, 12. Available at www.researchgate.net/publication/321807070_Effects_of_exercise_during_chemotherapy_on_chemotherapy-induced_peripheral_neuropathy_a_multicenter_randomized_controlled_trial

2 Krause, N. (2004) "Stressors arising in highly valued roles, meaning in life, and the physical health status of older adults." *Journal of Gerontology: Social Sciences 59B*, S287–S297.

CHAPTER 13

1 Bernardi, L., Sleight, P., Bandinelli, G. and Cencetti, S. (2001) "Effect of rosary prayer and yoga mantras on autonomic cardiovascular rhythms: Comparative study." *BMJ 323*, 7327, 1446–1449. Available at www.ncbi.nlm.nih.gov/pubmed/11751348

2 Stephens, M. (2017), op. cit.

3 Niventhita, L., Mooventhan, A. and Manjunath, N.K. (2016) "Effects of various prāṇāyāma on cardiovascular and autonomic variables." *Ancient Science of Life 36*, 2, 72–77.

4 Kuppusamy, M., Kamaldeen, D., Pitani, R., Amaldas, J. and Shanmugam, P. (2017) "Effects of Bhramari Pranayama on health—A systematic review." *Journal of Traditional and Complementary Medicine 8*, 1, 11–16.

5 Chakrabarty, J., Vidyasagar, M., Fernandes, D., Joisa, G., Varghese, P. and Mayya, S. (2015) "Effectiveness of *pranayama* on cancer-related fatigue in breast cancer patients undergoing radiation therapy: A randomized controlled trial." *International Journal of Yoga 8*, 1, 47–53.

6 Bernardi, L., Porta, C., Gabutti, A., Spicuzza, L. and Sleight, P. (2001) "Modulatory effects of respiration." *Autonomic Neuroscience: Basic & Clinical 90*, 1–2, 27–56.

7 Kuppusamy, M., Kamaldeen, D., Pitani, R. and Amaldas, J. (2016) "Immediate effects of *Bhramari Pranayama* on resting cardiovascular parameters in healthy adolescents." *Journal of Clinical & Diagnostic Research 10*, 5, CC17–CC19.

8 Shannahoff-Khalsa, D.S. and Kennedy, B. (1993) "The effects of unilateral enforced nostril breathing on the heart." *International Journal of Neuroscience 73*, 47–60.

9 Kaivalyadhama, S.M.Y.M. (1970) *Hathapradipika of Swatnaratna* II:16.

10 Rothenberg, R. (2019) *Restoring Prāṇa: A Guide to Prāṇāyāma and Healing through the Breath for Yoga Therapists, Yoga Teachers, and Health-Care Practitioners.* London and Philadelphia, PA: Singing Dragon.

11 Basovich, S.N. (2010) "The role of hypoxia in mental development and in the treatment of mental disorders: A review." *BioScience Trends 4*, 288–296.

12 Rothenberg, R. (2019) *Restoring Prāṇa: A Guide to Prāṇāyāma and Healing through the Breath*

for Yoga Therapists, Yoga Teachers, and Health-Care Practitioners. London and Philadelphia, PA: Singing Dragon.

13 Basovich, S.N. (2010) "The role of hypoxia in mental development and in the treatment of mental disorders: A review." *BioScience Trends* 4, 288–296.

14 Rothenberg (2019), op. cit.

15 The *Hatha Yoga Pradipika* is a classic 15th-century Sanskrit manual on *Hatha Yoga*, written by Svami Svatmarama, and is among one of the most influential texts.

16 Hölzel, B.K., Carmody, J., Evans, K.C., Hoge, E.A., *et al.* (2009) "Stress reduction correlates with structural changes in the amygdala." *Social Cognitive and Affective Neuroscience* 5, 1, 11–17.

17 Kerr, C.E., Jones, S.R., Wan, Q., Pritchett, D.L., *et al.* (2011) "Effects of mindfulness meditation training on anticipatory alpha modulation in primary somatosensory cortex." *Brain Research Bulletin* 85, 3–4, 96–103. Available at www.ncbi.nlm.nih.gov/pubmed/21501665

18 Khalsa, D.S., Amen, D., Hanks, C., Money, N. and Newberg, A. (2009) "Cerebral blood flow changes during chanting meditation." *Nuclear Medicine Communications* 30, 12, 956–961.

19 Mallison, J. and Singleton, M. (2017) *Roots of Yoga.* London, UK: Penguin, pp.228–258.

20 Saraswati Satyananda Sarasvati (1996) *Asana, Pranayama, Mudra and Bandha.* Munger, India: Bihar School of Yoga, p.426.

21 Le Page, J. and Le Page, L. (2014) *Mudras for Healing and Transformation.* Sebastopol, CA: Integrative Yoga Therapy.

22 We refer here to Patanjali's *Ashtanga Yoga* which specifies the *eight limbs of yoga: yama* (attitudes toward our environment), *niyama* (attitudes toward ourselves), *asana* (physical postures), *pranayama* (restraint or expansion of the breath), *pratyahara* (withdrawal of the senses), *dharana* (concentration), *dyana,* and *samadhi.*

23 Verbitskaya, E.V. (2015) "Meta-analysis: Problems with Russian publications." *The International Journal of Risk & Safety in Medicine* 27, Suppl. 1, S89–S90.

24 Lee, H.C., Khong, P.W. and Ghista, D.M. (2005) "Bioenergy based medical diagnostic application based on gas discharge visualization." *Annual International Conference of the IEEE Engineering in Medicine and Biology Society* 2, 1533–1536.

25 Korotkov, K.G., Matravers, P., Orlov, D.V. and Williams, B.O. (2010) "Application of electrophoton capture (EPC) analysis based on gas discharge visualization (GDV) technique in medicine: A systematic review." *Journal of Alternative and Complementary Medicine* 16, 1, 13–25.

26 Narayan, C.R., Korotkov, K.G. and Srinivasan, T.M. (2018) "Bioenergy and its implication for yoga therapy." *International Journal of Yoga* 11 2, 157–165.

27 Kumar, K.S., Srinivasan, T.M., Ilavarsu, J., Mondal, B. and Nagendra, H.R. (2018) "Classification of electrophotonic images of yogic practice of mudra through neural networks." *International Journal of Yoga* 11, 2, 152–156.

28 Sullivan, M. (2020) *Understanding Yoga Therapy: Applied Philosophy and Science for Health and Well-Being.* Oxfordshire: Routledge.

29 Texts in Appendix 2 were taken from Miller, R.C. (2015) *The iRest Program for Healing PTSD: A Proven-Effective Approach to Using Yoga Nidra Meditation and Deep Relaxation Techniques to Overcome Trauma.* Oakland, CA: New Harbinger Publications, Inc. and modified for the needs of our clients.

30 Miller (2015) *op. cit.*

31 Graham, L. (2013) *Bouncing Back: Rewiring Your Brain for Maximum Resilence and Well-Being.* Novato, CA: New World Library; Gerdes, L. (2008) *Limitless You: The Infinite Possibilities of a Balanced Brain.* Vancouver, Canada: Namaste Publishing; Segal, D. (2007) *The Mindful Brain: Reflection and Atonement in Cultivation of Well-Being.* New York: W.W. Norton.

32 Gendlin, E.T. (1982) *Focusing.* New York: Bantam Books.

33 Jasmin, K.M., McGettigan, C., Agnew, Z.K., Lavan, N., *et al.* (2016) "Cohesion and joint speech: Right hemisphere contributions to synchronized vocal production." *The Journal of Neuroscience* 36, 17, 4669–4680.

34 Kennedy, J. and Scott, A. (2005) "A pilot study: The effects of music therapy interventions on middle school students' ESL skills." *Journal of Music Therapy* 42, 4, 244–261.

35 Hertzell, J.F., Davis, B., Melcher, D., Miceli, D., *et al.* (2016) "Brains of verbal memory specialists show anatomical differences in language, memory and visual systems." *NeuroImage* 131, 181–192.

36 Acevedo, B.P., Pospos, S. and Lavretsky, H. (2016) "The neural mechanisms of meditative practices: Novel approaches for healthy aging." *Current Behavioral Neuroscience Reports 3*, 328–339.

37 Bernardi *et al.* (2001), op. cit.

38 Gao, J., Leung, H.K., Yan Wu, B.W., Skouras, S. and Sik, H.H. (2019) "The neurophysiological correlates of religious chanting." *Scientific Reports 9*, 1, 4262.

39 Rao, N.P., Deshpande, G., Gangadhar, K.B., Arasappa, R., *et al.* (2018) "Directional brain networks underlying OM chanting." *Asian Journal of Psychiatry 37*, 20–25.

40 Kalyani, B.G., Venkatasubramanian, G., Arasappa, R., Rao, N.P., *et al.* (2011) "Neurohemodynamic correlates of 'OM' chanting: A pilot functional magnetic resonance imaging study." *International Journal of Yoga 4*, 1, 3–6.

41 Mooventhan, A. and Khode, V. (2014) "Effect of Bhramari pranayama and OM chanting on pulmonary function in healthy individuals: A prospective randomized control trial." *International Journal of Yoga 7*, 2, 104–110.

42 Harne, B.P. and Hiwale, A.S. (2018) "EEG spectral analysis on OM mantra meditation: A pilot study." *Applied Psychophysiology and Biofeedback 43*, 2, 123–129.

43 Bhargav, H., Manjunath, N.K., Varambally, S. and Mooventhan, A. (2016) "Acute effects of 3G mobile phone radiations on frontal haemodynamics during a cognitive task in teenagers and possible protective value of Om chanting." *International Review of Psychiatry 28*, 3, 288–298.

44 The track can be obtained free from www.spiritvoyage.com and then looped to extend to 30 minutes.

45 Devanand, V. (no date) *Meditations and Mantras: An Authoritative Text*. New Delhi, India: Motilal Banarsidass Pub. Pvt. Ltd., p.63.

46 Frawley, D. (2010) *Mantra Yoga and Primal Sound*. Twin Lakes, WI: Lotus Press, p.158.

47 Sovik, R. (2006) *Moving Inward: The Journey to Meditation*. Honesdale, PA: Himalayan Institute Press, p.162.

APPENDIX 1

1   Kabat-Zinn, J. (2013) *Full Catastrophe Living: How to Cope with Stress, Pain and Illness Using Mindfulness Meditation*. London, UK: Piatkus.

APPENDIX 2

1   … indicates a pause.

Index